Quick Reference to
Therapeutic Nutrition

J. B. Lippincott Company Philadelphia
London Mexico City New York St. Louis São Paulo Sydney

LIPPINCOTT'S QUICK REFERENCES

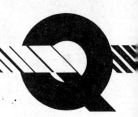

Quick Reference to

Therapeutic Nutrition

Barbara G. Morrissey, B.S., R.D., M.A.

Adjunct Professor of Nutrition and Diet Therapy,
College of New Rochelle School of Nursing,
New Rochelle, New York

Formerly, Clinical Dietitian,
Memorial Sloan–Kettering Cancer Center,
New York, New York, and The Hospital
for Special Surgery, New York, New York

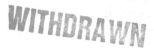

Sponsoring Editors: Paul R. Hill
                    Joyce Mkitarian
Manuscript Editor: Elizabeth P. Lowe
Indexer: Dorna Fowler
Art Director: Earl Gerhart
Cover Illustration: John Nearing Design
Designer: Carol C. Bleistine
Production Supervisor: N. Carolyn Kerr
Production Assistant: S. M. Gassaway
Compositor: International Computaprint Corporation
Printer/Binder: R. R. Donnelley & Sons Company

654321

Library of Congress Cataloging in Publication Data

Morrissey, Barbara G.
  Quick reference to therapeutic nutrition.
  (Lippincott's quick references)
  Bibliography: p.
  Includes index.
  1. Diet therapy—Outlines, syllabi, etc. I. Title.
[DNLM: 1. Diet therapy—Nursing texts.   2. Nutrition—
Nursing texts. WY 150 M883]
RM216.M546 1984   615.8'54'0202   83-9358
ISBN 0-397-54416-2

The author and publisher have exerted every effort to ensure that drug selection
and dosage set forth in this text are in accord with current recommendations and
practice at the time of publication. However, in view of ongoing research, changes
in government regulations, and the constant flow of information relating to drug
therapy and drug reactions, the reader is urged to check the package insert for
each drug for any change in indications and dosage and for added warnings and
precautions. This is particularly important when the recommended agent is a new
or infrequently employed drug.

To my husband, children, and parents for their patience
and encouragement while this book was being developed.

Preface

Quick Reference to Therapeutic Nutrition has been written to increase and update the clinical nurse's knowledge of nutrition and its interaction with other medical sciences. The nurse's knowledge of nutrition has always been important; however, it is becoming even more necessary now that the general public as well as health professionals have become more aware of the role of nutrition in promoting health. The client, then, is beginning to understand the principles of good nutrition and consequently he expects the hospital, clinical, and community nurse, as part of the health-care team, to answer his nutrition questions intelligently.

This book covers three major topics. The first two chapters discuss how individual nutritional status can be evaluated by the nurse or by other members of the health-care team through the assessment of simple and advanced anthropometric, physiological, biochemical, and clinical data. Additional emphasis is placed on how poor nutritional status may develop and the type of nutritional support that can be provided to improve the client's nutritional status, when indicated.

Chapters 3 through 9 identify diseases that can be controlled or aided by diet therapy. The role of diet in common disorders is presented, including its interaction in the development (etiology), progression (characteristics and symptoms), and treatment of the disease. The interaction of foods with common medications is discussed as well as the nutritional alterations that are necessary to alleviate symptoms, augment treatment, and enhance recovery. Treatment by diet is instituted by changing the method of feeding, increasing or decreasing specific nutrients, adapting food intakes, modifying meal plans, and altering food habits and other behavioral patterns. These chapters also emphasize the importance of adjusting these dietary alterations to a client's lifestyle to enhance compliance. Additionally, this section underscores how the nurse can enhance compliance by using her contact with the client to collect and report any subjective or objective information that may have nutritional implications.

The last two chapters of the book discuss the need for nutrient adjustment throughout the life cycle, with particular emphasis on nutrient adjustments and dietary adaptations during pregnancy and lactation.

Nurses today must have a basic understanding of all the parameters that influence body functions, and keeping up with all the current information is a formidable task. Consequently, this book has been written in outline and telegraphic form so that updated nutritional knowledge can be obtained quickly and efficiently.

Barbara G. Morrissey, B.S., R.D., M.A.

Acknowledgments

I wish to express my appreciation to the following people whose guidance, support, and knowledge made this book a reality:

My editors at J. B. Lippincott Company, Bernice Heller and Joyce Mkitarian.

My friends Mary June Cline, R.D., M.A.; Jan Wanake, R.D., M.A.; Maureen Leichman, R.N.; and Helen Borowitz.

Members of the health-care team who willingly shared their knowledge: David Madsen, Ph.D., Manager, Technical Development, Nutrition and Flow Control Division, Travenol Laboratories, Inc., Deerfield, Illinois; Mary Reinemann, R.D., Assistant Administrator of Patient Services, and Sister Elizabeth Looney, Director of Nutritional Services, Calvary Hospital, Bronx, New York; Michelle Fairchild, R.D., M.A., Memorial Sloan–Kettering Cancer Center, New York, New York; Thomas J. Sparacino, R.Ph., St. John's Riverside Hospital, Yonkers, New York; Patricia Krumholtz–Belkin, R.N., M.A., Skidmore College School of Nursing, New York, New York; Martin F. Stein, Jr., M.D., Director of Medicine, Chief, Nephrology Service, St. Joseph's Medical Center, Yonkers, New York; and Sheila Belle, M.S., R.D., Institute of Rehabilitation Medicine, New York University Medical Center, New York, New York.

contents

appendix IV

Recommended Daily Dietary
Allowances 550

appendix V

Exchange Lists for Meal Planning 554

appendix VI

Protein, Phosphorus, Sodium, and
Potassium Exchange Lists 563

appendix VII

Nutrient Composition of Selected
Parenteral Solutions 583

appendix VIII

Ideal Urinary Creatinine Values for
Adults 586

index 589

Quick Reference to
Therapeutic Nutrition

chapter 1

Assessment of Nutritional Status

Nutritional Status

The emphasis in this section (Chaps. 1 and 2) is on nutritional status: how poor nutritional status (malnutrition) develops, how the health team can assess an individual's nutritional status, and how members of the health team can effectively provide nutritional care that will maintain or restore a client's nutritional status.

Description

Nutritional status, or nutriture, is the degree to which an individual's physiological and psychological needs for nutrients are being met by the food he is consuming.

Classifications

Optimal nutritional status indicates that an individual is utilizing all the essential nutrients consumed at such efficiency that health and well-being are at the highest possible levels. Additionally, a nutrient reserve is available to nourish the body during times of stress.

Good nutritional status indicates that an individual's body is functioning on a day-to-day basis but that a nutrient reserve is lacking.

Poor nutritional status, or malnutrition, is a general term that indicates that an excess, deficit, or imbalance of one or more essential nutrients or calories exists. Consequently, growth, tissue synthesis, or body stores may be affected. There are classifications of malnutrition, as follows:

1

Marasmus

Marasmus is also called protein-energy malnutrition (PEM) or protein-calorie malnutrition (PCM).

Description

Marasmus is a nutritional deficiency related to severe deprivation of protein, vitamins, minerals, and calories.

Clinical Characteristics

See Table 1-1.*

Kwashiorkor (Hypoalbuminemic Malnutrition)

Description

Kwashiorkor is a nutritional deficiency related to a severe deprivation of good-quality protein; however, the caloric content of the diet may be nearly adequate.

Clinical Characteristics

See Table 1-1.

Marasmic Kwashiorkor

Description

Marasmic kwashiorkor is a nutritional deficiency that is related to both severe caloric deprivation and deprivation of good-quality protein.

Clinical Characteristics

Characteristics and clinical signs of both marasmus and kwashiorkor may be superimposed on one another at any stage of the undernourished condition (see Table 1-1).

Obesity (Overnutrition)

Description

Obesity is a nutritional condition related to excessive intake of fat, carbohydrate, and protein.

Clinical Characteristics

Weight is 20% or more above the ideal body weight (IBW) for an individual's age and sex. Excessive subcutaneous fat is present (see Structural Determinations in this chapter).

---

*See tables at the end of this chapter.

Etiology of Primary and Secondary Malnutrition

Primary Malnutrition

Environmental disasters (*e.g.*, droughts and war)
Individual food habits (*e.g.*, fad dieting)
Economics
Lack of education about nutrient needs
Maternal deprivation
Psychological disorders (*e.g.*, anorexia nervosa)
Increased needs (*e.g.*, pregnancy and illness)
Iatrogenic malnutrition

Secondary Malnutrition

Lack of sanitation may cause constant diarrhea
Maternal overfeeding
Psychological disorders (*e.g.*, bulimia)
Congenital defects (*e.g.*, inborn errors of metabolism)
Gastrointestinal disorders (*e.g.*, malabsorption)
Other disorders that impair utilization and excretion of nutrients (*e.g.*, diabetes mellitus and hypertension)

Primary Malnutrition

Primary malnutrition is marked by insufficient or unbalanced nutrient intake.

Secondary Malnutrition

In secondary malnutrition, nutrient intake may be sufficient, but utilization of nutrients is impaired by inadequate mastication, digestion, absorption, transport, or excretion (see etiology list).

Malnutrition Related to Increased Nutrient Requirements

Pregnancy and Lactation

Consult Chapter 10.

Metabolic Stress

Description

Stress refers to the hypermetabolic state (*e.g.*, increased basal metabolic rate or basal energy expenditure) associated with infection, trauma, therapeutic procedures (*e.g.*, surgical procedures), and certain chronic illnesses (*e.g.*, cancer).

Reactions to Stress

Individuals who experience stress-related conditions undergo synergistic reactions that involve the glands and hormones of the body. These reactions or adjustments occur in stages so that the body can gradually adjust to the changes introduced by stress. Without these hormonal and metabolic adjustments and effective medical and nutritional treatment, survival would be limited. Table 1-2 outlines the body's physiological adjustment to stress and its treatment. Nutritional requirements are increased more during stress than during simple starvation because there is a loss of two protein-conserving mechanisms normally brought into play during adaptation to starvation. One, *the metabolic rate tends to rise* rather than decrease as it would during starvation. Two, *the body cannot break down fat and utilize ketone bodies for energy as effectively;* therefore, protein, lean body tissue, becomes a major source of energy. The overall action of metabolism during stress is increased gluconeogenesis (formation of glucose from noncarbohydrate sources) and ureagenesis (formation or urea, a nitrogenous end product of protein metabolism). Ketogenesis (formation of ketone bodies from fat metabolism) does not occur to the same extent that it does in starvation. These changes in metabolism also create other nutrient imbalances, such as potassium, phosphorus, and zinc imbalances.

Iatrogenic Malnutrition

Iatrogenic malnutrition is health-team-induced malnutrition, especially that in hospitalized clients (Table 1-3).

Effect of Malnutrition on Drug Administration and Utilization

- Intramuscular injections may be more painful than normal if the amount of fatty tissue is decreased.
- Full absorption may not occur if the small intestines have been damaged by lack of nutrients. Villi will be shorter, and mucosa, thinner.

Additionally, diarrhea can enhance drug dilution and increase excretion before the drug can be absorbed. If this occurs, the individual will not receive the full benefits of the drug.

- Drugs may be diluted in the serum if overhydration, due to a change in colloidal (oncotic) osmotic pressure (low serum albumin concentrations), exists. Lower albumin levels may also decrease the number of receptor or binding sites on the albumin molecules, which will impair drug transport to the site of action.
- Liver function may be decreased. Consequently, possible decreased detoxification of the drug may induce adverse reactions or toxicity.
- Decreased cardiac output, due to decreased muscle and visceral protein, will cause decreased blood circulation and eventually decreased renal output. When this occurs, drug excretion will be impaired, which could induce drug toxicity.

Nutritional Status Evaluation (Nutritional Assessment)

Description

Nutritional status evaluation, or assessment, is essentially a process by which an individual's nutritional status is evaluated by collecting pertinent subjective and objective data and then comparing the data to a set of standards or percentiles. Assessment of the data identifies individuals who are malnourished and those at risk of developing nutritional inadequacies at intake, structural, biochemical, or clinical levels. Nutritional deficiencies or inadequacies, however, usually develop over a period of time, the normal progression being as follows:

1. Decreased nutrient intake induces mobilization of tissue reserves in an effort to maintain the necessary supply of nutrients to the cell. This is reflected in a reduced concentration of the nutrient in the blood or tissues as well as in decreased urinary or fecal excretion of the nutrient.

2. As tissue reserves are depleted, nutrient supplies to the cell are diminished. This leads to such biochemical modifications as changes in enzymes, coenzymes, and metabolites, which can be identified by blood and tissue evaluations.

3. Further progression of the nutrient deficiency or inadequacy is manifested in the anatomical modifications and clinical symptoms detectable in a thorough physical examination by an alert support team.

Who Should Be Nutritionally Assessed?

Ideally, all clients should be nutritionally evaluated in the office, clinic, or hospital. Lack of trained personnel and insufficient funds, however, often render the ideal prohibitively expensive. Even so, the personnel necessary and the cost involved in the treatment of disease and its complications are also prohibitive, so somewhere a balance must be achieved. The balance recommended here is a simple method of screening all persons in order to identify clients of high nutritional risk who may require advanced nutritional assessment and support. Often the staff nurse is responsible for this screening and for the reporting of any adverse findings to other health team personnel (*e.g.*, the dietitian or physician).

Methodology to Determine Nutritional Status

Simple Nutritional Evaluation Screening

Evaluate Subjective Information

An individual provides a member of the health team with information that cannot be measured objectively. It involves estimating intake determinations, as follows:

1. Evaluate information revealed by the client in the initial interview chart (Table 1-4).
2. Evaluate the client's own dietary assessment revealed in the food preference questionnaire (see sample).
3. Compare individual intake to recommended intake. Gross individual nutrient and caloric deficits revealed by eliciting information, as described above, can be measured by comparing individual intake to the intake recommended according to the Basic Four Food Groups, a simple nutritional tool (Tables 1-5, 1-6, 1-7, and 1-8). For instance, if an individual selects a variety of foods from each food group, chances are strong that he is not malnourished. However, if he fails to consume at least the minimum amounts from any of the four food groups, he may develop nutrient inadequacies over time. Additionally, there is no grouping for sweets, alcohol, or oils; consequently, if intake of these foods is not discussed individually with the client, caloric inadequacies may be overestimated. Therefore, using this tool as the only means of evaluating food intake demands caution because the information it elicits may be incomplete, biased, or only partially accurate.
4. Evaluate individual structural determinations, also called *anthropometric measurements*, such as height, usual weight, the maximum lifetime weight, and any recent weight loss.

Note. Another simple nutritional tool that may be used to compare individual nutrient intakes against recommended intakes, especially nutrient excesses, is the U.S. Dietary Goals (see Chap. 3). These dietary goals for the United States were released in April 1977 by the Senate Select Committee on Nutrition and Human Needs, and revised in December 1977. They are intended as a first step toward development of an agriculture and food policy for the country, with nutrition and health considerations in the forefront.

- *Goal 1:* To avoid overweight, consume only as much energy (calories) as is expended. If overweight, decrease energy intake and increase energy expenditure.

- *Goal 2:* Increase the consumption of complex carbohydrates and "naturally occurring" sugars from about 28% of energy intake to about 48% of energy intake.

- *Goal 3:* Reduce the consumption of refined and processed sugars by about 45% to account for about 19% of total energy intake.

- *Goal 4:* Reduce overall fat consumption from approximately 40% to about 30% of energy intake.

- *Goal 5:* Reduce saturated fat consumption to account for about 10% of total energy intake and balance that with polyunsaturated and monounsaturated fats, which should account for about 10% of energy intake each, making a total of 30% of energy intake.

- *Goal 6:* Reduce cholesterol consumption to about 300 mg/day.

- *Goal 7:* Limit the intake of sodium by reducing the intake of salt to about 5 g/day.

Food Preference Questionnaire

Name

Last   First   Middle initial

_____

Address

_____

_____

Telephone

_____

Sex _____   Age _____

Do you take any vitamins or minerals? Yes _____ No _____

If yes, which ones? _____ How often? _____ Dosage _____

Do you have any personal or religious dietary restrictions?

Kosher _____ Vegetarian _____

Other (specify) _____

(continued)

Do you take any other special food regularly? Yes _____ No _____

If yes, please list _____

Do you have any major food dislikes? Yes _____ No _____

If yes, please list

_____

If any of these foods cause an allergic reaction, please list

_____

_____

Note. The kind and amounts of food that you eat each day may play an important part in your physical and mental well-being. Therefore, foods may often be used as treatment to control or improve your physical or mental condition. If you have a physical or mental condition that can be treated by dietary alterations, it may mean that you will have to change some of your eating habits. In order to be provided with a meal plan that will be as close to your present habits as possible (*e.g.,* time of eating, foods preferred, quantity of foods preferred, place of eating), please answer the following questions as carefully as possible. Include sugar, milk, or cream used in beverages; butter or margarine used on bread or vegetables; dressing used on salads; and fried foods.

Time and Place of Eating	Kind of Food	Approximate Amount
Morning		
Time		
Place		
Noon		
Time		
Place		
Night		
Time		
Place		
Snacks		
Time		
Place		

(Adapted from Kaufman M: A food preference questionnaire for counseling patients with diabetes. J Am Diet Assoc 49:32, 1966)

Evaluate Objective Information

Objective information can be obtained from individual laboratory data and from other sources that can be measured by members of the health team and compared to a set of standards or percentiles. It involves making structural, physiological, biochemical, and clinical determinations.

Structural Determinations (Anthropometric Measurements)

1. Measure and weigh the client, who should be dressed in light clothing without shoes, on a beam scale at approximately the same time each day, preferably in the morning before breakfast. Record weight to the nearest ½ lb or 0.2 kg, for an adult, and then compare this height and weight to standard height and weight charts (*e.g.*, Metropolitan Life Insurance Company Height and Weight Charts and Build and Blood Pressure Study Average Weights); see Appendix I.

2. Determine the IBW for sex and height. Allow 100 lb for the first 5 feet for a medium-frame woman and 110 lb for a medium-frame man; allow 5 lb for each additional inch above 5 feet (subtract 5 lb for each inch under 5 feet); determine frame size (some examiners use wrist size as an estimate; others use hands, feet, elbow breadth, or bony chest breadth), and add 10% for a large frame or subtract 10% for a small frame (see Chap. 6, chart on Determination of Caloric Alteration Level and Appendix I, Metropolitan Life Insurance Company Height and Weight Charts).

3. Estimate degree of weight loss,* if applicable.

Formula for Weight Change

$$\text{Percent of IBW} = \frac{\text{Actual weight}}{\text{IBW}} \times 100$$

$$\text{Percent of usual body weight} = \frac{\text{Actual weight}}{\text{Usual weight}} \times 100$$

$$\text{Percent of weight change} = \frac{\text{Usual weight} - \text{Actual weight}}{\text{Usual weight}} \times 100$$

Example

$$\text{Percent of IBW} = \frac{110}{120} \times 100 = 92\%$$

$$\text{Percent of usual body weight} = \frac{110}{150} \times 100 = 73\%$$

$$\text{Percent of weight change} = \frac{150 - 110 = 40}{150} \times 100 = 27\% \text{ Recent weight change}$$

---

*   An individual may be deemed a nutritional risk if he has a 10-lb unintentional weight loss within 1 month or a 10% to 20% loss within 3 to 6 months.

Physiological and Biochemical Determinations
• Vital signs (pulse, blood pressure, respiration, and temperature). For example, fever increases the basal metabolic rate (BMR) approximately 7% for each degree rise in body temperature above 98.6°F or 13% for each degree above 37°C. Consequently, caloric requirements are increased.
• Blood Analysis
    1. Complete blood count (CBC) (hemoglobin [Hgb], hematocrit [HCT], and white blood counts [WBC]). For example, decreased hemoglobin levels (normally 12–17 g/dl) indicate that supplements of iron, protein, pyridoxine, and ascorbic acid may have to be administered. Additionally, fluid intake will need to be increased.
    2. Constituents analyzed by the sequential multiple autoanalyzer (SMA). See Figure 1-1. *Note.* Constituents examined may vary from laboratory to laboratory and with individual diagnosis. For example, serum albumin (SA) is a transport protein for numerous substances, including drugs, and the main determinant of plasma osmotic pressure. Normal levels range from 3.6 to 5.5 g/dl (mild depletion, 3.3–3.5 g/dl; moderate, 2.8–3.2 g/dl; severe, <2.7 g/dl). When they are reduced below 3.5 g/dl, clinical signs of kwashiorkor may be evident. If poor nutritional status is evident by other assessment analysis as well, extensive nutritional support (*i.e.*, high intake of calories and protein) will be indicated.
• Urine Analysis (specific gravity, glucose, acetone, albumin, *p*H, and color). For example, normally the quantity of acetone found in the urine is minute (0.003–0.015 g/24 hr); consequently, when higher levels are present, it may represent a physiological disorder (*e.g.*, dehydration, starvation); hypermetabolic stress; nutrient inadequacies or excesses (*e.g.*, high-protein, low-carbohydrate diet); or diabetes mellitus. Nutritional care plans will be altered according to the disorder. High intake of macronutrients is indicated in hypermetabolic stress in order to enhance lipogenesis and impair lipolysis. Balanced intake of macronutrients is indicated for diabetes mellitus (see Chap. 5).

Clinical Determinations
Consult Table 1-9. See chapters on specific disorders for other nutritional implications and nutritional alterations that can be determined by simple nutritional evaluation screening.

Identify Individuals Who Will Need Advanced Nutritional Evaluation

Such individuals include those who
• Are malnourished upon admission

- Have an unintentional weight loss of 10 lb or 10% to 20% of their body weight within recent months
- Are anorexic
- Have been admitted to the hospital for frequent illnesses
- Are admitted for major surgery that will require a long recovery period
- Have a hypermetabolic disease (*e.g.*, cancer)
- Will require extensive drug, radiation, or other treatment after hospitalization
- Have a primary or secondary nutrient deficiency that has been induced by their inability to ingest, digest, absorb, transport, or utilize nutrients (*e.g.*, pancreatic disease or inflammatory bowel disease)
- Have serum albumin concentrations of less than 3.5 g/dl
- Have a lymphocyte count of less than 1500 cells per cubic millimeter when the WBC is evaluated.

Advanced Nutritional Evaluation Screening

Evaluate Subjective Information

1. Evaluate information revealed by the individual in the 24-hour recall, dietary record, or diet history (Table 1-10).
2. Estimate caloric and nutrient intake by comparing individual intake to the nutrient composition of various foods listed in reliable food composition tables. Compare individual intake to recommended intake established in the recommended daily allowances (RDAs; see Table 1-10 and Appendix IV). Exact determinations (*e.g.*, nutrient deficiencies or excesses), however, must not be established until the advantages and disadvantages of these nutritional tools have been taken into consideration (see Table 1-10).

Evaluate Objective Information

Intake Determinations

1. Measure, weigh, control, and record all foods consumed.
2. Collect, analyze, and record all nutrients excreted.
3. Compare findings to established food composition tables and the RDAs. See Appendix IV. *Note.* Procedure is done when a severe metabolic condition is suspected.

Structural Determinations (Anthropometric Measurements)

1. Body composition is measured by densitometry, dilution methods, and total body potassium measurements. Consult advanced texts.
2. Subcutaneous fat stores are measured by triceps skinfold measurements (Table 1-11 and Fig. 1-2).

CHEMISTRY

ROUTINE ☐ EMERGENCY ☐ OR in AM ☐

SPECIMEN ▲ BLOOD ☐ URINE ☐ CSF ☐ BODY FLUIDS ☐

ACCESS NO. DONE BY DATE DONE

BASIC ADMISSION PROFILE	
CARDIAC PROFILE	
LIVER PROFILE	
RENAL PROFILE	
GLUCOSE 70 - 110 mg/dl	
BUN 5-25 mg/dl	
CREATININE 0.5 - 1.5 mg/dl	
URIC ACID 3.5 - 7 mg/dl	
NA 135 - 148 mEq/L	
K 3.5 - 5.3 mEq/L	
CL 95 - 105 mEq/L	
CO$_2$ 24 - 31 mEq/L	
SGOT 10 - 30 U/L	
LDH 109 - 220 U/L	
CPK 36 - 188 U/L	
AMYLASE 45 - 200 units	
LIPASE 0 - 1.5 units	
ACID P/TASE 0 - 2.0 units	
CHOLESTEROL up to 250 mg/dl	
TRIGLYCERIDES 10 - 190 mg/dl	
TOTAL PROTEIN 6 - 8 g/dl	
ALBUMIN 3.5 - 5.5 g/dl	
ALK P/TASE 36 - 120 U/L	
BILIRUBIN TOTAL 0.1 - 1.7 mg/dl	
BILIRUBIN 1 min. < 0.5 mg/dl	
CALCIUM 8.5 - 10.5 mg/dl	
PHOSPHORUS 2.5 - 4.5 mg/dl	
LITHIUM < 1.5 mEq/L	
MAGNESIUM 1.8 - 3.0 mg/dl	
Fe 55 - 165 ug/dl	
TIBC 250 - 450 ug/dl	
% SATURATION $> 16\%$	
CSF GLUCOSE 40 - 80 mg/dl	
CSF PROTEIN 15 - 45 mg/dl	

Fig. 1–1. Constituents analyzed in blood by the sequential multiple autoanalyzer (SMA).

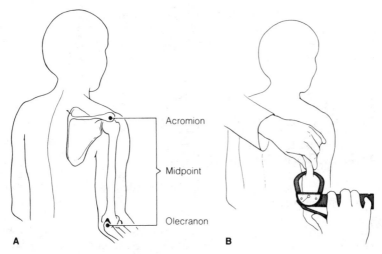

Fig. 1–2. Arm anthropometry. (*A*) Measuring upper right arm midpoint. (*B*) Applying caliper to measure skinfold thickness. (Courtesy of Medical Illustrations, The Ohio State University)

3. Lean body mass is estimated by mid-arm-muscle circumference (see Table 1-11 and Fig. 1-2).

Physiological or Biochemical Determinations

The major purpose of advanced physiological and biochemical assessments is to detect subclinical inadequacies so that early nutritional intervention can be initiated for individuals at "nutritional risk" prior to onset of overt clinical signs.

- Blood Analysis
  1. Complete blood count, including total lymphocyte determinations (Table 1-12)
  2. Constituents analyzed in SMA (see Fig. 1-1 and Table 1-12)
     a. Albumin, if not analyzed during simple nutritional evaluation screening
     b. Serum transferrin (TFN)
     c. Total iron binding capacity
- Urine Analysis (see Table 1-12)
  1. Urinary urea nitrogen (UUN)
  2. Urinary creatinine–creatinine height index (CHI; see Appendix VIII)
- Integumentary Determinations. Skin test antigens (see Table 1-12)

Clinical Determinations

Consult Table 1-9. Clinical signs of malnutrition may be nonspecific for they may be caused by multiple nutrient inadequacies (*e.g.*, glossitis may be induced by a niacin deficiency as well as a riboflavin deficiency). Clinical data alone, therefore, are not sufficient evidence on which to base extensive nutritional support, unless they are confirmed by biochemical or dietary data and physician examinations.

Nurses' Responsibilities in Evaluating Nutritional Status

Initiate Good Evaluation

Nurses in doctors' offices, community nursing services, and outclient clinics should *recognize clients who may be at nutritional risk*. After recognition, nurses should initiate nutritional care, if the physician recommends care, by advising the client to seek nutritional consultation at a health center that provides *qualified* nutritional advice and instruction.

Nurses in the hospital should follow through on the physician's request for a nutritional evaluation by the dietitian. Nurses, who are the only health-team members available to perform nutritional assessments, should develop a strong knowledge of nutrition, including how to use nutritional tools. Additionally, they should attend workshops that teach nutritional assessment techniques.

Participate in Evaluation

- Observe, note, and report any clients who refuse to eat or any who are not eating enough (*e.g.*, clients who consistently leave certain groups of foods such as salads, bread and butter, or milk on their trays).
- Record all intake and output data necessary for nutritional evaluation (*e.g.*, food intake, diuresis, vomiting, and diarrhea).
- Collect nutrition-related data (*e.g.*, 24-hr urine samples) when requested.
- Make sure prescribed special diets, supplements, and so on are being administered.
- Provide emotional support, especially when advanced nutritional evaluations are necessary or when an individual's dietary intake has been altered.
- Weigh the client every day and report weight loss or gain so that the physician and dietitian can evaluate the effectiveness of the nutritional care plan.
- If advanced dietary intake records are necessary, encourage the individual to participate in the food recording. Use the trust the client

has put in you to have him realize the importance this procedure bears to his overall health. If the nurse is the only interviewer, she can obtain dietary intake determinations more effectively if she

1. Develops a rapport with the individual before asking questions that the individual may find threatening
2. Provides a pleasant environment while interviewing the client
3. Obtains an advanced knowledge of how to use nutritional tools when recording and analyzing food intakes (see Tables 1-5, 1-6, 1-7, 1-8, and 1-10), and evaluates the advantages and disadvantages before using individual tools (see Tables 1-5 and 1-10)
4. Uses proper interviewing techniques that will improve communication such as
   a. Using language the learner understands, not professional jargon
   b. Considering the learner's intelligence level
   c. Using nonverbal techniques when indicated
   d. Evaluating the client's attitudes toward food as a means of pleasure and treatment
   e. Avoiding moralistic judgments, giving constructive rather than destructive criticisms
   f. Summarizing information obtained and given

Coordinate Evaluations

- Organize and contribute to health-team conferences. Obtain and report information such as usual weight, recent weight, and any new laboratory data or treatment plans that may influence nutritional status
- Incorporate nutritional assessment information into overall holistic client care by developing a strong attitude toward food as treatment and then making sure it is delivered and consumed properly

Reinforce and Follow Up Evaluation

- Observe and report any clinical signs (*e.g.*, sparse hair) that indicate a decline in nutritional status; this decline may be due to the disease progression or complications, iatrogenic malnutrition, or an inadequate nutritional care plan
- Motivate food consumption by relating improved nutritional status to enhanced recovery, when applicable. Reinforce dietary instructions when appropriate (see chapters on particular disorders)

Table 1–1
Clinical Characteristics of Marasmus and Kwashiorkor

Clinical Signs	Marasmus	Kwashiorkor
Growth failure	Common	Common
Edema	Absent	Very common
Mental changes	Uncommon but severe if marasmus present in infants over long periods	Very common
Hepatomegaly	Common	Very common
Hair changes	Common	Very common (*e.g.*, red pigment)
Dermatosis (flaky)	Rare	Common
Anemia	Common	Common
Subcutaneous fat	Absent	Reduced but present
Weight loss	Severe	Severe but may be masked by edema
Appetite	Good	Poor
Infection	Common	Very common
Diarrhea	Uncommon	Very common
Wound healing	Fair in short-term stress, poor in long-term stress	Poor

Table 1–2 17

Table 1–2
Metabolic and Hormonal Response to Stress

Metabolic Reactions	Hormonal Reactions	Clinical and Biochemical Signs	Clinical Treatment
Stage I (1–48 hr or longer, depending on severity of trauma)			
↓ BMR ↓ BP ↑ Diuresis	Initiated by the CNS ↑ Catecholamine release ↓ Insulin secretion	↑ Weakness and fatigue ↓ BP that can lead to shock ↑ Diuresis	Medical treatment that reduces the stress (*e.g.*, relieves pain and replaces blood loss)
Stage II (48 hr–3 wk, depending on severity of trauma)			
↑ BMR (catabolism) ↑ Increased heart rate, which restores BP ↑ Gluconeogenesis at the expense of lean body tissue	↑ ADH secretion, which stimulates water retention ↑ ACTH production, which stimulates aldosterone secretion; consequently, Na retention enhanced and K excretion enhanced ↑ ACTH production also stimulates the release of glucocorticoids (*e.g.*, cortisol), which enhances gluconeogenesis, lipolysis, and muscle proteolysis ↑ Catecholamine release (*e.g.*, epinephrine and norepinephrine) enhances lipolysis, glyco-	Edema Increased BP Oliguria Hypokalemia and possibly hyponatremia Hyperglycemia Glycosuria Negative nitrogen balance Hyperlipidemia or hyperketonemia Weight loss (may be masked by edema) Sepsis Increased lactic acid levels Respiratory failure that can lead to pneumonia and death	Medical, surgical, or drug treatment to abate trauma Nutritional support: replace electrolytes, water, and glucose; other nutritional support of little help until trauma is treated Once trauma subsides (usually in 3 to 4 days with medical treatment), other nutritional support regimens such as parenteral or enteral solutions should be individualized according to tolerance and extent of body wasting (see Chap. 2)

(continued)

Table 1–2
Metabolic and Hormonal Response to Stress (continued)

Metabolic Reactions	Hormonal Reactions	Clinical and Biochemical Signs	Clinical Treatment
Stage II (48 hr–3 wk, depending on severity of trauma) *(continued)*			
	genolysis, and glucagon secretion; consequently, insulin secretion or sensitivity impaired, which ultimately reduces protein and fat synthesis		If trauma is elective (*e.g.*, elective surgery), nutritional support before trauma is induced may reduce extent of body wasting
Stage III (3 wk–6 mo, depending on severity of trauma)			
Normal BMR	↓ ADH, ACTH, catecholamines and glucagon	Muscle synthesized	Medical treatment continued
Normal BP	↑ Insulin release and sensitivity	Visceral function returned to normal	Nutritional support: progression from parenteral solutions (if applicable) to high-caloric, high-protein oral feeding (depends on severity of trauma; see Chap. 2 and Table 2-1 for energy and nutrient needs of adults under stress
Normal colloidal osmotic pressure for increased protein synthesis enhances albumin production		Nitrogen in balance or positive	
		Fatty tissue increased	
Lean body and adipose tissue replaced as insulin secretion normalizes		Weight gain	
		Client desires nourishment	

↑ = increased; ↓ = decreased; BMR = basal metabolic rate; BP = blood pressure; CNS = central nervous system; ADH = antidiuretic hormone; ACTH = adrenocorticotropic hormone; Na = sodium; K = potassium

Table 1-3 19

Table 1-3
Causes and Prevention of Iatrogenic Malnutrition

Health-Team Practices That May Enhance or Induce Poor Nutritional Status	Health-Team Practices That May Prevent or Alleviate Poor Nutritional Status
1. Weight and height are not obtained or recorded upon admission or during convalescence.	1. Obtain and record height and weight upon admission and frequently during convalescence; additionally, record "usual" weight and recent weight loss information.
2. Frequent rotation of staff may interrupt personal contact with clients; thus poor food consumption will not be recognized.	2. Nursing supervisors and head dietitians should assign personnel to one floor whenever possible.
3. Food intake and output are often not observed or recorded.	3. The head nurse should instruct staff nurses to observe and record clients' food and liquid intake. This is especially important when the client is receiving oral supplements or is on a "special diet." In all cases, however, it should be kept in mind that food is treatment; consequently, if several groups of foods are left on the tray, daily nutrient and caloric deficiencies will develop.
4. Meals or supplemental feedings are often withheld for diagnostic tests or treatment.	4. The nurse should note on the client's record that he has not consumed his meal at the usual time.
5. Members of the hospital team often fail to recognize that food refusal is one way a client can maintain his identity or some control over his affairs.	5. Members of the health team should recognize that a client's refusal to eat is not always related to unpalatable food. Instead, many underlying reasons may account for a refusal to eat. The nurse or physician should request clerical, social, or psychiatric consultations.
6. Simple requests for food likes and dislikes are often ignored.	6. Record simple food requests (*e.g.*, client prefers coffee to tea). These notes are important; when requests are consistently ignored, the client begins to feel like a "number," not a person, and he begins to wonder what other mistakes are being made in his overall treatment. The result is anxiety and anger.

(continued)

Table 1-3
Causes and Prevention of Iatrogenic Malnutrition (continued)

Health-Team Practices That May Enhance or Induce Poor Nutritional Status	Health-Team Practices That May Prevent or Alleviate Poor Nutritional Status
7. Drug–nutrient interactions are often overlooked.	7. Physicians should prescribe increased nutrient intake when medications interrupt nutrient utilization. Additionally, they should advise the nurse and client when the medications should be taken (*e.g.*, with or without food) in order to minimize gastrointestinal discomforts.
8. The nutritional status of a client is often not considered a factor in the success of recovery, especially when an individual undergoes surgical procedures.	8. Physicians should prescribe nutritional support therapy before or after surgical procedures when the client is deemed a nutritional risk. The nurse's responsibility to the client on nutritional support is to make sure that the client receives the treatment.
9. Physical impairments (*e.g.*, dentures, immobilized limbs, or poor eyesight) may be overlooked as the reason that a client's food consumption is poor.	9. The head nurse in most hospitals is responsible for the proper delivery of nourishment to all clients, especially those that may need feeding assistance. Guidelines to be implemented when a client cannot or will not feed himself are as follows: • Serve the tray last, but keep hot food hot and cold food cold while the tray is being held • Alternate foods • Provide a relaxed atmosphere: Do not appear rushed • Avoid treating the client like a baby • Keep the cover on, between bites • Encourage food consumption but *do not scold* • Encourage client to feed himself whenever possible: if the client is blind, self-feeding can be enhanced if foods are arranged clockwise on the plate and their positions described to the client *(continued)*

Table 1–3 21

Table 1-3
Causes and Prevention of Iatrogenic Malnutrition (continued)

Health-Team Practices That May Enhance or Induce Poor Nutritional Status	Health-Team Practices That May Prevent or Alleviate Poor Nutritional Status
10. Insufficient dietary instructions are given before discharge.	10. The physician is responsible for requesting special dietary instructions when the client is admitted if he knows that a special diet will be needed upon discharge. The dietitian is responsible for instructing the client gradually so that the dietary alterations are thoroughly understood. The nurse is responsible for reinforcing dietary instructions when she is near the client or when she delivers the tray.
11. Poor communication among health team members leads to incomplete nutritional management of the client.	11. Physicians, nurses, dietitians, and other members of the health team should learn to communicate and share involvement in the means of preventing and treating disease. The nurse has a special role in this communication for she has the closest contact with all health-team members and the client. Communication and coordination, however, are not solely the responsibilities of the nurse; it is also the duty of other staff members to reveal to the nurse how their services and treatments can contribute to complete client care and then be *available to provide these services when requested.*

Table 1–4
Initial Interview Chart and Related Nutritional Implications

Components	Related Nutritional Implications
Name	
Sex	The sex of an individual determines his standard caloric and nutrient requirements.
Age	The age of an individual determines his caloric and nutrient needs. *Note.* Usually caloric and nutrient needs *decrease* with age because basal metabolic rate and lean body mass decrease.
Ethnic and religious background	The ethnic or religious beliefs of a person may alter his intake of certain foods and nutrients.
Occupation	The occupation of a person may reflect his caloric requirements.
Housing and family	A person's place of residence can determine his ability to prepare, store, and procure food. Individuals in families usually eat more nutrient-dense, mixed dishes than do persons living alone.
Diagnosis	Individuals under severe physiological stress have increased caloric and nutrient needs.
Mental status	Psychological stress can impair or enhance food consumption. Additionally, it can increase caloric and nutrient requirements.
Medical history	An individual with a chronic illness has twice the likelihood of being a nutritional risk that an individual admitted for the first time has.
Medications	Medications can interact with nutrients, impairing their ingestion, digestion, absorption, transport, and utilization.
Allergies	Particular food allergies may enhance adverse symptoms (*e.g.*, diarrhea after milk ingestion).
Mastication or swallowing difficulties	Ingestion of certain nutrients may be impaired (*e.g.*, complex carbohydrates) unless the consistency of the diet is adjusted.

(continued)

Table 1–4 23

Table 1–4
Initial Interview Chart and Related Nutritional Implications (continued)

Components	Related Nutritional Implications
Special diet	If an individual has previously been or is presently on a prescribed special diet, he may know a great deal about what foods he can consume, or he may have many misconceptions that need correcting. Gradual instruction should begin as soon as possible.
Appetite	Poor appetite enhances the likelihood of being a nutritional risk.
Skin conditions	Skin conditions can be induced by nutrient inadequacies (*e.g.*, dry skin).
Structural determinations (height and weight)	Height and usual weight, maximum lifetime weight, and recent weight loss can affect caloric needs and provide an estimate of nutritional status.
Problem list	If an individual states that he frequently has adverse symptoms such as vomiting and diarrhea, nutrient inadequacies may exist.
Special requests	If an individual requests to see a social worker or clergyman, he may have emotional or financial needs that have impaired food consumption.
Attending physician	The name of the attending physician to be notified may reveal what nutritional alterations may be necessary (*e.g.*, individuals admitted for a GI surgical procedure may need a clear liquid diet).

Table 1–5
The Basic Four Food Groups

Group	Major Nutrients Supplied	Examples of Foods and Serving Sizes
Milk and cheese	Protein Vitamins A, B_6, B_{12} Calcium Riboflavin	1 8-oz cup of milk 1 cup of plain yogurt 2-inch cube of cheddar or Swiss cheese 1½ cups of ice cream 2 cups of cottage cheese

Meat, poultry, fish, beans	Protein
	Vitamins B_6, B_{12}, B_1, Niacin
	Iron
	Phosphorus
		1½–2 oz of cooked meat, poultry, fish
		  without bone
		2 eggs
		1 cup of cooked dried beans, peas, soy-
		  beans, lentils
		4 tbsp of peanut butter
		½–1 cup of nuts, sesame seeds, sunflower
		  seeds

Fruits and vegetables	Vitamin A Vitamin C Potassium	½ cup of cooked fruit or vegetable ½–¾ cup of fruit or vegetable juice 1 whole orange, 1 whole tomato, 1 medium potato

Bread and cereal (whole-grain, enriched, or fortified products)	Carbohydrate
	B-vitamins
	Phosphorus
		1 slice of bread
		½ cup of cooked or ¾ cup of uncooked
		  cereal
		½ cup of cooked macroni, noodles, rice,
		  spaghetti

(Adapted from US Department of Agriculture, Home and Garden Bulletin No. 228)

Table 1-6 25

Table 1–6
Suggested Number of Servings From the Basic Four Food Groups

Food Group	Suggested Daily Servings From Each Food Group			
	Adults	Adolescents	Infants and Children	Pregnant and Lactating Women
Milk	2	4	3	4
Meat/meat alternative	2	2	2	2–3
Fruits and vegetables	4	4	4	4
Bread and cereal	4	4	4	4

Note. The Basic Four Food Groups, however, do not include foods such as fats, sweets, and alcohol, all of which provide calories and some nutrients (*e.g.,* vitamin E in oils), but very few. Because Americans consume a great quantity of these foods, however, they should be kept in mind when analyzing dietary intake for nutrient inadequacies and nutrient excesses. Recently the Basic Five Food Group, or the Daily Food Guide, has been introduced to include these foods, but it is not usually used to analyze the nutrient contribution of a dietary intake because the fifth group contains very few nutrients.

Table 1–7
Major Nutrients Contained in a Diet Planned According to the Basic Four Food Groups

Adult Plan	Grams	Approximate Measure	Energy (kcal)	Protein (g)	Calcium (mg)	Iron (mg)	Vitamin A (IU)	Thiamine (mg)	Riboflavin (mg)	Niacin (mg)	Vitamin C (mg)
Milk group, 2 servings of milk	488	2 glasses (1 pt)	330	17	570	0.4	740	0.14	0.82	0.4	4
Meat group,* 2 servings of meat, fish, or poultry		1 avg serving, 3½ oz									
	100	cooked, lean only	295	24	11	2.2	178	0.16	0.21	6.0	
Egg	50	1 medium	80	6.5	27	1.2	590	0.06	0.15	0.1	2
Fruits and vegetables group, 4 or more servings											
Vegetables											
Deep green or yellow†	100	½ cup cooked	29	2.0	5	1.1	3900	0.07	0.11	0.6	29
Potato	100	1 medium, baked	93	2.6	9	0.7	Trace	0.10	0.04	1.7	20
Other‡	100	½ cup cooked	42	2.1	22	0.8	220	0.07	0.06	0.7	13
Fruits											
Citrus or tomato§	185	6 oz juice	55	1.1	20	0.7	519	0.09	0.04	0.7	50
Other¶	100	1 avg serving	75	0.7	13	0.7	550	0.04	0.05	0.5	11
Bread and cereal group, 4 or more servings											
Bread, white, enriched	70	3 slices	180	6.0	57	1.8	Trace	0.18	0.15	1.8	Trace

(continued)

Table 1-7 27

Table 1-7
Major Nutrients Contained in a Diet Planned According to the Basic Four Food Groups (continued)

Adult Plan	Grams	Approximate Measure	Energy (kcal)	Protein (g)	Calcium (mg)	Iron (mg)	Vitamin A (IU)	Thiamine (mg)	Riboflavin (mg)	Niacin (mg)	Vitamin C (mg)
Cereal, whole-grain or enriched	30	⅔ cup flakes	70	1.8	5	0.6	Trace	0.09	0.03	0.6	
Total nutrients in foundation diet			1250	64	740	10.2	6700	1.00	1.66	13.1	130
Recommended allowances											
Man, 70 kg, moderately active, 23–50 years old			2700	56	800	10	5000 (1000 RE)	1.4	1.6	18**	60
Woman, 55 kg, moderately active, 23–50 years old			2000	44	600	18	4000 (800 RE)	1.0	1.2	13**	60

* Average of 10 100-g servings of lean, edible portion of meats, including beef, lamb, pork, poultry, and fish

† Average of 10 100-g servings, one each of asparagus, broccoli, Brussels sprouts, carrots, green snap beans, green lettuce and romaine, spinach, yellow (winter) squash, and sweet potato

‡ Other vegetables: average of 10 100-g servings of beets, cauliflower, celery, corn, green peas, lima beans, onions, summer squash, turnips, and zucchini

§ Daily average based on 3 servings of orange juice, 2 servings of grapefruit juice, 3 servings of tomato juice, and 2 servings of fresh raw tomatoes

¶ Other fruits: daily average based on 1 average serving each of fresh apple, banana, peach, pear; 1 serving each of canned applesauce, apricots, peaches, and pineapple, plus 1 serving of dried or stewed prunes

** Includes niacin, as such, and from tryptophan conversion

(Calloway DH, Carpenter KO: Nutrition and Health. Philadelphia, Saunders College Publishing, 1981)

Table 1–8
Less Studied Nutrients in a Menu Based on the Basic Four Pattern*

Food	Grams	Phosphorus (mg)	Sodium (g)	Potassium (g)	Magnesium (mg)	Zinc (mg)	Vitamin E (IU)	Free Folacin (mcg)§	Vitamin B6 (mg)	Vitamin B12 (mcg)	Pantothenic acid (mg)
Milk group											
Milk	244	227	122	352	32	1.0	0.1	12	0.10	1.0	0.83
Cheddar cheese	30	143	210	25	14	0.9	0.1	<1	0.02	0.3	0.15
Meat group											
Chicken	100	257	78	381	20	1.8	0.4	4	0.30	0.4	0.90
Egg	50	102	61	64	6	0.7	0.2	25	0.06	1.0	0.80
Fruits and vegetables group											
Green beans	100	32	1	152	20	0.3	0.1	7	0.07		0.14
Summer squash	100	25	1	141	16	0.2	<0.1	2	0.06		0.17
Potato	100	65	4	503	20	0.2	<0.1	12	0.09		0.25
Tomato, raw	100	18	3	227	10	0.2	1.0	18	0.10		0.25
Orange juice, fresh	100	16	1	186	10	<0.1	<0.1	35	0.03		0.16
Apple, raw	100	10	1	110	8	<0.1	0.31	3	0.03		0.10
Bread and cereal group											
Bread, enriched, white	70	68	335†	73	15	0.5	0.1	8	0.03	trace‡	0.30
Corn flakes	30	14	300†	36	5	0.1	<0.1	4	0.02		0.06
Total		977	1137†	2250	176	6	2.7	130	1	3	4

(continued)

Table 1-8 29

Table 1-8
Less Studied Nutrients in a Menu Based on the Basic Four Pattern* (continued)

Food	Grams	Phosphorus (mg)	Sodium (g)	Potassium (g)	Magnesium (mg)	Zinc (mg)	Vitamin E (IU)	Free Folacin (mcg)§	Vitamin B_6 (mg)	Vitamin B_{12} (mcg)	Pantothenic acid (mg)
Recommended allowance											
Men		800	1–3	2–6	350	15	10	400	2.2	3.0	4–7
Women		800	1–3	2–6	300	15	8	400	2.0	3.0	4–7

* Compositional data for these nutrients (except for phosphorous and potassium) are not as reliable as one would wish and are tabulated only to indicate the order of magnitude of a nutrient. Methods are poor for the vitamins and minerals vary by a factor of 10 to 100, depending on soil composition and processing contaminants.
† Sodium added to these cereal products in manufacture. Other foods would have salt added in cooking. The expected daily total would be about 5 g of sodium, with these additions and use of salted butter or margarine.
‡ Vitamin B_{12} due to added milk in recipe
§ World Health Organization recommendation for *free* folacin; NRC RDA is 400 mg *total* folacin.
(Calloway DH, Carpenter KO: Nutrition and Health. Philadelphia, Saunders College Publishing, 1981)

Table 1–9
Significant Clinical Signs in Nutritional Evaluations

Body Area	Clinical Signs That May Indicate Poor Nutritional Status	Nutritional Implications
Hair	Dull, dray, sparse, or shedding	Multiple nutrient inadequacies may be present (*e.g.*, protein and vitamin deficiencies)
Face	Swollen or edematous	Protein deficiency (albumin) or sodium excess with resultant water retention may be present
Eyes	Pale	Iron and protein inadequacies
	Pale	Iron deficiency
	Red	Vitamin B complex inadequacies, especially of riboflavin
Lips	Swollen, red cracks at the sides (cheilosis)	Vitamin B complex inadequacies, especially of riboflavin
Tongue	Bright red or swollen	Vitamin B complex inadequacies or GI disorders
	Pale	Iron deficiency
	Papillary hypertrophy	Multiple nutrient inadequacies
Teeth	Carious or missing	Excessive intake of carbohydrate (sucrose) or alcohol, poor hygiene, or multiple nutrient inadequacies (*e.g.*, calcium)
Gums	Bleeding	Vitamin C deficiency with resultant true or conditioned scurvy

(continued)

Table 1–9 31

Table 1–9
Significant Clinical Signs in Nutritional Evaluations (continued)

Body Area	Clinical Signs That May Indicate Poor Nutritional Status	Nutritional Implications
Abdomen	Edematous	See Face
Skin	Dry, flaking, or scaly	Vitamin A or B-complex deficiencies
	Petechiae (small black spots or hemorrhages under the skin)	Vitamin C deficiency
	Poor turgor or tone; pressure sores	Multiple nutrient inadequacies, especially of protein and vitamin C
	Xanthomas (fat deposits under the skin, around joints, and under the eyes)	Increased serum levels of LDLs or VLDLs with resultant hyperlipoproteinemia
Nails	Brittle, ridged, or spoon-shaped	Iron deficiency
Extremities	Muscle wasting	Macronutrient inadequacies (carbohydrate, fat, and protein) with resultant marasmus
		Protein deficiency with resultant kwashiorkor
	Edematous	See Face
Nervous system	Mental confusion or irritability	Chronic nutrient inadequacies, especially B-complex (*e.g.*, thiamine) deficiencies; excessive intake of alcohol or drugs

Table 1-10
Tools Used to Estimate Caloric and Nutrient Intake in Advanced Nutritional Evaluations

Nutrition Tool	Procedure	Advantages	Disadvantages
24-hour dietary recall	Individual recalls everything he has eaten within the last 24 hours. This information is recorded on a questionnaire or told to an interviewer who records the information.	It detects an exogenous lack of nutrients within an individual's dietary habits. It is a simple procedure for most individuals and interviewers. Memory is more accurate within 24 hours than after more time elapses.	Some people feel that their food intake patterns are inadequate owing to economics, lack of knowledge, or illness so that they simply do not tell the truth. Some people simply do not recall what they ate the previous day. What is recalled may be atypical of the usual intake (*e.g.,* client may be ill or celebrating).
Food diary or record	Individual is asked to record what, how much, how often, with whom, where, and why he eats. Information is recorded immediately following a meal. Records are kept for 3 days to 1 week, with one weekend day included (see Chap. 6, chart on One Entry in a Daily Food Diary).	Individual becomes aware of his eating patterns. Lifestyle is revealed. Psychological reasons for eating are discovered by the individual and interviewer. Individual usually cooperates since the recording time is short.	It has the same disadvantages as 24-hour recall. Snack foods are often excluded, especially those consumed in front of the refrigerator. It is expensive and needs a trained interviewer to analyze the results.
Dietary history	A typical pattern of food intake and composition is not-	It probes the food habits of an individual over a long peri-	It has the same disadvantages as other dietary intake

(continued)

Table 1-10 33

Table 1-10
Tools Used to Estimate Caloric and Nutrient Intake in Advanced Nutritional Evaluations (continued)

Nutrition Tool	Procedure	Advantages	Disadvantages
	ed over a period of time (*e.g.*, 6 months) by an individual and a trained interviewer.	od of time, which provides a more accurate estimate of the balance and quantities of nutrients consumed. Increased information is obtained on lifestyle (*e.g.*, cultural background, shopping habits, and cooking facilities).	assessments. Individual tires of recording and forgets or simply invents the records.
Food composition tables*	Foods taken in by the individual are compared by a trained professional to the caloric and nutrient values of identical foods listed in these handbooks.*	Food and nutrient lists are more extensive than those in the Basic Four Foods Group (*e.g.*, oils, sweets, snack foods, and baby foods are listed). Consequently, nutrient calculations are more accurate.	Caloric and nutrient content of some foods are not listed (*e.g.*, cultural foods, "health" foods, and mixed dishes). Individuals make mistakes while converting household measures into metric weights (*e.g.*, converting ounces into grams). Nutrient calculations do not take into account variations in laboratory measurement techniques; seasonal, processing, and preparation differences in foods; and individual physiological

(continued)

Table 1-10
Tools Used to Estimate Caloric and Nutrient Intake in Advanced Nutritional Evaluations (continued)

Nutrition Tool	Procedure	Advantages	Disadvantages
Recommended daily allowances (RDAs)	Food intake recorded by individuals is compared by trained personnel to the RDAs for 29 nutrients (see Appendix IV).	They are good for planning and obtaining food supplies for groups, especially public assistance programs (*e.g.,* WIC). They are good for establishing guidelines for new food products, nutrition education programs, and nutritional labeling. *Note.* The U.S. RDAs found on food labels are based on the highest nutrient requirements of the RDAs in most instances.	availability of nutrients because much of the information is unknown. They have the same disadvantages as the food composition tables. *They are recommendations, not requirements.* They provide a margin of safety for most individuals; consequently, two thirds of the nutrient recommendations are closer to the requirements for healthy individuals. They are not based on the needs of individuals under the stress of illness; they are only based on the needs of healthy individuals living under normal stress in the U.S. Recommendations for carbohydrates, fat, and some trace elements are not included.

* Found in *Composition of Foods*, USDA Handbook No. 8; *Nutritive Values of American Foods*, Handbook No. 456; *Food Values of Portions Commonly Used* by Pennington and Church (consult References)

Table 1-11 35

Table 1-11
Anthropometric Measurements Used in Advanced Nutritional Evaluations

Anthropometric Measurement	Procedure	Advantages	Disadvantages
Triceps skinfold measurement (TSF)	Measurements are obtained at the triceps (mid-point) of the non-dominant arm by a Lange caliper (see Fig. 1-2). Measurements should be taken by the *same person* 3 times. Individual measurements should then be compared to normal standards or percentiles (see Appendix III).	Measures subcutaneous *fat* stores. Useful as a screening tool for large populations. Identifies weight loss in an individual over time (*e.g.*, good diagnostic tool for identifying iatrogenic malnutrition). Identifies individuals who may be nutritional risks*	Different fat distributions among individuals. Does not evaluate other body constituents (*e.g.*, water). Measurements, due to human error, often inconsistent. Comparison standards or percentiles not accurate for everyone. Expensive and uncomfortable when steel calipers used.
Mid-arm-muscle circumference measurement (MAMC)	A centimeter tape, made of nonstretchable material, is used to measure upper-arm circumference at the mid-point (see Fig. 1-2). Total mid-arm circumference measurement minus the individual's triceps skinfold measurement is then used to measure mid-upper-arm-*muscle* circumference.	Estimates somatic (skeletal) protein changes. Useful tool for estimating *lean body mass*. Identifies individuals who may be nutritional risks* Painless and inexpensive	Different total fat to muscle mass among individuals (*e.g.*, athletes *vs.* others). Measurements, due to human error, often inconsistent. Variations in upper-arm anthropometric parameters not always related to nutritional status (*e.g.*, change with age and energy expenditure (exercise).

(continued)

Table 1–11
Anthropometric Measurements Used in Advanced Nutritional Evaluations (continued)

Anthropometric Measurement	Procedure	Advantages	Disadvantages
	That is, arm-muscle circumference (mm) = arm circumference (mm) −(3.14 × triceps skinfold thickness [mm]) Individual measurements should then be compared to normal standards or percentiles (see Appendix III).		Edema with some treatments (*e.g.*, drugs and surgical removal of the breast)

* In general, persons are deemed nutritional risks if they fall within the following standards or percentiles:
Standards: 80%, mild risk; 70%, moderate risk; 60%, severe risk
Percentiles: 15%, mild to moderate risk of becoming depleted; 5%, severe nutritional risk

Table 1–12 37

Table 1–12
**Physiological and Biochemical Measurements
Used in Advanced Nutritional Evaluations**

Measurements	Procedure	Advantages	Disadvantages
Blood analysis*			
Total lymphocyte count (TLC) Normal levels, 1500–3000 mm³; mild depletion, 1500–1800 mm³; moderate depletion, 900–1400 mm³; severe deple- tion, lower than 900 mm³	Total lymphocyte counts are obtained from white blood count differentials (CBC). $$TLC = \frac{\% \text{ lymphocytes} \times WBC}{100}$$	Lymphocyte counts are a good indicator of immuno- competence. Low concentrations may indi- cate that malnutrition exists subclinically, since they are an indicator of visceral, not somatic, protein stores. Inexpensive, a normal routine blood analysis	Lymphocyte counts measure infection; therefore, higher levels will be seen in viral infections; these higher readings may mask lower levels that may indicate that malnutrition is present.
Transferrin			
β-1 globulin (protein) binds and transports iron in plasma. Normal levels, 205–410 mg/dl; mild depletion, 180–200 mg/dl; moderate depletion, 160–180 mg/dl; severe deple- tion, 150 mg/dl	Levels (TFN) measured directly from serum or calculated by measuring total iron-binding capacity (TIBC): TFN = (TIBC × 0.8) − 43 Total iron-binding capacity (mcg/dl): mild depletion, 182– 214 mcg/dl; moderate deple- tion, 181/152 mcg/dl; severe depletion, 151 mcg/dl	Indirect measurement of avail- ability of protein (amino acids) Transferrin half-life considera- bly shorter than that of al- bumin; consequently, it is more valid when estimating *present* nutritional status Sensitive to short-term inten- sive dietary manipulation,	Expensive Variations other than malnu- trition may affect concen- tration

(continued)

Table 1–12
**Physiological and Biochemical Measurements
Used in Advanced Nutritional Evaluations** (continued)

Measurements	Procedure	Advantages	Disadvantages
Transferrin (continued)			
		thus it is a good indicator of nutritional support effectiveness	
		Test for iron as well as visceral protein deficiency	
Urine Analysis			
Urinary urea nitrogen (UUN) is an estimate of the body's nitrogen balance	Dietary nitrogen formula: 6.25 g of protein (approximate amount found in 1 oz of meat) = 1 g of nitrogen	Excellent indication of the extent of lean body mass, energy expenditure, and rate of proteolysis	Individual does not comply or urine tests are forgotten
Normal nitrogen balance, urinary nitrogen = dietary nitrogen intake	From a 24-hr urine specimen, amount of urea (nitrogen) is calculated by: UUN g + 3 g (amount of nitrogen lost in feces and sweat)	Negative balance, over time, indicates nutritional support necessary	Test not valid unless all specimens available
Positive nitrogen balance, urinary nitrogen is less than dietary intake	Normal healthy individuals should be in *nitrogen balance*, meaning they excrete the same amount of nitrogen as taken in	Support aims to acquire nitrogen balance or positive balance since 1 g of nitrogen = 30 g of lean body mass	Organ dysfunctions can interfere with reading
Negative nitrogen balance, urinary nitrogen exceeds dietary intake			
Urinary creatinine Normal levels: Male, 20–26 mg/kg/day; female, 14–22	All urine excreted within a 24-hour period is collected to	A good indicator of lean body mass	Individual does not comply or urine tests forgotten

(continued)

Table 1–12 39

Table 1–12
**Physiological and Biochemical Measurements
Used in Advanced Nutritional Evaluations** (continued)

Measurements	Procedure	Advantages	Disadvantages
Urine Analysis *(continued)*			
mg/kg/day (abnormal levels in Appendix VIII)	determine the release of creatinine (anhydride of creatine) from muscle. Creatinine excretion is then compared to normal standards. Individuals of the same age and sex have a constant excretion of creatinine from day to day (see Appendix VIII). Formula: creatinine height index (CHI) = $$\frac{\text{Actual urinary creatinine}}{\text{Ideal urinary creatinine}} \times 100$$	Excreted by the kidney at a constant rate, when anabolism and catabolism are in equilibrium Lower levels indicate lean tissue (muscle) depletion	Test not valid unless all specimens available CHI standards compiled from small population If kidney is not functioning properly, readings inaccurate Expensive; trained personnel need to collect and analyze data
Integumentary Determinations			
Skin test antigens Normal, sensitivity higher than 5 mm/24 hr after injection; moderately disposed, immune system responds only to one antigen; severe, all tests negative	Skin tested with up to 8 antigenic solutions (*e.g.*, *Candida*, mumps, and streptokinase); 24–48 hours after testing, a red area, around the tested site, appears if reaction positive; this area can be measured in mm and compared to normal standards, which should be 5 mm or more	Good indicator of cell-mediated immunity Identifies possible nutritional risks if other determinations, such as low levels of albumin (<3.0 g/dl) and decreased body weight (<85% of standard), also evident	Drugs, as well as stress of illness (*e.g.*, sepsis), can suppress cellular immune response, as well as malnutrition

* Additional constituents in blood that can be evaluated to estimate visceral protein levels are thyroxine, prealbumin, and retinol binding protein.

Bibliography

Adams CF: Nutritive Value of American Foods: In Common Units, US Department of Agriculture Handbook No. 456. Washington, DC, US Government Printing Office, 1975

Beisel WR, Wannemacher RW: Gluconeogenesis, ureagenesis and ketogenesis during sepsis. JPEN 4:277, 1980

Bishom CN, Bowen DE, Ritchey SJ: Norms for nutritional assessment of American adults by upper arm anthropometry. Am J Clin Nutr 34:2530, 1981

Bistrian BR: Letters: Anthropometric norms used in assessment of hospitalized patients. Am J Clin Nutr 33:2211, 1980

Blackburn GL: Nutritional assessment: An overview. Clinical Consultations in Nutritional Support 1:10, 1981

Blackburn GL, Bistrian BR, Marni BS et al: Nutritional and metabolic assessment of the hospitalized patient. JPEN 1:11, 1977

Blackburn GL, Maini BS, Piece EC: Nutrition in the critically ill patient. Anesthesiology 47:181, 1977

Butterworth CE: The skeleton in the hospital closet. Nutrition Today 9:4, 1974

Butterworth CE, Blackburn GL: Hospital malnutrition. Nutrition Today 10:8, 1975

Calloway DH, Carpenter KO: Nutrition and Health. Philadelphia, Saunders College Publishing, 1981

Caly JC: Helping people eat for health: Assessing adults' nutrition. Am J Nurs 77:1605, 1977

Cronk CE, Roche AF: Race- and sex-specific reference data for triceps and subscapular skinfolds and weight/stature. Am J Clin Nutr 35:347, 1982

Derelian D, Schoefer D: Clinical use of the "four food groups." Nutrition & the MD 7:1, 1981

Doyle Pharmaceutical Company: Nutrition in trauma and stress. Minneapolis, Doyle Pharmaceutical Company, 1979

Flear CTG, Bhattacharya SS, Singh CM: Solute and water exchanges between cells and extracellular fluids in health and disturbances after trauma. JPEN 4:99, 1980

Frisancho AR: New norms of upper limb fat and muscle areas for assessment of nutritional status. Am J Clin Nutr 34:2540, 1981

Frisancho AR, Flegel PN: Elbow breadth as a measure of frame size for US males and females. Am J Clin Nutr 37:311, 1983

Garn SM, Pesick SD, Hawthorne VM: The bony chest breadth as a frame size standard in nutritional assessment. Am J Clin Nutr 37:315, 1983

Gray FG, Cray LK: Anthropometric measurements and their interpretation: Principles, practices, and problems. J Am Diet Assoc 77:534, 1980

Green ML, Harry J: Nutrition in Contemporary Nursing Practice. New York, John Wiley & Sons, 1981

Henneman A, Houfek JF, Morin P et al: Teaching nutritional assessment to nursing students. J Am Diet Assoc 78:498, 1981

Howard RB, Herbold NH: Nutrition in Clinical Care. New York, McGraw-Hill, 1978

Jensen TG, Dudrick SJ: Implementation of a multidisciplinary nutritional assessment program. J Am Diet Assoc 79:258, 1981

Kamath S, Malasamos L, Barkauskas V et al: Health Assessment. St Louis, CV Mosby, 1977

Kaminski MV, Ruggiero RP, Mills CB: A guide to diagnosis and treatment of the hypermetabolic patient. J Fla Med Assoc 66:390, 1979

Kaufman M: A food preference questionnaire for counseling patients with diabetes. J Am Diet Assoc 49:32, 1966

Krause MV, Mahan LK: Food, Nutrition and Diet Therapy, 6th ed. Philadelphia, WB Saunders, 1979

Pennington JAT, Church HN: Food Values of Portions Commonly Used, 13th ed. Philadelphia, JB Lippincott, 1980

Randall HT: Fluid and electrolyte requirements in surgical patients: Clinical application. Surg Clin North Am 56:1034, 1976

Ross Laboratories: A nursing role in nutritional assessment. Columbus, Ohio, Ross Laboratories, 1978

Saudek CD, Felig P: The metabolic events of starvation. Am J Med 60:117, 1976

Seltzer MH, Bastidas JA, Cooper DM et al: Instant nutritional assessment. JPEN 3:157, 1979

Senate Committee on Nutritional and Human Needs: Dietary Goals for the United States, 2nd ed. Washington, DC, US Government Printing Office, 1977 (Pub No 052-070-04376-8)

Thiele VP: Clinical Nutrition, 2nd ed. St Louis, CV Mosby, 1980

Tobias AL, Van Itallie TB: Nutritional problems of hospitalized patients. J Am Diet Assoc 71:253, 1977

Watt BK, Merrill AL: Composition of Foods, US Department of Agriculture Handbook No. 8. Washington, DC, US Government Printing Office, 1963

Weissberger LE, Sowa D, Weddle D: Clinical nutritional assessment: A two-month evaluation. J Am Diet Assoc 81:58, 1982

Williams CO: Malnutrition. Lancet 2:342, 1962

Williams SR: Nutrition and Diet Therapy, 4th ed. St Louis, CV Mosby, 1981

Wilmore DW: Hormonal responses and their effect on metabolism. Surg Clin North Am 56:999, 1976

Wretlind A: Parenteral nutrition. Nutr Rev 39:257, 1981

chapter 2

Nutritional Care Plans

Types of Nutritional Care Plans

Normal or Regular Diets

Normal or regular diets, prescribed in a hospital, are calorically adequate and nutrient-balanced. The balance yields all the known chemical elements needed for physiological and psychological well-being, if consumed. If nutritional restoration is required during stress, however, the normal diet may have to be supplemented.

Therapeutic Diets

Therapeutic diets use nutrients as a factor in the prevention, control, and reversal of adverse effects induced by disease or by the metabolic effects of stress. Therapeutic diets may have altered nutrient intake, altered nutrient ratios, or altered food consistency (*e.g.*, liquid diets [including enteral supplements], soft diets, or nutrients in solution [parenteral solutions]). Additionally, the frequency of the meal plan may be altered.

Goals of Nutritional Care Plans

1. Prevent, control, or decrease the clinical symptoms of diseases that are related to primary or secondary nutritional inadequacies; this may be accomplished by providing nutritional care and education within the community
2. Enhance the individual's ability to tolerate and respond to surgical and medical treatments, including drug therapy

3. Enhance recovery, decrease convalescent time, and prevent the morbidity and mortality associated with the complications of decreased nutritional status such as pressure sores, poor wound healing, sepsis, fistulas, pneumonia, and psychological disturbances

An individualized nutritional care plan must address several factors. General factors are listed in Tables 2-1 and 2-2.* Specific factors include the following:

- Energy nutrient and electrolyte requirements, determined by
  1. Age and stage of development (especially important when determining the nutritional needs of children)
  2. Nutritional status prior to trauma
  3. Present nutritional status
  4. Extent of hypercatabolic state and how long the hypercatabolic state may last
  5. Anticipated treatment of illness (*e.g.*, radiation; see Tables 2-1 and 2-2)
- Tolerance, determined by
  1. Individual's sense of taste (palatability)
  2. Individual's ability to ingest, absorb, and utilize required nutrients and calories without adverse complications (*e.g.*, diarrhea)
- Administration route required, determined by
  1. Medical condition
  2. Nutritional assessment data
  3. Clinical condition

These factors commonly affect the client's willingness to eat, ability to eat, or ability to eat enough to restore, maintain, or enhance his nutritional status during hypercatabolic stress:

- Cost, determined by
  1. Benefits *versus* palatability (*e.g.*, intact nutrients *vs.* purified nutrients)
  2. Benefits *versus* risks (*e.g.*, will a tube feeding enhance recovery as well as parenteral solutions, which may induce risks such as sepsis?)
- Composition of feedings, determined by
  1. Caloric and nutrient requirements, tolerance, medical condition, or prognosis
  2. Administration route required
  3. Advantages and disadvantages including
     a. Particle size, which will affect osmolality
     b. Ease of digestion
     c. Nutrient balance

---

*See tables at the end of this chapter.

    d. Risk of complications such as overhydration or dehydration
    e. Cost
    f. Hygienic safety
    h. Shelf life
    i. Ease of preparation

The remainder of the chapter classifies and describes feedings used in nutritional care plans.

Regular or Oral Feedings

Description

Regular feedings contain foods that have intact nutrients in their natural forms (Table 2-3). Regular feedings are always preferred over other feedings for they "nourish the spirit" as well as the body, prevent atrophy of the gastrointestinal tract, stimulate peristalsis, and stimulate enzyme, hormone, and mucosal cell production. (In other words, when the gut works, use it.)

Indications

Regular feedings are administered when the client
- Is well nourished on admission
- Is undergoing minor surgery and medical treatment
- Will not need extensive medical or drug treatment during or after hospitalization
- Is able to ingest and chew foods without any oral cavity difficulties

Contraindications

Regular feedings are not administered when the client
- Is malnourished on admission unless oral enteral supplements augment the regular diet
- Has any of the adverse symptoms or dysfunctions listed under indications for enteral feedings

Composition

The composition of regular feedings in most types of trauma, especially surgery, usually progresses from a clear liquid consistency to foods with regular texture (Table 2-4; for advantages and disadvantages of regular oral feedings, see Table 2-3).

Table 2–4
Calories and Macronutrients in Progressive Hospital Diets

Diet	Calories	Protein (g)	Fat (g)	Carbohydrate (g)
Clear liquid diet	400–500	5–10	0	100–120
Full liquid diet	1300–1500	45	65	150
Soft diet	1800–2000	60–80	80–100	200–250
Regular diet	2000–2500	60–80	80–100	200–300

Nurses' Responsibilities to Hospitalized Clients on Normal or Therapeutic Oral Feedings

Before the Meal

1. Involve the client in his own meal planning.

    a. Explain the selective menu so that he can choose foods he enjoys, but guide him a little so that he chooses a variety of foods with nutrient density, not four desserts.

    b. If the client is on a therapeutic diet, explain abbreviations (*e.g.*, SF means salt free).

    c. If traditional foods that he enjoys are not listed, instruct him to write in his choice, next to comparable foods (*e.g.*, rice next to potatoes). Use discretion in this policy, however, for some foods might not be available, which will frustrate and anger the client when they do not arrive.

    d. Help him select a meal plan that suits his normal lifestyle (*e.g.*, if he prefers a larger lunch than dinner, help him select hot foods at lunch; however, if he prefers 6 small, rather than 3 large, meals, inform the dietitian so that snacks can be provided.

2. Develop a strong attitude toward food as treatment so that you can extend this attitude to your client. Relate food as a means of treatment to regained strength and decreased convalescent time. Never use the sentence, "You must eat because food is good for you." This statement has no utility.

3. If a client has special needs or is on a therapeutic diet, inform the dietitian upon his admittance, so that dietary instructions can be given during the client's hospital convalescence.

4. Prepare the client for meals.

    a. Position the client properly (*e.g.*, raise the bed or sit him in a chair) so that utensils can be manipulated and swallowing is enhanced.

    b. Allow him to freshen up before meals (*e.g.*, offer him a washcloth for his face and hands). Also, make dentures available, when applicable.

    c. Make the room as pleasant as possible (*e.g.*, remove bed pans and raise curtains).

    d. Suggest that pleasant visitors remain during the meal, if possible.

During the Meal

1. If nursing service is responsible for tray delivery

    a. Make sure trays are clean when delivered (*e.g.*, coffee has not been spilled).

    b. Make sure all utensils are available.

    c. Make sure only the condiments allowed are on the tray (*e.g.*, remove salt packets if the client is on a low-sodium dietary regimen).

    d. Make sure hot foods are hot and cold foods are cold.

2. After the meal is delivered

    a. Help clients who need assistance (*e.g.*, open milk cartons or cut meat for those with impaired hands).

    b. Feed clients who need to be fed (see proper feeding procedures listed in Table 1-3).

3. Encourage consumption of a variety of foods by appealing to client's senses of taste and smell (*e.g.*, you might say, "This meat smells delicious").

4. Encourage the consumption of fluids. This is especially important in bedridden individuals for they often refuse fluids so that they will not have to use the bed pan as frequently. Record fluid intake and output.

5. If supplements are part of the meal (*e.g.*, Sustacal puddings), make sure they are served.

6. If a client is on dietary alterations, point out the important dietary adaptations that have been made in his meal plan (*e.g.*, portion sizes, limitation, or addition of some foods).

After the Meal

1. Pick up empty trays quickly. Stale foods leave undesirable odors, which persist until the next mealtime.

2. Record all inadequate food intake or difficulties with food (including likes and dislikes) for the dietitian and ask that she visit or revisit the individual.

3. Report severe lack of food intake to the physician.

4. Listen to questions clients who are on altered dietary regimens ask. If you can answer the questions accurately, do so in non-dogmatic fashion; if not, write a note on the client's chart or ask the dietitian to see the client.

Client Instruction and Follow-up Care

Instructing, evaluating progress, and assessing compliance of clients on therapeutic dietary regimens and of those who are at risk of developing nutritional deficiencies should be, and usually is, the dietitian's responsibility. In certain circumstances (*e.g.*, rural areas) a dietitian may not be available; consequently, treatment by diet, including instruction and enhancing an individual's dietary compliance, becomes the nurse's responsibility. If she wishes to perform this responsibility efficiently, however, or simply reinforce advice from other members of the health team, she must acquire two skills:

1. A strong knowledge of nutrition that she can adapt to dietary alterations
2. A working knowledge of the methodology involving
   a. Tools used for nutritional instruction (*e.g.*, exchange lists for meal planning)
   b. The sequence of instruction used to enhance the client's understanding of the dietary regimen and his compliance with it

Sample Sequence and Methodology to Obtain Dietary Compliance When Introducing a New Dietary Prescription

Visit 1

The physician should inform the client that he is prescribing a nutritional care plan that will relieve or prevent adverse symptoms or help control the progression of the disease. The physician, after seeing the client, should then request that the dietitian or nurse begin instructing the client on how to make these dietary alterations.

Visit 2

The dietitian or nurse should learn what foods the client normally eats by having him fill out a food preference questionnaire (see Chap. 1) or keep a dietary record for 3 days before his next visit (refer to Daily Food Diary in Chap. 6). This procedure may also be helpful if the client has been on the prescribed regimen previously, for often clients do not understand some of the important points of the nutritional care plan. In the meantime, before the client's next visit, reassess the interview chart in order to acquaint yourself with his lifestyle. Also, evaluate any anthropometric measurements or laboratory data that may be affected by dietary indiscretions or alterations. Additionally, obtain booklets, published by specific organizations (*e.g.*, American Heart Association) that pertain to his disease. Make these accessible for reference at the next visit.

Visit 3

Silently examine the client's food preference questionnaire or dietary record sheet and then discuss some of the dietary adaptations that will be necessary on his nutritional care plan (*e.g.*, limiting sodium) and the rationales (*e.g.*, how certain food limitations accelerate drops in blood pressure). The depth of this discussion should depend upon your client's motivation, understanding, and ability to procure and prepare food. *Note.* Including family members in this discussion may also be helpful, especially those who procure and prepare the client's food. After this discussion, let the client reexamine his food record and analyze what food adjustments he thinks he can make without too much difficulty, before the next visit. For example, he may see that he needs to limit or eliminate salt at the table, but he may not recognize that any other adjustments are necessary (*e.g.*, limiting ham consumption). If this is the case, advise him to make this adjustment before his next visit. Do not discuss any further limitations at this time. However, if the client seems exceptionally motivated and asks for more detailed information on necessary alterations, show him the booklets you have available and let him borrow them to read before the next visit.

Visit 4

After the client has seen the physician, reevaluate his chart, if possible. If not, ask him about any changes in his condition (*e.g.*, is his blood pressure lower?). If there are changes that indicate good dietary compliance, compliment him and then recount the rationales that connect dietary compliance to relief of symptoms and disease control. If the client is enthusiastic, discuss booklets that explain his nutritional care plan (only those that are within his level of understanding). If he is not ready for this, however, simply discuss portion control (*e.g.*, show him how much 1 oz of meat is). Food models or paper food models are especially helpful. However, if the client has already read the booklets, assess his understanding and answer any questions. Additionally, discuss how exercise can augment diet therapy in many disease conditions. If the client is receptive, have him keep a record of his exercise patterns before the next visit.

Visit 5

If the client continues to be motivated and shows objective signs of compliance (*e.g.*, weight loss), introduce him to other methods of controlling what he eats, such as reading labels on packages to see what foods may contain hidden sources of the food or nutrient he must eliminate or limit, what methods of food preparation are preferred, and how to choose foods from a restaurant menu that are acceptable on his nutritional care plan (*e.g.*, initially advise him to eat only plain food and then graduate him to mixed dishes). However, if his compliance or understanding is slow, try other methods of instructing such as pictures, packages, and traditional recipes but never scold. *Note.* This is only a sample sequence. It is not a rigid plan, and it must be adjusted to each individual and each health team. Regardless of the progression or the type of plan used for nutritional instruction, however, throughout this learning period, it is always the responsibility of the nurse to

1. Weigh the client
2. Assess all other factors in developing a nutritional care plan (see chapter on specific diseases and disorders)
3. Collect and assess all necessary laboratory data (*e.g.*, urine), when applicable
4. Assess the progression or reversal of complications
5. Assess the increase or decrease in drug dosage
6. Praise the client who has tried hard to learn new skills that will enhance his nutritional status

Enteral Nutritional Support

Description

Enteral feedings contain intact nutrients or nutrients that can be easily digested or absorbed by the gastrointestinal tract. They are liquid or blenderized sustenance that can be consumed orally as a source of complete nutrition or used to supplement regular diets in order to maintain optimal nutritional status. Additionally, some formulas can be passed through a tube when the client will not eat, cannot eat, or cannot eat enough regular food. These liquids can be prepared at home, from natural foods, in a food processor or blender, or they can be made commercially. Feedings made commercially are nutritionally complete liquid diets that contain intact nutrients or nutrients that have been purified and hydrolyzed (predigested). Formulas made of purified nutrients or synthetically made nutrients are called "chemically defined" or "elemental" diets.

Indications

Enteral feedings are administered when the client's

- Medical or psychological condition suggests that a nutrient inadequacy will develop without the initiation of nutritional maintenance and restoration
- Nutritional assessment data manifest
  1. A 10-lb unintentional loss of usual weight within 1 month
  2. A 10% to 20% loss of body mass within 3 to 6 months

3. Albumin levels below 3.5 g/dl
4. A lymphocyte count below 1,500 mm³
- Clinical condition has impaired ability to consume, absorb, or utilize nutrients; psychological and physiological disorders that lead to such impairments include
    1. Unwillingness of the client to eat (*e.g.*, because of anorexia nervosa or another mental disorder)
    2. Inability of the client to eat (*e.g.*, because of medical or dental conditions that cause chewing difficulties, such as oral surgery, stroke, fractured jaw, or cancer of the head and neck)
    3. Inability of the client to eat enough (*e.g.*, because of hypermetabolic conditions such as cancer, burns, or major surgery; use of medications that impair ingestion [such as antimetabolites], digestion [such as analgesics and corticosteroids], or absorption and utilization [such as antacids, laxatives, and antibiotics]; malabsorption conditions, such as celiac sprue, Crohn's disease, severe ulcers, and stomach or bowel obstructions)

The site of tube insertion may be changed according to the disorder being treated (Fig. 2-1). These changes may induce the "dumping syndrome" or other complications that may necessitate using parenteral solutions rather than enteral feedings. However, parenteral solutions should not be instituted until enteral feedings through adjusted sites have been tested.

Fig. 2-1. Types and sites of gastric feeding.
Intragastric (nasogastric, NG). A tube is passed through the nose or mouth into the stomach and secured in place. (A tube passed through the mouth is more correctly called an *orogastric* tube. An orogastric tube is ordinarily inserted at mealtime and removed following the meal.) Intragastric tube preferred for short-term gavage feeding; easily inserted by physician or trained nurse, remains in place between feedings. (Some clients are taught to insert their own tube; they may remove the tube between meals.) Variations include nasopharyngeal and nasojejunal feeding tubes.
Esophagotomy. A temporary or permanent opening (*stoma*) is constructed at one of several sites to allow a tube to be introduced through the skin into the esophagus. Feeding tube is usually removed between meals. *Advantages.* Dependable for long-term feeding, allows concealment of apparatus, easy to handle.
Gastrostomy. A temporary or permanent stoma is constructed allowing food to be introduced through the skin directly into the stomach. Preferred for long-term gavage feeding of children and for long-term feeding of adults when use of esophagus is contraindicated. *Disadvantages.* Partial undressing necessary at mealtime; skin care may pose problems.
Jejunostomy. A stoma is constructed which gives direct access to the jejunum. This method of feeding may be used when the stomach must be bypassed. *Disadvantages.* High incidence of dumping syndrome and diarrhea; adequate nutrient intake difficult to maintain. (Suitor CW, Hunter MF: Nutrition: Principles and Application in Health Promotion. Philadelphia, JB Lippincott, 1980)

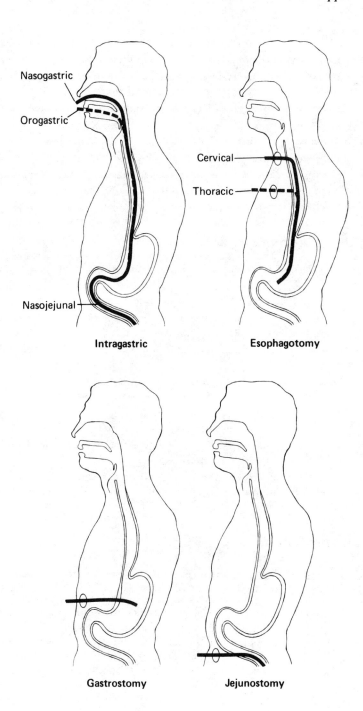

Intragastric

Nasogastric

Orogastric

Nasojejunal

Esophagotomy

Cervical

Thoracic

Gastrostomy

Jejunostomy

Contraindications

Enteral feedings are not administered when the client

- Has an impaired ability to digest or absorb nutrients (*e.g.*, has impaired mucosa, enzyme, or hormone production)
- Has severe intestinal disorders that will only heal with complete rest (*e.g.*, fistulas)
- Is vomiting frequently
- Has severe and persistent diarrhea
- Has a respiratory disease or nasal or skull fracture, unless a site other than the nasal site is used for infusion of the feeding
- Is removing the tube frequently either by choice or inadvertently

Route of Administration

Before selecting the route of administration, consider the following factors:

- How long the client will require enteral feedings
- How well the client will psychologically accept one type of enteral feeding (*i.e.*, oral *vs* tube feeding) over the other
- The client's past and present nutritional status (*e.g.*, nitrogen balance and weight loss)
- The amount of calories and protein the client will require to meet his metabolic needs (*e.g.*, obtain positive nitrogen balance)
- The client's ability to ingest oral feedings (*e.g.*, will simple oral supplements meet his requirements or will he require tube feedings?)
- The technical and physiological dangers that may accompany the particular feeding route of infusion
- The client's clinical condition (*e.g.*, individuals with a stomach removed will not tolerate hyperosmolar formulas; they will develop the "dumping syndrome" [see Chap. 7])

Sites and Types

Oral Feeding Supplements or Oral Defined-Formula Feedings (ODF)

Oral enteral feedings contain intact nutrients or feedings with synthetic nutrients that can be made palatable by adding flavorings. These are recommended for use only when the gastrointestinal tract is intact. These feedings usually supplement regular feedings, or they may be added to regular foods to prevent nutrient deficits (see Table 2-5 and Appendix II for composition of feedings).

Tube Feedings

Enteral feedings used in tubes are liquids composed of intact nutrients or predigested nutrients. The most common route of formula infusion is the nasogastric route; however, when this route is not indicated, other routes of infusion may be used (see Fig. 2-1 for other sites of infusion and Table 2-5 and Appendix II for composition of feedings).

Details of tube placement, infusion of the formula (*e.g.*, bolus *vs* continuous drip), and monitoring of individual tolerance of enteral feedings are beyond the scope of this handbook. However, some discomforts and clinical symptoms that result from improper techniques are presented in Table 2-6. Nurses interested in details of proper techniques should consult advanced nursing manuals.

Infusion Rate

Oral Enteral Supplements

Enteral feeding supplements should be given in small quantities or in diluted concentrations until the client is able to tolerate the osmolality of the feeding. Adverse symptoms that will develop without this precaution are severe cramping, diarrhea, and nausea and vomiting.

General Infusion Rate

Day 1

Dilute feeding to one quarter the usual concentration in order to dilute the osmolality of the formula. Infuse only 50 ml to 100 ml at a time for bolus feedings or 20 ml to 70 ml/hr for continuous drip.

Days 2 to 3

Increase the strength of the formula to one half the desired concentration. Increase the infusion rate by 25 ml each feeding or 50 ml to 90 ml/hr.

Days 4 to 5, or Until Tolerance

Increase the infusion rate gradually until 300 ml to 400 ml of formula (100% concentration) or 15 ml to 30 ml/min are tolerated every 3 hours (6–8 feedings/day) by bolus feeding or 125 ml/hr are tolerated by continuous drip. Tolerance can be monitored by fluid intake and output records, urine glucose tests, and the client's clinical condition.

Specific Infusion Rate

Check manufacturer's recommendations. See Table 2-7 for a sample plan.

Composition

Generally, when the individual is able to tolerate the full concentration of enteral feedings, he receives 1800 kcal to 3000 kcal and 1800 ml to 3000 ml of fluid. However, this is only a generalization, because macronutrients, micronutrients, nutrient digestibility (intact nutrients *vs* purified nutrients), and fluid contents of enteral feedings vary from formula to formula. See Table 2-5 and Appendix II. Moreover, they are not specific energy intakes; the nutrient needs of individuals with varied diseases and metabolic requirements differ.

Factors in Selecting an Enteral Formula

- The overall caloric, nutrient, and electrolyte needs of the client according to sex, age, activity, and metabolic state
- The infusion rate and flow rate
- The osmolality of the formula
- The palatability of the formula when applicable
- The cost of the formula (*e.g.*, intact *vs* purified nutrients)
- The hygienic safety and shelf-life of the formula
- The medical condition and the treatment, including medications being used and the possibilities of nutrient–drug interactions
- The client's present and previous intolerances to various foods (*e.g.*, allergic reactions to milk or eggs)

For the composition of specific types of enteral formulas, consult Table 2-5 and Appendix II. For advantages and disadvantages of enteral formulas, consult Table 2-5. For the nurses' responsibilities to clients on tube feedings or enteral oral supplements, consult Table 2-6.

Parenteral Nutritional Support

Description

Parenteral nutritional support is the infusion of large amounts of basic nutrients and electrolytes, in solution, through a peripheral or central vein in order to maintain or restore tissue synthesis, immunocompetence, and weight.

Indications

Parenteral solutions are administered to maintain homeostasis (*e.g.*, glucose, fluid, and electrolyte balance) preoperatively and postoperatively, or when a client is not receiving enough nourishment by other feeding methods to prevent starvation or restore nutritional status.

Psychological and physiological disorders that may necessitate the administration of these solutions include

- Unwillingness of the client to eat (*e.g.*, because of anorexia nervosa)
- Inability of the client to eat (*e.g.*, because of shock, coma, stroke, Crohn's disease, fistulas, GI obstructions, short bowel syndrome immediately following surgery, idiopathic diarrhea in infants, malabsorption syndromes, or respiratory difficulties)
- Inability of the client to eat enough
  1. Clients with nutritional assessment profiles below 85% of standard or lower than the 15th percentile
  2. Clients undergoing chemotherapy or radiation that may interfere with GI function
  3. Clients with hypercatabolic conditions such as sepsis, burns, or cancer
  4. Clients who are malnourished on admission who will not receive food for 7–10 days after treatment
  5. Infants having a long-standing inability to thrive

Most physicians prefer to use enteral or oral feedings and parenteral solutions, concomitantly, if the gut maintains any function, for this methodology of feeding prevents atrophy of the GI tract.

Contraindications

Parenteral nutritional support solutions are not administered when the client

- Is in a metabolic state not conducive to protein utilization (*e.g.*, wound has not been tended) because if increased nitrogen is given during the peak of trauma, more urea will be synthesized (putting greater stress on the kidneys and liver)
- Is in hepatic coma, unless specialized solutions are infused (*e.g.*, branched-chain amino acids)
- Is in kidney failure because increased fluids may not be excreted and overhydration will occur; also protein renal load may be exceeded, unless special solutions are infused
- Has pathogenic hyperlipidemia, lipid nephrosis, or acute pancreatitis unless lipid emulsions are excluded
- Is in hyperosmolar coma or has hypoglycemia as the result of diabetes
- Has severe cardiovascular or pulmonary complications
- Is severely septic, burned, or cachexic, unless special precautions are taken, because the risks from the procedure may exceed the nutritional benefits derived
- Is terminally ill, unless this type of nutritional support improves his feeling of well-being

Route of Administration

Before selecting the route of administration,

- Estimate how long the client will need parenteral nutritional support
- Estimate how well the client will psychologically accept one type of parenteral administration route over the other
- Assess the client's past and present nutritional status (*e.g.*, nitrogen balance and weight loss)
- Estimate the amount of calories and protein the client will need to reach nitrogen balance or positive nitrogen balance and weight gain
- Evaluate the client's ability to supplement parenteral solutions with oral or tube feedings
- Estimate the technical and physiological dangers that may accompany the parenteral administration route (*e.g.*, estimate the dangers of sepsis by evaluating the extent of hypercatabolic stress and its effect on immunocompetence)

Sites and Types

Peripheral Vein

Solutions that are infused through the peripheral veins must be isotonic to the blood. Consequently, only low concentrations of carbohydrate and amino acids can be administered, for they are hypertonic. Fat, however, can be used in larger concentrations, for it is isotonic.

The peripheral veins used for infusion of nutritional solutions are the radial, basilic, and cephalic veins and the veins on the dorsum of the hand (if large enough). Consult chart on Generalized Infusion Rates of Parenteral Nutritional Solutions and Tables 2-8 and 2-9 for more detailed information on the infusion rate, nutrient and caloric composition, and advantages and disadvantages of specific parenteral solutions.

Central Vein

Solutions that are infused through the central veins may be hypertonic to the blood because the increased blood flow in the superior vena cava will rapidly dilute the concentration of the solutions. Therefore, these solutions contain higher concentrations of carbohydrate and amino acids. Additionally, fat may be "piggy-backed" with the carbohydrate and amino acid solutions when additional calories are necessary.

The central veins commonly used for nutritional infusion are the subclavian vein in adults and the jugular vein in infants. Consult chart on Generalized Infusion Rates of Parenteral Nutritional Solutions and Tables 2-8 and 2-9 for more detailed information.

Generalized Infusion Rates of Parenteral Nutritional Solutions

Progression of Infusion	Volume of Solution Infused (ml)
Day 1	1000
Day 2	2000
Day 3	3000
or	
Degree of Stress	
Mild	1000
Moderate	2000
Severe	3000

Infusion Techniques

The techniques of peripheral or central vein nutritional infusions involve a central venous catheter or, in a peripheral vein, a cannula; infusion equipment; preparation of solutions; and monitoring of administration. In general, monitoring entails checking the composition of the solution, the rate of infusion, and the total amount of nutrients given, including water, and noting toxic symptoms that indicate an imbalance. Monitoring also entails following the nutritional status of the client, as evidenced by body weight; anthropometric measurements; vital signs (blood pressure, respiration, pulse, and temperature); laboratory data (*e.g.*, blood and urine glucose levels, plasma protein levels, and urinary nitrogen levels); and immunocompetence (*e.g.*, lymphocyte count), when indicated.

Often the staff nurse is responsible for administering and monitoring this nutritional support. In order to reduce complications, however, a team approach is more appropriate. The team should include knowledgeable and skilled personnel (physicians, nurses, dietitians, and pharmacists) who can deliver these solutions to the client in a way that promotes optimal benefits and minimizes complications. In order to accomplish these goals, the team's responsibility is to

- Determine how often catheters should be changed
- Decide what techniques should be implemented in order to minimize complications (*e.g.*, sepsis and thrombophlebitis)
- Decide what solutions are appropriate to meet the client's hypermetabolic needs (this includes determining the quantities and ratios of nutrients incorporated and how they effect the osmolality of the formula)

Since a specialized team usually is responsible for the composition, administration, and monitoring of parenteral solutions, the staff nurse's responsibilities to clients on these formulas is to support both the client and the nutritional support team (see Nurses' Responsibilities to Individuals on Parenteral Nutritional Support, p. 60). Nurses desiring more information on responsibilities of the support team should consult advanced parenteral support manuals.

The infusion rate of parenteral nutritional support solutions will depend on the client's tolerance to the solutions. Therefore, the infusion rate listed in the chart on Generalized Infusion Rates is a guide rather than a definitive schedule. The rate will also depend upon the route of administration, with less volume usually being infused through the peripheral veins.

Composition

Peripheral Vein Solutions

Peripheral vein solutions generally are designed to provide sufficient calories, in the form of carbohydrate or fat, to spare enough protein, in the form of amino acids, to prevent excessive lean tissue catabolism. The macronutrients contained in these solutions are the same components as those found in central vein solutions except that their concentration is lower (*e.g.*, 5% dextrose solution) so that they remain nearly isotonic to the blood. Micronutrients and electrolytes are added to these solutions in amounts that meet individual requirements. Consult Tables 2-8 and 2-9 and the macronutrient components used in parenteral solutions for more detailed information on the specific composition of components used in peripheral nutritional support solutions.

Central Vein Solutions

Central vein solutions generally are designed to provide total nutritional support according to present scientific knowledge. Ultimately, when the full concentration of the total central vein nutritional support infusion is tolerated, the client will receive 1500 to 3000 kcal per 3000 ml. The calorie content is determined by the percentage of dextrose and amino acids added to the solution and the amount of fat "piggy-backed" or added by a separate infusion line. The usual amount of fat added is one unit of 10% fat emulsion (500 ml). The value is 1.1 kcal/ml. The protein value is approximately 1 g of nitrogen to every 150 to 200 g of nonprotein calories, usually dextrose. The protein value can be increased, however, by changing the nutritional composition and fluid content of the infusion. Micronutrients (vitamins and minerals) and electrolytes added to the solution or given intramuscularly include all those known to be essential at the present time.

Factors in Selecting a Parenteral Formula

See Factors in Selecting an Individualized Nutritional Care Plan and Factors in Selecting an Enteral Formula, above. Note that palatability need not be considered in selecting a parenteral solution.

Specific composition is, however, important.

Caloric Content

Consult Table 2-8 and Appendix II.

Carbohydrate Content

The carbohydrate used in parenteral solutions is dextrose. Intravenous dextrose is a monohydrous dextrose rather than an anhydrous dextrose; 1 g provides 3.4 kcal rather than the usual 4.0 kcal/g. Failure to take this into consideration can overestimate the caloric content of carbohydrate in the solution by 15%. (*Note*. A 5% dextrose solution has an osmolality of 250 mOsm/liter.)

Protein Content

The protein source used in parenteral solutions is amino acids. These amino acids are based on the pattern of amino acids found in egg and potato. Some newer solutions now being researched, however, contain high concentrations of branch-chain amino acids (*e.g.*, valine, leucine, and isoleucine), rather than aromatic amino acids. (*Note*. Crystalline amino acid solutions on an average yield 1 g of nitrogen for every 5.9 g of amino acids rather than the average yield of 1 g of nitrogen for every 6.25 g of intact proteins found in foods. This is only an average, however, for the nitrogen yield as a percent by weight of protein varies with the type of protein [crystalline amino acids] used in the solution. See Table 2-8.)

Fat Content

The fat used in parenteral solutions is an emulsion. Usually it is a mixture of soybean oil (Inralipid) or safflower oil (Liposyn), egg yolk, phospholipid, and glycerol. This emulsion is not clear; it looks like milk. Fat cannot be added to the dextrose and amino acid solution because it coalesces with the formula. Additionally, dilution with the formula may break the emulsion. The maximum amount of fat recommended for an adult is 2.5 g/kg of IBW; it should not exceed 60% of the total caloric intake. The recommended amount for children is 250 ml/day with the maximum being 4 g/kg of IBW or less than 60% of the total calories.

Electrolyte, Vitamin, and Mineral Content

The major electrolytes (sodium, potassium, calcium, magnesium, chloride, and phosphate) must always be a part of any complete parenteral nutritional support solution, regardless of the duration of therapy. Ideally, they should be added and decreased according to the individual's needs. Additionally, all the essential vitamins, minerals, and trace elements should be added to the solution just before infusion. In severe stress, the requirements for vitamins and minerals may be three times the recommended daily allowances. Vitamins and minerals not added to the solution just before infusion are vitamin K, folic acid, vitamin B_{12}, and iron. These nutrients are not added to the solution because they interact with other vitamins or minerals, causing nutrient imbalances, or they precipitate with other vitamins and minerals and impair availability. Instead, they should be administered intramuscularly. However, for clients in whom musculature is poor, iron and folic acid may be added to the solution.

Fluid Content

The fluid-to-kilocalorie value in parenteral solutions is presently approximately 1 ml to 1 kcal. Some researchers, however, believe that this amount of fluid and dextrose may cause electrolyte imbalances, deranged liver function, and hyperglycemia. To eliminate these adverse effects, they recommend a mixture of amino acid solution (AAS) (10%), 500 ml; dextrose solution (20%), 1000 ml; and 500 ml of fat emulsion. This would allow 2.2 liters of solution rather than 3 liters, and the protein ratio would be 1.5 to 2.5 g/kg/day rather than 1 g/kg/day.

Consult the manufacturer's literature for detailed information on types and amounts of nutrients provided in the solution. (See Table 2-9 and Appendix VII.)

Advantages and Disadvantages of Parenteral Nutritional Solutions

Consult Table 2-9.

Nurses' Responsibilities to Individuals on Parenteral Nutritional Support

Participate in and Coordinate Care

- Reassure the client by emphasizing that this nutritional support will make him more comfortable or enhance his recovery.
- Check the infusion site for signs of inflammation or infection. Check the rate of infusion frequently, and make adjustments as necessary. If the prescribed amount of solution is not consumed in one feeding, however, do not try to catch up. Report all adverse findings to the nutritional support team or physician.
- Take measures to maintain the client's oral cavity. See Table 2-6.
- Take measures to prevent pressure sores, which develop with ease in the nutritionally deficient client but heal with great difficulty.
- Monitor the data collected. See Infusion Techniques, above. Report adverse findings to the nutritional support team or physician.

• Assist the support team when the client is being weaned from parenteral nutritional support. Weaning is necessary after parenteral support because

1. Secretory activity is low (*e.g.*, secretion of saliva)
2. Levels of enzyme secretions in the GI tract are low (*e.g.*, impaired secretions of disaccharidases, including lactase, and peptidases)
3. GI tract muscles are often atrophied
4. Peristalsis is inactive
5. Hypoglycemia may occur if solutions are stopped too rapidly

Reinforce and Follow Up Care

If the client is going home on parenteral nutritional support care, reinforce the instructions given and assist him when he is reading and trying to understand nutritional parenteral support manuals. Reassure the client and members of his family that a near normal lifestyle can be maintained while he is on this nutritional care. Additionally, reassure the family and client that professional help will always be available as needed.

Table 2–1
Energy and Nutrient Needs of a Healthy Adult and an Adult Under Metabolic Stress

Healthy Adult	Adult Under the Stress of Illness

Caloric Requirements
 	
25–35 kcal/kg/day
Example. 70 kg × 30 kcal = 2100 kcal
OR
 	
To determine the daily caloric needs for an adult, use the formula that incorporates an individual's basal daily caloric needs and his degree of activity (see Chap. 6, chart on Determination of Caloric Alteration Level, and Table 6-9).
	Mild stress (with decreased activity), 20–35 kcal/kg/day
	Moderate stress, 45–50 kcal/kg/day
	Severe stress (*e.g.*, burns), 60–70 kcal/kg/day
	For every degree of rise in body temperature (Fahrenheit), add 500–600 extra kcal
	OR
	
	To determine amount of exogenous calories needed under stress of illness, use following formula:
	1. Determine basal daily caloric needs, indicated by the basal metabolic rate (BMR; see Chap. 6, chart on Determination of Caloric Alteration Level)
	2. Determine minimal needs related to physical activity, called resting metabolic expenditure (RME)
	   a. In minimal stress, add 10%–15% more calories to the basal daily caloric needs
	   b. In severe stress, add 20%–80% more calories to the basal daily caloric needs (see Table 2-2)
	3. Estimate total exogenous caloric needs by adding 50% more calories to the RME caloric needs
	Example. If an individual's RME caloric needs are 1800, add 50% more calories to his RME caloric needs (900 kcal) during stress, and he will require 2700 kcal per day.
	
	(continued)

Table 2-1 63

Table 2-1
**Energy and Nutrient Needs of a Healthy Adult
and an Adult Under Metabolic Stress** (continued)

Healthy Adult	Adult Under the Stress of Illness
Caloric Requirements (continued)	*Note.* It is estimated that the human body stores approximately 165,900 endogenous kcal in the form of fat, lean tissue, and glycogen; however, this endogenous supply can be depleted rapidly when the individual loses 1 lb per day or a total of 3500 kcal daily (1 lb = 3500 kcal).
Protein Requirements 0.8 g/kg/day *Example.* 70 kg × 0.8 g = 56 g protein/day or 56 g protein ÷ 6.25 = 8 g nitrogen/day. This is the amount estimated to be needed to keep a 70-kg individual in nitrogen balance.	Mild stress, 0.8–1 g/kg/day Moderate Stress, 1 g–2 g/kg/day *Example.* 70 kg × 1 g protein = 70 g protein/day or 70 kg × 2 g protein = 140 g protein/day Severe stress (*e.g.*, burns or infections), as high as 3 g/kg/day *Example.* 70 kg × 3 g protein = 210 g protein/day because increased protein is needed to replace the nitrogen lost during the catabolism of lean body tissue in hypermetabolic stress.
Carbohydrate Requirements 50%–60% of total kcal, with complex carbohydrate making up the greatest quantity of intake whenever possible. Refined sugars should be consumed only in small quantities.	50%–60% of total kcal or more, if fat is not tolerated or cannot be administered because carbohydrate is needed to spare protein for tissue synthesis. Simple sugars may be better absorbed because they require less digestion than complex carbohydrates.

(continued)

Table 2-1
**Energy and Nutrient Needs of a Healthy Adult
and an Adult Under Metabolic Stress** (continued)

Healthy Adult	Adult Under the Stress of Illness
Fat Requirements	
25%–35% of total kcal Total fat intake should be divided into moderate amounts of saturated, monounsaturated, and polyunsaturated fat. At least 2% of the dietary fat intake must be polyunsaturated fat, or an essential fatty acid deficiency will develop.	25%–35% of total kcal, if tolerated; division should be same as for healthy individuals. Fat is beneficial in parenteral feedings for it is nearly isotonic to the blood. Some polyunsaturated fat must be consumed, or an essential fatty acid deficiency will develop over time. If fat, in the form of long-chain triglycerides (LCTs) is not tolerated, medium-chain triglycerides (MCTs) may be substituted. Consult Table 8-2 for the composition, advantages, and disadvantages of MCT commercial formulas.
Vitamin Requirements	
Two thirds of the recommended daily allowances (RDAs) (see Appendix IV); a variety of nutrient-dense foods eaten daily will usually provide these requirements without the need for supplements.	100% of the RDAs daily + supplements, depending on the extent of trauma and vitamin utilization (*e.g.*, nutrient–drug interactions), because special emphasis must be placed on vitamin balance during disease and on replacing vitamins lost owing to disease symptoms (*e.g.*, diarrhea and vomiting)
Mineral Requirements	
Two thirds of the recommended daily allowances (RDAs) (see Appendix IV); a variety of nutrient-dense foods eaten daily will usually provide these requirements without the need for supplements.	100% of the RDAs daily + supplements, depending on the extent of trauma and mineral utilization (*e.g.*, nutrient–drug interactions) because special emphasis must be placed on mineral balance during disease and on replacing minerals lost owing to disease symptoms (*e.g.*, diuresis) *Note.* Levels of supplements of fat-soluble vitamins and minerals, especially trace minerals, must be monitored for toxic effects.

(continued)

Table 2–1 65

Table 2–1
**Energy and Nutrient Needs of a Healthy Adult
and an Adult Under Metabolic Stress** (continued)

Healthy Adult	Adult Under the Stress of Illness
Fluid Requirements	Fluid requirements may be increased to more than 3000 ml per day because fluid is needed to replace fluids lost by disease symptoms (*e.g.*, vomiting), excrete increased urea, lower body heat, and increase blood volume. Increased fluids will also help prevent urinary tract infections and renal stones that may develop during immobilization. Fluid intake and output should be monitored in all cases of trauma. Monitoring is especially important when the individual is on enteral or parenteral feedings or in coma; formulas may be too diluted or too concentrated (see Tables 2-5, 2-6, 2-7, 2-8, and 2-9 and chart on Generalized Infusion Rates of Parenteral Nutritional Solutions). Additionally, the sensation of thirst may be altered.
Adult, 1 ml/kcal/day or 30–35 ml/kg/day Infant, 150 ml/kg/day Child, 50–60 ml/kg/day *Example.* 70 kg × 35 ml = 2450 ml of fluid/day; to meet this requirement, 6–8 cups of fluid per day are recommended. Intake is usually regulated by thirst. *Note.* 60% of the adult body and 75% of an infant's body are composed of water.	

Table 2–2
Calculated Daily Caloric Requirements for Average Male Surgical Client (70 kg)

Condition	Normal BMR*	Actual Resting Expenditure[†]		Calculated Daily Calorie Intake
		BMR (%)	Cal	RME + 50%
Normal	1800	0	1800	2700
Postoperative	1800	+20	2160	3240
Multiple fracture	1800	+40	2520	3780
Major sepsis	1800	+80	3240	4860
Major burn	1800			

* The basal metabolic rate (BMR) is the rate of energy utilization in the body during absolute rest but while the subject is awake.
† The resting metabolic rate (RME) is the energy required to support the needs of a hospitalized patient. The resulting requirement is a balance between the increase due to disease or injury and the decrease that normally occurs with depletion from partial starvation and immobilization.
(Reprinted with permission from Protein for the hospitalized patient. Nutritional Thinking in Action. Columbus, Ohio, Ross Laboratories, 1978)

Table 2–3 67

Table 2–3
Composition, Advantages, and Disadvantages of Progressive Hospital Diets

Diet	Composition	Advantages	Disadvantages
Clear liquid	Clear transparent liquids, including tea, coffee (black), carbonated beverages, gelatin, bouillon, consommé, water, ice, Popsicles, and (in some hospitals) clear juices such as apple juice	Prevents dehydration Relieves thirst Cleanses the GI tract before surgery Provides glucose for CNS function Provides electrolytes (*e.g.*, sodium) Stimulates peristalsis Promotes a gradual return to oral feedings following IV feedings	Lacks nutrients to replenish body stores (*e.g.*, iron) Lacks nutrients needed for tissue synthesis (*e.g.*, protein) Does not meet BMR or RME caloric needs (see tables 2-1, 2-2, and 2-4)
Full liquid	Foods that liquefy at room or body temperature, including all those allowed on the clear liquid diet plus milk and liquid milk products (*e.g.*, yogurt, ice cream, custards, and cream soups), and fruit and vegetable juices that do not contain pulp Additionally, full liquid diets can be made from regular whole foods that have been blenderized with extra fluids.	Prevents dehydration Provides electrolytes, especially potassium Provides protein and ascorbic acid for tissue synthesis Can be made to meet BMR and RME caloric needs (see Tables 2-1, 2-2, and 2-4) Provides a source of nutrition for the client who is acutely ill, unable to swallow solid or semisolid foods, or unable to chew without fatigue	Lacks iron for hemoglobin synthesis High in milk sugar (lactose), which induces gas, bloating, and diarrhea in individuals who have a lactose deficiency Low in fiber, which induces constipation High in fat, which may induce atherosclerosis if used for extended periods

(continued)

Table 2–3
Composition, Advantages, and Disadvantages of Progressive Hospital Diets (continued)

Diet	Composition	Advantages	Disadvantages
Full liquid (*continued*)	Feedings are usually divided into 6 small meals a day in order to meet caloric and other nutrient needs (see Tables 2-1, 2-2, and 2-4).	Bridges gap between the clear liquid and soft diet during convalescence	High in calcium, which may precipitate kidney stones or the milk alkali syndrome when used in conjunction with antacids (see Chaps. 7 and 8 and Table 7-1)
Soft diet	Easily digested foods soft in consistency and easy to chew including all those allowed on the clear and full liquid diet plus cooked and canned fruits without seeds; tender-chopped or strained vegetables; cooked and dry refined cereals; enriched and refined breads; tender or ground meats, fish, and poultry; eggs; soft and mild cheeses (*e.g.*, cottage cheese); butter or fortified margarine; soups and plain desserts (*e.g.*, angel food cake) Foods avoided are those that contain harsh fibers and stimulating seasonings (*e.g.*, chili)	Provides a source of nutrition for clients with acute infections, chewing or swallowing difficulties (*e.g.*, stroke clients), mild GI disturbances, and cardiac disturbances Provides most of the calories and nutrients included on a regular diet (see Table 2-4) Provides a psychological boost to the client, especially if ground foods are placed under or near whole foods on the menu Serves as an intermediate step between the full liquid and regular diet	Low in fiber, which induces constipation Unpalatable if no seasonings are added (*e.g.*, salt) Psychological problems may develop when "baby foods" used; avoid whenever possible substitute whole foods that have been blenderized

(continued)

Table 2–3 69

Table 2–3
Composition, Advantages, and Disadvantages of Progressive Hospital Diets (continued)

Diet	Composition	Advantages	Disadvantages
Regular diet (also called general, full, or house diet)	All foods that have intact nutrients in their natural form including all soups, salads, refined or unrefined breads and cereals, whole fruits and vegetables, all types of meats and fish, and desserts that contain cream, seeds, or nuts Diet is nutritionally adequate (see Tables 2-1, 2-2, and 2-4) Individual should be allowed a choice from the available food categories	Provides all the nutrients necessary for maintenance and restoration, if consumed Attractive colors and texture Can be provided for various ethnic groups Psychologically the individual feels he is recovering Additionally, when the individual is allowed to select foods he prefers from the selective menu, his spirit is nourished as well as his body	Individual with poor eating habits will continue to choose foods not nutritionally balanced If individual does not select or eat foods from all the available categories of foods (*e.g.,* fruits) he will lack essential calories and nutrients Large meals may discourage some individuals from food consumption.

Table 2–5
Composition, Advantages, and Disadvantages of Enteral Feeding Formulas

Composition	Advantages	Disadvantages
Naturally Balanced Complete Formulas		
Contain intact nutrients, in a balanced ratio, that come from natural foods such as eggs, milk, oils, meat, vegetables, fruits, and grains. They may be blended together at home or made commercially. Commercial examples. Compleat B and Formula 2	High nutritive density; caloric content averages 1 kcal/ml Consistent nutrient content Isotonic to the GI tract Promotes normal insulin response Promotes natural GI tract functions (*e.g.*, peristalsis) Psychologically acceptable Palatable (can be flavored and colored to taste) Inexpensive and easy to prepare Fewer septic complications than other nutrition-support solutions (*e.g.*, parenteral solutions)	Nutrient inadequacies may develop if a variety of nutrient-dense foods is not added to homemade formulas; commercial formulas, however, are nutritionally balanced Dehydration or overhydration may develop if client does not consume adequate amounts or dilute the formula properly, when applicable If particle size is not small enough or liquid is not sufficient, tube will become occluded Certain types of foods, when mixed together, will curdle (*e.g.*, acidic foods added to milk-based foods) Formulas that contain excessive amounts of eggs or milk may induce allergic reactions or lactose-intolerance symptoms (see Chap. 7) Feedings may become contaminated if not handled, refrigerated, and heated properly. Commercial formulas have a lower incidence of contamination

(continued)

Table 2–5 71

Table 2–5
Composition, Advantages, and Disadvantages of Enteral Feeding Formulas (continued)

Composition	Advantages	Disadvantages
Milk-Based and Nonmilk-Based Formulas		
A balance of protein, carbohydrate, and fat. Protein sources in milk-based formulas are nonfat and whole milk. Protein sources in nonmilk-based formulas are Na + Ca caseinate and soy protein. Fat sources are corn oil, soy oil, or medium-chain triglyceride oil (fractionated coconut oil). Carbohydrate sources are corn syrup, sucrose, or lactose. Vitamin and mineral supplements may be added. Commercial examples. Milk-based, Meritene, Sustacal pudding, Forta pudding; Nonmilk-based, Sustacal liquid, Sustacal HC, Ensure, Ensure Plus, Isocal HCN	High nutritive density; caloric content averages 1 kcal/ml (*e.g.*, Sustacal liquid), 1.5 kcal/ml (*e.g.*, Sustacal HC), or 2 kcal/ml (*e.g.*, Isocal HCN) Consistent nutrient content Can be used either to supplement the caloric intake of a regular diet or to provide complete nutrition by mouth or tube Palatable (client can choose the color and taste he prefers) Easy to prepare Maintains the integrity of the gut mucosa Highly concentrated formulas (*e.g.*, 2 kcal/ml) enhance caloric intakes when fluids are restricted	Fixed-nutrient composition requires a specific volume to supply adequate nutrition and is contraindicated in renal, hepatic, or cardiac disease Milk-based formulas contain high contents of lactose, which can induce cramping and diarrhea in lactose-intolerant individuals These have higher osmolality than do balanced complete formulas (see elemental diets) They are more expensive than home-prepared formulas They contaminate rapidly when not refrigerated Clients on highly concentrated formulas must be monitored for signs of dehydration, hyperglycemia, and excessive nitrogen retention
Modular Feedings or Incomplete Nutrient Supplements or Feedings		
Generally contain a high quantity of one nutrient but lack or have inadequate amounts of other essential nutrients.	Can be mixed with other supplements or with regular foods to increase the caloric or nutrient content of these feedings	Excessive quantities of one nutrient, especially purified sugar, often causes osmotic diarrhea

(continued)

Table 2–5
Composition, Advantages, and Disadvantages of Enteral Feeding Formulas (continued)

Composition	Advantages	Disadvantages
Modular Feedings or Incomplete Nutrient Supplements or Feedings (continued)		
The imbalance is reached by using purified or synthetically made nutrients Commercial examples. High carbohydrate feedings, Cal-Power, Hy-Cal, Polycose; high protein feedings, Casec, Pro Mix; high fat feedings, Lipomul-Oral, Microlipid, MCT oil	Can be used to increase the carbohydrate content of the diet, which spares protein for tissue synthesis, without increasing the protein content Beneficial in diseases of kidney and liver Can provide fat in the form of MCT when long-chain triglycerides cannot be absorbed or utilized Can be modified to meet almost any disease condition	Feedings must be chosen with care to meet individual needs, or serious nutrient imbalances may develop Some formulas are not palatable, especially those that contain hydrolyzed proteins (*e.g.,* amino acids) They are more expensive than are other complete supplements
Chemically Defined or Elemental Formulas or Diets		
Nutrient-balanced complete feedings. The nutrients, however, have been purified, hydrolyzed, or synthetically made by commercial methods. Proteins are in the form of free amino acids or small peptides. Carbohydrates are in the form of dextrins, corn syrup, modified corn-starch, glucose, or oligosaccharides. Fats are in the form of MCT oils or soy oils and safflower oils. The latter two oils provide linoleic acid Vitamins and minerals are added to meet recommended needs Commercial examples. Vivonex, Vipep, Flexical, Vital, and Criticare HN	High in nutritive and caloric density; caloric content is 1 kcal/ml Balanced mixtures of amino acids in patterns that increase protein synthesis and tissue repair Require little or no digestion; consequently, rest the GI tract Have very little residue or lactose so can be used in intestinal malabsorption diseases Some contain linoleic acid so essential fatty acid deficiencies do not develop Lessen stress ulceration and bleeding in the GI tract Easy to store	Small particles cause hyperosmolality (osmolality is expressed as milliosmoles [mOsm] per kilogram of solvent). The osmolality of normal body fluids is approximately 300 mOsm/kg. Formulas that contain a higher osmolality than normal consequently cause a rush of water to the intestines when they are administered, in an attempt to dilute the solute. This causes fermentation in the intestines with resultant clinical signs of bloating, cramping, and watery diarrhea Constipation may develop over time because the formula has a minimal residue content *(continued)*

Table 2–5 73

Table 2–5
Composition, Advantages, and Disadvantages of Enteral Feeding Formulas (continued)

Composition	Advantages	Disadvantages
Chemically Defined or Elemental Formulas or Diets (continued)		
	Easier to administer than homemade formulas for they have small particles, which seldom clog tube	They are unpalatable; therefore, they usually have to be administered by tube They are expensive They become contaminated if not refrigerated
Specialized Formulas		
Have molecules added or deleted to relieve the symptoms or progression of specific diseases		
Commercial examples. Amin-Aid, contains all 8 essential amino acids plus histidine, partially hydrogenated soy oil, and maltodextrins	Amin-Aid provides all amino acids needed for protein synthesis without providing nonessential amino acids, which would increase urea load that must be excreted by kidney Has a high caloric-to-fluid content of 2 kcal/ml; therefore, spares protein for tissue synthesis	Formula does not contain vitamins, digestible bulk, fibrous material, or electrolytes. Therefore, the client must be monitored closely for signs of nutrient or electrolyte imbalances They have a high osmolarity They are high in carbohydrates They are unpalatable and thus must usually be administered by tube They are expensive
Hepatic Aid contains a relatively high branched-chain amino acid content and a relatively low aromatic amino acid content, plus partially hydrogenated soy oil, lecithin, monodiglycerides, maltodextrins, and sucrose Trauma Cal also contains a high concentration of branched-chain amino acids	Branched-chain amino acids (*e.g.*, leucine, isoleucine, and valine) are metabolized in muscle, not liver, as are aromatic amino acids; therefore, liver is allowed to rest (consult Chap. 8 for more information on use of branched-chain amino acids in liver disease)	

Table 2–6
Nurse's Responsibilities in Tube Feedings or Enteral Oral Supplements

Discomforts	Possible Rationales for Discomforts	Nursing Procedures That May Alleviate Discomforts
Psychological Disturbances		
Fear, anger, hostility, and depression	Perception that his condition is declining	Assure client, when applicable, that these feedings are usually temporary measures used to help him regain his strength, which ultimately reduces convalescent time.
	Fear of physical discomfort (*e.g.,* choking or being unable to breathe when the tube is inserted)	Assure client that this is a relatively painless procedure. Encourage him to swallow water, if allowed, or to swallow frequently while the tube is being inserted.
		Let him choose which nostril will be used for insertion. Hold his hand when tube is being inserted. This creates a nearness that is relaxing.
	Fear that he has lost all control over his life, including the ability to select his own foods or enjoy a meal	Allow client to choose his own formula from those allowed, whenever possible (*e.g.,* Meritene *vs* Sustacal).
		Encourage pleasant family members to eat with him.
		Serve tube feedings from a tray, if possible.

(continued)

Table 2–6 75

Table 2-6
Nurse's Responsibilities in Tube Feedings or Enteral Oral Supplements (continued)

Discomforts	Possible Rationales for Discomforts	Nursing Procedures That May Alleviate Discomforts
Psychological Disturbances *(continued)*		
		Explain what foods are in the feeding so he can acquire a visual image. *Note.* This image may also stimulate saliva. If this procedure is not effective, allow him to savor food, without swallowing, if he desires.
	Loss of body image (*e.g.,* males often correlate these feedings with "baby foods"; therefore, feel they have lost their masculinity)	If the client is a male or an adolescent, explain that these feedings were originally designed for astronauts. Encourage muscular activity. Moderate physical activity often enhances relaxation and a feeling of well being.
Physiological Disturbances		
Drying of the oral cavity and tooth decay	Lack of salivary gland stimulation	See procedures used to alleviate a client's feeling of losing control, noted above. Give client ice cubes to suck or sugarless gum to chew if he is coherent. Discuss the use of an artificial saliva substitute with the physician. Help the client cleanse his teeth often unless contraindicated by oral surgery.
Nasal crusting and ulceration	Nasal care overlooked	Cleanse and lubricate nares frequently. Change tape that anchors tube frequently.

(continued)

Table 2-6
Nurse's Responsibilities in Tube Feedings or Enteral Oral Supplements (continued)

Discomforts	Possible Rationales for Discomforts	Nursing Procedures That May Alleviate Discomforts
Psychological Disturbances (continued)		
Coughing or choking	Tube may irritate the client, causing him to cough or choke	Check position of the tube. Suggest a smaller tube if sensation is excessive. Encourage client to clear throat to relieve anxiety.
Aspiration	Tube positioned incorrectly during insertion or dislocation between feedings	Check tube for placement initially and *before each feeding*. Use a stethoscope to listen for "rumbling" and "bubbling" sounds in the stomach.
	Induction of gastric retention when stomach or intestinal emptying times impaired	If gastric retention is suspected (*e.g.*, stomach distention is evident), aspirate gastric contents before feeding. If more than 100 ml–150 ml is aspirated, report findings to physician.
	Positioning of client incorrect during initial insertion or during subsequent feedings (malpositioning increases risk of aspiration because tube has a tendency to kink, which, in turn, causes precipitation of food, viscosity, and improper flushing)	Roll up the bed so that the patient is reclining at a 30°–45° angle. If the bed cannot be adjusted, place him on his side.
Vomiting	Induced by gag reflex while tube is being inserted	Encourage client to swallow frequently during the insertion procedure.
	Incorrect position of client during tube insertion or during follow-up feedings	See Aspiration, above, for proper positioning.
		(continued)

Table 2-6
Nurse's Responsibilities in Tube Feedings or Enteral Oral Supplements (continued)

Table 2-6 77

Discomforts	Possible Rationales for Discomforts	Nursing Procedures That May Alleviate Discomforts
Physiological Disturbances *(continued)*		
Vomiting *(continued)*	Improper position of tube	See Aspiration for effective procedures to check tube placement.
	Gastric retention	Aspirate gastric contents before additional feedings, especially after initial feedings, if gastric retention is suspected. Report delayed emptying to the physician, if applicable.
		Allow client to rest for at least ½ hour after tube insertion (see Generalized Infusion Rate and Tables 2-5 and 2-7).
	Feeding too soon or too rapidly after tube insertion	Suggest switching from bolus feedings to infusion pump feeding.
	Using too large a tube for feeding	Suggest using a smaller tube.
	Using unclean equipment	Rinse tubes before and after all feedings. Amount of water ranges from 30 ml to 50 ml depending on individual hydration assessment.
		Change tubes frequently, every 2–3 days. Change the infusion line (above feeding tube) daily.
	Contamination of formula	Check date of formula. Discard any open formula that has been left more than 24 hours.

(continued)

Table 2–6
Nurse's Responsibilities in Tube Feedings or Enteral Oral Supplements (continued)

Discomforts	Possible Rationales for Discomforts	Nursing Procedures That May Alleviate Discomforts
Physiological Disturbances *(continued)*		
Vomiting *(continued)*	Formula too cold	Refrigerate all open formula. Check temperature of formula. *Serve only room temperature formula.* Continuous drip feedings can be placed in ice packs in order to prevent spoilage. Suggest switching from enteral feedings made at home to commercial formulas. Home feedings have a higher contamination rate.
	Anxiety, which can increase intestinal transit time	Help client relax.
Diarrhea	Feeding *hyperosmolar* (high concentrations of solutes to fluids, especially of glucose) formulas too rapidly, with consequent development of "dumping syndrome" and resultant osmotic diarrhea (consult Chap. 7)	Check manufacturer's recommended infusion rate. Check formula for liquid contents and recommended dilution. Check to see that adequate amounts of water have been used to rinse the tubes.
	Feeding concentrated milk formulas to individuals with impaired lactase activity	Check the lactose content of the formula and report diarrhea to dietitian. Discuss changing to a similar formula without lactose (*e.g.*, use Ensure instead of Meritene; see Appendix II for other lactose-free formulas).

(continued)

Table 2-6 79

Table 2-6
Nurse's Responsibilities in Tube Feedings or Enteral Oral Supplements (continued)

Discomforts	Possible Rationales for Discomforts	Nursing Procedures That May Alleviate Discomforts
Diarrhea (continued)	Feeding formulas with too high a concentration of long-chain triglycerides to individuals with malabsorption disorders (steatorrhea, the end result)	Report the development of steatorrhea to the physician and dietitian. Discuss using a formula with less fat or one that contains MCT oil (see Chap. 8 and Tables 8-1 and 8-2).
	Feeding too concentrated a formula too soon or too rapidly	See Vomiting. Check to see that adequate amounts of water have been used to rinse the tubes.
	Using too large a tube for feeding	Suggest using a smaller tube.
	Using unclean equipment	See Vomiting.
	Contamination of formula	See Vomiting.
	Too low a concentration of sugar in formula	Suggest using antidiarrheal medications to the physician.
		Discuss formula change with the dietitian and physician. Laxatives may be used, if prescribed by the physician, rather than changing the formula.
Constipation	Formula too concentrated	Check dilution recommended on commercial formulas and water content of home-prepared formulas. Check amount of water being used to rinse tubes.
	Chemically defined formulas being administered for too long a time. (low fiber)	Discuss a formula change with physician and dietitian.

(continued)

Table 2–6
Nurse's Responsibilities in Tube Feedings or Enteral Oral Supplements (continued)

Discomforts	Possible Rationales for Discomforts	Nursing Procedures That May Alleviate Discomforts
Physiological Disturbances *(continued)*		
Dehydration or overhydration	Infusion of formulas that have too high or too low a fluid-to-solute ratio	Check formula for fluid contents and dilution recommendations.
	Excessive or inadequate amount of water being used to rinse tubes	Check how often and how much water was used to rinse tubes.
	Sodium content of formula too high or too low (too much causes overhydration; and too little, dehydration [thirst mechanism may be impaired])	*Keep accurate intake and output records.* Assess client's thirst whenever possible. Weigh client, frequently, in order to prevent edema development. Check for other signs of overhydration or dehydration such as dry skin. Report all findings and records to the physician and dietitian. Discuss a formula change or increased or decreased dilution of formula. Also discuss the possibility of increased dietary restriction. For instance, kidney complications may have developed (see Sodium content, above.)
	Protein content of formula too high or too low (too much causes dehydration; and too little, overhydration with resultant edema)	
	Tubes too small or too large	Check tubes for excess residue and clogging. If tube is clogged, formula may be too concentrated for the size of the tube. Before discussing a formula or tube size change, however, check the

(continued)

Table 2–6 81

Table 2–6
Nurse's Responsibilities in Tube Feedings or Enteral Oral Supplements (continued)

Discomforts	Possible Rationales for Discomforts	Nursing Procedures That May Alleviate Discomforts
Physiological Disturbances *(continued)* *Dehydration or overhydration (continued)*		tube for proper placement (it may be kinked) and cleanliness of the tube.
Hypokalemia	Diuretic therapy Excessive insulin Excessive GI losses	Administer potassium Replace GI losses
Weight gain or loss	Formula too concentrated or too diluted May lack caloric requirements needed to meet the metabolic requirement of stress Omitted feedings or excess residue left on the tube or in the syringe after feeding	Weigh client frequently and report any changes to the physician and dietitian. Discuss a change in the volume, concentration, or number of feedings. Check the nurses' notes regarding the number of feedings accurately administered. Check tube and syringe for signs of residue. Check the amount of water being used to rinse the tube.
Hypoglycemia or hyperglycemia	Too high or too low a concentration of glucose Insulin activity impaired by release of "stress" hormones	Check urine, frequently, for any signs of sugar. Report any signs of sugar to the physician. Clinically assess client for symptoms of either hypoglycemia or hyperglycemia. Check with physician to see if formula changes or insulin adjustments may be necessary.

Table 2-7
Sample Initial Support Plan for Continuous-Drip Nasogastric Tube Feeding of Flexical

	Strength	Volume	Kcal	Protein (g)	Fat (g)	CHO (g)	Approximate Osmolality
Day 1 70 ml/hr	0.25	1680	420	9.5	14	64	138
Day 2 70 ml/hr	0.50	1680	840	18	28	128	275
Day 3 90 ml/hr	0.50	2160	1080	24.3	36.7	166.3	275
Day 4 100 ml/hr	0.75	2400	1800	40.5	61.2	277.2	413
Day 5 125 ml/hr	1.00	2700	2700	67.5	102	462	550

(Reprinted with permission. Letsou AP, Ma KM, Stollar CA, Hain WF: A Guide to Nutritional Care. Evansville, IN, Mead Johnson Nutritional Division, Mead Johnson and Company, 1981)

Table 2–8
Caloric and Macronutrient Composition of Selected Parenteral Nutritional Support Solutions (24-Hour Supply)

Nutritional Support Components	Crystalline Amino Acids	Carbohydrate	Fat	Total Kilocalories per Liter of Solution
Peripheral Vein Protein-Sparing Solution				
Dextrose (5%) in water D₅W (5% or 5 g dextrose/dl)		50 g/1000 ml (1 g dextrose = 3.4 kcal)		50 g dextrose/liter = 170 kcal
Crystalline amino acids (3.5%) (3.5% or 3.5 g amino acids/dl)	35 g/1000 ml (1 g amino acids = 3.6–4 kcal; 5.9 g amino acids = 1 g nitrogen)			35 g amino acids/liter = approximately 140 kcal* and 5.9 g nitrogen/liter
Unit of 10% fat emulsion = 500 ml, caloric value[†]			50 g/500 ml = 550 kcal	1 unit of fat emulsion = 550 kcal 1 liter = 1100 kcal
Peripheral Vein Complete Nutritional Support Solution[‡]				
Crystalline amino acid solution (3.5%) +	35 g/1000 ml			35 g amino acids/liter = approximately 140 kcal* and 5.9 g nitrogen
Dextrose solution (20%) D₂₀W (20% or 20 g dextrose/dl) (Final osmolality decreases when fat is added)		200 g/1000 ml		200 g dextrose/liter = 680 kcal

Table 2–8 83

Table 2-8
**Caloric and Macronutrient Composition of Selected
Parenteral Nutritional Support Solutions (24-Hour Supply)** (continued)

Nutritional Support Components	Crystalline Amino Acids	Carbohydrate	Fat	Total Kilocalories per Liter of Solution
Peripheral Vein Complete Nutritional Support Solution (continued)				
Fat emulsion (10%) 500 ml† 1 unit = 500 ml			50 g/500 ml	500 ml fat emulsion = 550 kcal Total kcal/day for 2000 ml of amino acid solutions (3.5%) and 20% dextrose combined = 680 kcal and 35 g amino acids (5.9 g nitrogen). Infusing a fat unit in addition brings the volume to 2500 ml and the caloric value to 1230 calories
Central Vein Complete Nutritional Support Solution				
Crystalline amino acid solution (5.5%) (5.5% or 5.5 g amino acids/dl) +	55 g/1000 ml			55 g amino acids/liter = approximately 220 kcal* and 9.32 g nitrogen

(continued)

Table 2-8 85

Table 2-8
**Caloric and Macronutrient Composition of Selected
Parenteral Nutritional Support Solutions (24-Hour Supply)** (continued)

Nutritional Support Components	Crystalline Amino Acids	Carbohydrate	Fat	Total Kilocalories per Liter of Solution
Central Vein Complete Nutritional Support Solution *(continued)*				
Dextrose solution (30%) $D_{30}W$ (30% or 30 g dextrose/dl)		300 g/1000 ml		300 g dextrose/liter = 1020 kcal
Fat emulsion (10%) 500 ml[†]			50 g/500 ml	500 ml fat emulsion = 550 kcal Total kcal/day for 2000 ml of amino acid solutions (5.5%) and 30% dextrose combined = 1020 kcal and 55 g amino acids (9.32 g nitrogen). Infusing a fat unit (500 ml) in addition brings the volume to 2500 ml and the caloric value to 1570 calories

* Amino acids are not infused to supply calories. They are administered to maintain or prevent catabolism of lean body mass. Consequently, they should not be considered a significant source of calories or energy.
† 1 ml = 1.1 kcal.
‡ The word *complete* does not mean that the infusions supply total nutritional needs for the hypermetabolic individual, only that protein *and* calories are included.
(David C. Madsen, PhD, Biochemist: personal communication)

Table 2–9
Advantages and Disadvantages of Parenteral Nutritional Support Solutions

Components	Advantages	Disadvantages*
Peripheral Vein Protein-Sparing Solution		
Glucose solution D₅W (5% dextrose in water)	Partially spares protein Nearly isotonic to the blood Provides glucose for the central nervous system Inexpensive	Permits extensive loss of lean body mass over time Caloric content not sufficient to meet normal body needs; consequently, cannot meet hypermetabolic needs (see Table 2-1)
Amino acid solution (AAS) Crystalline amino acids (3.5%)	Use of a glucose-free solution decreases the release of insulin, which enhances lipolysis. Consequently, the free fatty acids and ketone bodies released from adipose tissue into the blood are used for energy rather than protein from lean tissue catabolism. Provides a source of nitrogen, which helps maintain nitrogen balance Amino acids, at this concentration, are nearly isotonic to the blood	Carbohydrate-free therapy requires careful monitoring of blood and urine sugar levels Solution not used to provide calories; therefore, not to be used in individuals with limited fat stores as a source of calories May raise blood urea nitrogen levels. Consequently it is contraindicated in renal disorders. Drugs and other mixtures cannot be added to protein solutions. More expensive than dextrose solutions.
Peripheral Vein Total Nutritional Support Solution†		
Amino acid solution (3.5%) + dextrose solution (20%; 10% concentration) + fat emulsion (10%)	Meets nutritional requirements fairly well, with only mild to moderate nutritional deficits	See Amino Acid and Dextrose Solution Disadvantages

(continued)

Table 2-9 87

Table 2-9
Advantages and Disadvantages of Parenteral Nutritional Support Solutions (continued)

Components	Advantages	Disadvantages*
Peripheral Vein Total Nutritional Support Solution*† *(continued)		
Electrolytes are added according to individual needs.	See Amino Acid Solution and D$_5$W solution above	Must administer fat separately, cannot be added to amino acids or dextrose solutions
	Advantages to adding fat emulsions are that carbohydrates or proteins; consequently they enhance weight gain.	Fats may not spare protein as well as carbohydrate if used as the total source of calories
	Lipids are isotonic to blood.	Fat elevates serum cholesterol levels.
	Lipids do not raise insulin levels.	Fat may induce nausea, headaches, and fever
	Lipids contain linoleic acid, which prevents essential fatty acid deficiencies.	
		Expensive and needs expert monitoring for complications, including local sepsis, thrombophlebitis, and overhydration, especially when fluids are also consumed orally
***Central Vein Total Nutritional Support Solution*‡**		
Amino acid solution (8.5%)	Central vein total nutritional support solutions (also called *total parenteral nutrition* [TPN] or hyperalimentation) have all the advantages of total nutritional support solutions administered peripherally	Have all the disadvantages listed for Total Peripheral Solutions
Dextrose solution (50%)		Higher concentrations of dextrose, administered rapidly, can induce hyperglycemia, glycosuria, excess CO_2 production, water retention and/or osmotic diuresis
(These solutions become concentrations of AAS, 4.5%, and dextrose, 25%, when added together and diluted.)		
Fat emulsion (500 ml)		

(continued)

Table 2–9
Advantages and Disadvantages of Parenteral Nutritional Support Solutions (continued)

Components	Advantages	Disadvantages*
Central Vein Total Nutritional Support Solution‡ *(continued)*		
Electrolytes, vitamins, and minerals are added according to individual needs.	Supply the caloric requirements of a hypermetabolic individual (a total of 3000–5000 kcal/day can be administered, especially when fat emulsions are used) Are able to restore lean body mass and adipose tissue when tissue wasting has occurred Can modify solutions to promote normal growth and development in infants and children	Hyperosmolar coma can develop if hyperglycemia and dehydration are excessive Prerenal azotemia or hyperammonemia may develop if excessive amounts of amino acids infused Hyperlipidemia or fatty liver may develop if excessive amounts of fat infused Essential fatty acid (EFA) deficiencies may occur if too little fat administered over time If feeding is too fast, hyperglycemia or hypoglycemia may develop Additionally, hypoglycemia may develop if feeding is discontinued too rapidly If feeding is too slow, nutrient deficiencies may be induced If solutions are not properly prepared or handled, bacterial contamination may be excessive

* Most expensive of all solutions. The risk of complication with parenteral solutions is substantial. Only some of the complications are given here. If more information is desired, consult parenteral solution manuals and advanced nutritional, nursing, and medical textbooks

† The word *total* does not mean that the solution supplies all the nutritional needs of the hypermetabolic individual.

‡ This solution is only one sample of macronutrient percentages; percentages may be altered according to the disease condition and individuals metabolic needs.

Bibliography

Abbott Laboratories: Advances in peripheral vein parenteral nutrition. Physicians Monograph. North Chicago, IL, Abbott Laboratories, Hospital Products Division, 1980

Abbott Laboratories: Nutritional assessment and intravenous support: Indications for parenteral nutrition. Physicians Monograph. North Chicago, IL, Medical Directions, Inc., Abbott Laboratories, 1978

Aronson V, Fitzgerald B: Guidebook for Nutrition Counselors. North Quincy, IL, The Christopher Publishing House, 1978

Blackburn GL, Copeland EM, Rankin GB: Feeding the malnourished patient. Patient Care 15:50, 1981

Blackburn GL, Flatt JP, Clowes GHA, et al: Peripheral intravenous feeding with isotonic amino acid solutions. Am J Surg 125:447, 1973

Chernoff R: Nutrition support: Formulas and delivery of enteral feeding. Enteral formulas I. J Am Diet Assoc 79:426, 1981

Chernoff R: Nutrition support: Formulas and delivery of enteral feeding, Delivery systems II. J Am Diet Assoc 79:430, 1981

Doyle Pharmaceutical Company: Publications Program on Tube Feeding. Minneapolis, MN, Doyle Pharmaceutical Company, 1979

Feldtman RW, Andrassy RJ: Meeting exceptional nutritional needs. Postgrad Med 64:64, 1978

Guild RT, Gerda JJ: Total parenteral nutrition. J Fla Med Assoc 66:401, 1979

Heymsfield SB, Bethel RA, Ansley JD et al: Enteral hyperalimentation: An alternative to central venous hyperalimentation. Int Med 90:63, 1979

Howard RB, Herbold NH: Nutrition in Clinical Care. New York, McGraw-Hill, 1978

Korczowski MM, Coevern SV: Strengthen the nurse's role in nutritional counseling. Nursing and Health Care 2:210, 1981

Krause MV, Mahan LK: Food, Nutrition, and Diet Therapy, 6th ed. Philadelphia, WB Saunders, 1979

Letsou AP, Ma KM, Stoller CA, et al: A Guide to Nutritional Care. Evansville, IN, Mead Johnson and Company, Nutritional Division, 1981

Mead Johnson and Company, Nutritional Division. The Enteral Nutritional Management System. Evansville, IN, Mead Johnson and Company, 1981

Paul GJ: Total parenteral nutrition: A guide for its use. Am J Gastroenterol 72:186, 1979

Pennington J: Nutritional Diet Therapy. Palo Alto, Bull Publishing, 1978

Ross Laboratories: Dietary modifications in disease: Progressive hospital diets. Columbus, OH, Ross Laboratories, 1978

Ross Laboratories: Protein for the hospitalized patient. Nutritional Thinking in Action. Columbus, OH, Ross Laboratories, 1978

Senate Committee on Nutritional and Human Needs: Dietary Goals for the United States, 2nd ed. Washington, DC, US Government Printing Office, 1977

Shils ME: Enteral nutrition by tube. Cancer Res 37:2432, 1977

Suitor CW, Hunter MF: Nutrition: Principles and Application in Health Promotion. Philadelphia, JB Lippincott, 1980

Travenol Laboratories Inc: Insights into Parenteral Nutrition. Deerfield, IL, Travenol Laboratories, Inc, 1976

Suggested Reading

Green ML, Harry J: Nutrition in Contemporary Nursing Practice. New York, John Wiley & Sons, 1981

Hunt SM, Groff JL, Holbrook JM: Nutrition and Clinical Practice. New York, John Wiley & Sons, 1980

Shils ME: Guidelines for total parenteral nutrition. JAMA 220:1721, 1972

Sowers MF, Litzinger L, Stumbo P et al: Development and critical evaluation of the food nomogram. J Am Diet Assoc 79:536, 1981

Thiele VF: Clinical Nutrition, 2nd ed. St Louis, CV Mosby, 1980

William SR: Nutrition and Diet Therapy, 4th ed. St Louis, CV Mosby, 1981

chapter 3

Cardiovascular System

Coronary Heart Disease (CHD)

Description

In coronary heart disease, the channels of the coronary arteries become too narrow to carry the amounts of blood needed by the heart. Narrowing of the coronary arteries is caused by atherosclerosis (see below).

Types

- *Myocardial infarction (MI)*. Necrosis of the heart muscle due to interruption of its blood supply; caused by partial or complete obstruction of a coronary artery
- *Angina pectoris.* Episodes of transient chest pains resulting from temporary decreases in the blood supply to the heart muscle (myocardium); caused by obstruction or constriction of the coronary arteries
- *Coronary insufficiency.* Inadequate coronary flow; also known as unstable angina (cardiac ischemic pain coming on frequently and severely, including pain not provoked by exertion); probably represents new occlusion or near-occlusion of a major coronary vessel, compromising blood supply to an area of myocardium
- *Congestive Heart Failure (CHF).* A type of CHD because it is a complication that often develops after an MI; the weakened myocardium is unable to maintain an adequate output to sustain a normal blood circulation; the resulting fluid imbalances cause pulmonary edema to develop, which induces labored breathing with resultant added stress on the laboring heart

Incidence

- National number 1 killer; an estimated 4.4 million Americans afflicted
- 1.5 million heart attacks per year; 550,000 fatal

Etiologic Risk Factors

Personal Characteristics (Risk factors that cannot be altered)

Male

Advanced age

Black—hypertension

Familial hyperlipidemia (Type 1)*

Diabetes mellitus*

Hypertension (10%–15% of the population)*

Electrocardiographic abnormalities*

Environmental Factors (Risk factors that can be altered by dietary and behavioral changes)

Stress

Cigarette smoking

Sedentary living

Obsessive–compulsive, competitive personality (Type A)

Food habits: High intake of calories, refined sugars, fats, especially saturated fats, cholesterol, salt, and alcohol†; low intake of potassium

---

* These disorders cannot be cured, but they may be controlled by altering behavioral and dietary patterns and by drug therapy.
† High intake of these substances may induce obesity, hypertriglyceridemia, hypercholesterolemia, hyperuricemia, diabetes mellitus, and hypertension.

Drug Therapy

Drug therapy during the acute phase of the illness is beyond the scope of this handbook. See Tables 3-3 and 3-11* for medications used in chronic care.

Diet Therapy

Acute Phase

Goals in a Coronary-Care Unit

- Maintain and gradually improve nutritional status in order to prevent further tissue destruction and aid in repair of damaged tissue

---

* See tables at the end of this chapter.

- Adjust fluid and electrolyte balance, especially sodium and potassium, to reduce edema (excessive sodium limitation, however, may induce shock, and client must be monitored)
- Minimize cardiac work (myocardium and digestive oxygen demands) and pressure by
  1. Altering food consistency (*e.g.*, serve bland, cooked, soft, low-roughage foods instead of spicy, raw, fibrous foods)
  2. Decreasing the amount of energy required to prepare and consume (chew) foods (*e.g.*, serve ground foods, but not baby foods, or cut up foods before serving)
  3. Decreasing gastrointestinal distention (*e.g.*, serve six small, rather than three large, meals a day, decrease total daily food volume by limiting "empty" calorie intake such as those in rich desserts, decrease total meal volume by limiting fluid intake during meals), which enhances displacement of the diaphragm toward the heart. Additionally, decreased distention may prevent symptoms of indigestion and heartburn, symptoms that may frighten the client.

Nutritional Care Plan

A sample progressive nutritional care plan for a coronary-care unit is provided in Table 3-1.

Chronic or Rehabilitative Phase

The two etiologic risk factors most frequently identified in clients who develop cardiovascular disease are hypertension and atherosclerosis. These two disorders may be identified as separate entities, have a synergistic effect (hypertension→ artherosclerosis→ MI), or occur concomitantly in clients with cardiovascular disease. Physicians treating clients with or at risk of developing cardiovascular disease, therefore, may prescribe regimens that will help control hypertension and atherosclerosis. (In this handbook, however, these regimens are considered as separate entities for purposes of clarity.)

For diet therapy, see nutritional care plans advised for clients with hypertension, hypercholestrolemia, and hypertriglyceridemia.

Hypertension

Description

Hypertension is high arterial blood pressure due to sustained resistance of the blood vessels to the forward flow of blood (Table 3-2). Generally, mild hypertension is defined as a diastolic blood pressure (BP)

Table 3–2
**Upper Limits of Normal
Blood Pressure by Age Group**

Age Group (years)	Blood Pressure (mm Hg)
Infants	90/60
3–6	110/70
7–10	120/80
11–17	130/80
18–44	140/90
45–64	Normotensive, 120/80
	Borderline or labile,* 140/90
	Hypertensive, 150/95
65 and older	160/95

* Subject to free and rapid change
(Adapted from Batterman B: Hypertension. Part I: Detection and evaluation. Cardiovasc Nurs 11:38, 1975)

between 90 mm Hg and 104 mm Hg, moderate hypertension as a diastolic BP between 105 mm Hg and 114 mm Hg, and severe hypertension as a diastolic BP above 115 mm Hg.

Essential hypertension is hypertension of unknown cause. It is also called *idiopathic hypertension.* Secondary hypertension is hypertension associated with a specific disease, such as primary aldosteronism, Cushing's disease, renal disease, pheochromocytoma (tumor of adrenal medulla), and possibly obesity. Certain drugs (*e.g.*, oral contraceptives and alcohol) may also induce hypertension.

Incidence

In all, 23 to 60 million Americans, or 10% to 20% of the adult population, are hypertensive, depending upon the blood pressure levels considered by the clinician to be diagnostic and the age groups included in various surveys.

- Essential hypertension, 90% of total
- Secondary hypertension, 10% of total

Etiologic Risk Factors in Essential Hypertension

Etiologic risk factors with nutritional implications include obesity; high intake of saturated fat, alcohol, and sodium; and low intake of potassium (see list of Etiologic Risk Factors in Cardiovascular Disease).

Drug Therapy

Medications are prescribed when the client does not comply with dietary recommendations, when dietary treatment is ineffective, or in conjunction with diet therapy.

Medications are usually prescribed in steps or concomitantly. *Stepped care* (SC) implies that if one drug does not lower diastolic BP to 90 mm Hg or below, additional medications should be prescribed (*e.g.*, beta blockers) to obtain the most effective individual control. This methodology of care also has a "step-down" provision, *i.e.*, if BP is well controlled for a suitable length of time (6–12 mo), it is appropriate to reduce medications step by step in an attempt to control the pressure with as little medication as possible. Additionally, diet therapy may be used as a substitute for or in addition to drug therapy, whenever feasible.

Medications presently prescribed are presented in Table 3-3.

A recent study, the Multiple Risk Factor Intervention Trial (MRFIT), has indicated the need to reassess the current widespread, routine, and aggressive SC use of antihypertensive drugs for all hypertensive clients including mildly hypertensive clients. This treatment had been advocated by the findings of the Hypertension Detection and Follow-up Program (HDFP). The MRFIT study was a seven-year randomized primary prevention trial that was designed to test the value of reductions in cigarette smoking, hypercholesterolemia, and hypertension by special intervention (SI) programs as compared with the usual sources of care (UC) in the community in the progression of coronary vascular disease. Thirteen thousand men aged 35 to 57 years who were at increased risk of death from CHD (*e.g.*, who smoked more than 30 cigarettes per day or had cholesterol levels higher than 295 mg/dl or diastolic BP above 90 mm Hg) participated in the study.

The findings were as follows:

- Coronary mortality, 7.1% lower in the SI group, was not statistically significant. However, most authorities think that this was because the UC clients and their physicians were influenced by the recently launched vigorous public health programs intended to reduce smoking, lower blood pressure, and lessen dietary intake of fat and cholesterol in the general population. Consequently, the UC clients were practicing the same health care practices as the clients who were exposed to SI care.
- The group of clients with initial diastolic BP of 90 mm Hg to 94 mm Hg who were treated intensively with antihypertensive drugs (the SI group) had significantly higher coronary and total mortality rates than did the group treated less intensively (the UC group). No difference was observed in those with diastolic BP of 95 mm Hg to 99 mm Hg, and more intensive therapy was shown to be valuable for those whose diastolic BP was at or above 100 mm Hg. Of addi-

tional concern was the higher coronary death rate in the group of more intensively treated SI hypertensive clients who had an abnormal baseline resting electrocardiogram (ECG).

In light of these surprising findings, many physicians are now practicing a more conservative approach to drug therapy for hypertensive patients. This conservative approach is as follows:

- Providing selective and quick SC drug therapy for those at high risk (*e.g.*, those with a diastolic BP of 100 mm Hg or above)
- Strongly encouraging all clients, regardless of risk status as long as they are under medical surveillance, to follow non–drug therapies that are likely to lessen the cardiovascular disease progression. Non–drug therapy treatments advocated are diet therapy (*e.g.*, weight reduction programs for the obese, mild sodium restriction for all [reduce sodium intakes from 4–5 g to 2–3 g per day], moderate alterations in total fat intakes [reduce total fat intake from 40% to 30%–35% of total energy intake and reduce saturated fat intake, which includes fats that contain cholesterol, to 10% of total fat intake]); moderate exercise and relaxation programs; and behavioral programs that help the client abstain from cigarette smoking

Diet Therapy

Goals
- Lower blood pressure by
    1. Reducing caloric consumption to achieve weight reduction (see Chap. 6)
    2. Reducing sodium consumption reduces fluid volume by decreasing retention of excess sodium and water in extracellular compartments; also enhances the antihypertensive effect of diuretics
    3. Changing the potassium-to-sodium ratio; increase consumption of potassium and decrease consumption of sodium
    4. Changing the polyunsaturated-fat–to–saturated-fat ratio may be helpful according to recent research. That is, increase polyunsaturated fat intake in order to enhance production of prostaglandins (*e.g.*, PGE_2 and PGI_2) that may inhibit platelet aggregation and relax vascular smooth muscle
- Encourage lifelong compliance with dietary modifications by adapting dietary adjustments to individual lifestyle
- Decrease the cost and side-effects of treatment by reducing the dosage or eliminating the need for medications, including potassium supplements

Table 3-5
Mortality Experience Among Treated Hypertensive Insured Men*

Pressure (mm Hg)	Increased Chance of Death Compared to Normal (%)
Systolic	
≤ 127	2
128–137	10
138–147	13
148–157	66
≥ 158	101
Diastolic	
≤ 83	4
84–87	24
88–92	24
93–97	67
≥ 98	102

* 1979 Build and Blood Pressure Study, which included a highly selected sample of 20,000 insured men who had received treatment before they applied for insurance between 1954 and 1972. Even though they were under medical treatment, they were otherwise in good health. (Ad Hoc Committee of the New Build and Blood Pressure Study, Association of Life Insurance Medical Directors of America and Society of Actuaries, 1979)

Nutritional Care Plan

- Factors in Developing a Nutritional Care Plan for Hypertension
  1. Interview Chart (Components With Special Significance)
     a. Ethnic and religious background. Jewish and Chinese clients may consume more sodium
     b. Household. Persons living alone may eat more highly processed, quick-to-prepare, and fast foods. These often contain more sodium and less potassium (Tables 3-6 and 3-7)
     c. Diagnosis. Severity of disease and other complications (*e.g.*, hyperlipidemia) influence dietary restrictions
     d. Medications. Diuretics lower sodium levels; many other medications contain sodium
     e. History of modified diets. Helps nurse judge client's knowledge of present dietary restrictions and degree of compliance
  2. Nutritional Assessment (Data With Special Significance)
     a. Diet history. Condiments used at the table (*e.g.*, salt); seasonings used in food preparation (*e.g.*, salt, monosodium glutamate [MSG], soy sauce); snack foods consumed; and fruits and vegetables consumed

b. Vital signs. Blood pressure. Severity of hypertension determines modification of diet (*e.g.*, mild sodium restriction to severe restriction).

c. Anthropometric measurements. Height and weight determines need for, and extent of, caloric restriction

d. Laboratory data

(1) Blood. Serum lipid levels, potassium, blood urea nitrogen, and creatinine (latter two important in diagnosing secondary hypertension)

(2) Urine. 24-hr urinary sodium determines sodium restriction; 24-hr urinary potassium and kallikrein excretions may also determine dietary intake

e. Clinical evaluations

(1) Extent of obesity. Determines caloric restriction needed

(2) Edema of abdomen or limbs. Determines sodium restriction

(3) Symptoms of hypokalemia or hyperkalemia. Determine need for potassium supplements or restriction (see Signs and Treatment of Hypokalemia and Hyperkalemia)

Signs and Treatment of Hypokalemia and Hyperkalemia

Hypokalemia	Hyperkalemia
Laboratory Findings	**Laboratory Findings**
Serum potassium (K) below 3.5 mEq/L Electrocardiographic changes	Serum potassium (K) above 5.5 mEq/L Electrocardiographic changes
Clinical Findings	**Clinical Findings**
Frequently none until K levels are extremely low	Frequently none until K levels are dangerously high
Skeletal Muscle Effects	**Skeletal Muscle Effects**
General muscle weakness Muscle cramps, paresthesias, difficult respiration	General muscle weakness Paresthesias, difficult speech, and difficult respiration
Cardiac Effects	**Cardiac Effects**
Tachycardia with cardiac dilatation → heart block → cardiac arrest Faint heart sound, weak pulse, hypotension	Bradycardia → heart block → cardiac arrest Decreased pulse rate Peripheral vascular collapse

Hypokalemia	Hyperkalemia

GI Smooth Muscle Effects

Hypokalemia:
Diminished peristalsis, which leads to vomiting, distention, anorexia, paralytic ileus

Hyperkalemia:
Diminished peristalsis, which leads to nausea or diarrhea

Nervous System Effects

Hypokalemia:
Listlessness
Lethargy

Hyperkalemia:
Irritability
Mental confusion

Excretory Effects

Decreased urinary output

Treatment

Hypokalemia:

Medications

Potassium-sparing diuretics
KCl supplements (see Table 3-3)

Hyperkalemia:

Medications

Potassium-losing diuretics
KCl supplements discontinued

Dietary (Hypokalemia)

Foods, high in potassium, low in sodium (see Conversion Table for Sodium-Restricted Diets and Table 3-7)

Dietary (Hyperkalemia)

Foods, low in potassium.
Foods high in potassium (*e.g.*, certain fruits and vegetables) can be leached. To leach, soak the food extensively in water and then drain. Potassium is excreted in the water, which is then discarded (see Conversion Table for Sodium-Restricted Diets and Table 3-6)

(Adapted from Lewis CM: Nutrition and Diet Therapy: Self-Instructional Units. Philadelphia, FA Davis, 1976)

Consult Chapter 2 for more details on developing a nutritional care plan. Consult Chapter 1 for more details on nutritional assessment data.

- Nutritional Care Plan Alterations for Essential Hypertension
  1. Caloric alterations
     a. Intake of high-calorie foods is restricted
     b. Eating patterns are adjusted (*e.g.*, by behavioral modifications)

    c. Exercise patterns are adjusted (consult Chap. 6 for details on how to adjust body weight)

2. Sodium alterations (Table 3-8). The extent of the alteration (the dietary prescription) is determined by

    a. Progression of the disease, as measured by blood pressure levels, extent of edema, extent of cardiac involvement

    b. Adjunctive treatment, such as administration of antihypertensive medications, especially diuretics

    c. Sodium content in natural foods. Sodium, a mineral, is the most prevalent extracellular cation in all plant and animal tissue; consequently, it is found in all natural foods. It is estimated that 20% to 30% of the daily sodium intake is contributed by sodium occurring naturally in foods.

    d. Sodium added to food. Table salt (sodium chloride) is composed of 40% sodium and 60% chloride. Therefore, when salt is added to foods for taste, preservation, and so on, sodium is also added in very high percentages (see Conversion Table for Sodium-Restricted Diets). It is estimated that 20% to 40% of the daily sodium intake is contributed by salt that individuals add with a salt shaker, and 40% to 60% is contributed by sodium added to foods in commercial food processing. Salt substitutes are sometimes prescribed (Table 3-9).

Conversion Table for Sodium-Restricted Diets*

Mineral	Molecular Weight
Sodium (Na)	23

Sample: Moderate Sodium-Restricted Diet Approximately 2.5 g salt (1000 mg or 44 mEq Na)[†]

1. To convert weight of salt to weight of sodium, multiply weight of salt by 0.4 (NaCl contains about 40% Na by weight)
Example: 2.5 g salt $\times$ 0.4 = 1000 mg Na

2. To convert weight of sodium to milliequivalents, divide the number of milligrams of sodium by the molecular weight
Example: 1000 mg Na $\div$ 23 = 44 mEq Na

    * Milliequivalents of potassium can be calculated by the same method using its molecular weight of 39

    † Physicians often prescribe a 2-g salt diet; however, food tables express the content of salt in food as milligrams of sodium. The laboratory, in contrast, expresses the amount of salt in milliequivalents of sodium. Therefore, it is important that the nurse be able to convert the figures readily.

    (Adapted from Suitor CW, Hunter MF: Nutrition: Principles and Application in Health Promotion. Philadelphia, JB Lippincott, 1980)

3. Sodium–potassium ratio alterations (see chart on p. 102). Rationale for decreasing sodium intake and increasing potassium intake in the treatment of hypertension

   a. Increasing potassium intake in the form of foods or supplements (*e.g.*, 80 mEq of potassium chloride per day as Slow-K) may reduce blood pressure by increasing sodium excretion, decreasing renin secretion, decreasing sympathetic nerve activity, or directly dilating the arteries.

   b. Reducing sodium intake and increasing potassium intake from foods may reduce the necessity of potassium supplements and potassium-sparing diuretics (Table 3-10).

   c. Hypokalemia symptoms, including tachycardia, that are induced by the use of nonpotassium-sparing diuretics (*e.g.*, thiazides) may be prevented.

   d. Reducing sodium intake may enhance the antihypertensive effect of the diuretic drug. Consequently, the drug dosage may be reduced (see Tables 3-7, 3-8, and 3-10 for foods high in potassium and low in sodium).

- Nutritional Care Plan Alternations in Secondary Hypertension

   1. Same as for essential hypertension.

   2. Primary disease may call for additional dietary alterations. For example, renal disease necessitates protein alterations.

Table 3–9
Salt Substitutes

Product	Ion Exchange
Adolph's	Potassium chloride
Featherweight	Potassium chloride
Neocurtasal	Potassium chloride
Selora	Potassium chloride
Nu-Salt	Potassium chloride
Co Salt	Potassium chloride and ammonium chloride
Morton-Lite Salt*	Potassium chloride, 50%, sodium chloride 50%

* 1 teaspoon (5 g) = 1300 mg of potassium and 975 mg of sodium

Examples.
Diamond Crystal Iodized Salt. 1 teaspoon = 1955 mg of sodium and approximately 1.5 mg of potassium (0.01% in a 1-lb, 10-oz box)
Nu-Salt. 1 packet (1 g) = 19 μ of sodium, 830 mg of potassium chloride, 167 mg of dextrose, and 3.3 mg of potassium bitartrate
Note. Commercial salt substitutes should be prescribed by a physician. Most salt substitutes are mineral bases consisting of salts other than sodium chloride and taste similar to table salt. These mineral bases, in excess, may be dangerous to the kidney (potassium) or the liver (ammonium). They should also be used sparingly or food will taste bitter.

Estimated Ratio of Sodium to Potassium Content in the Total Diet in Three Selected Age Groups

Sodium	Potassium	Age
0.5	>1	Infancy (6 mo)
0.9	1	Toddler (2 yr)
1.5	<1	Adult (15–20 yr, male)

(The sodium-to-potassium ratio of the infant diet is approximately the same as the desirable ratio estimated from The Estimated Safe and Adequate Daily Dietary Intake (ESADDI) of these minerals established by the National Academy of Sciences National Research Council. The adult diet deviates most from the desired ratio)

Estimated Total Dietary Intakes of Sodium and Potassium per 1000 kcal for Selected Age Groups

Sodium (mg)	Potassium (mg)	Age Group
802–1008	1759–1913	6 mo
1235–1388	1319–1491	Toddler (2 yr)
1716–1757	1168–1200	Adult (15–20 yr, male)

(Sodium and potassium exogenous intakes and ratios adapted from the FDA Total Diet Study analysis of sodium and potassium intakes for selected age groups since 1977 [except for 1979])

Atherosclerosis

Description

Atherosclerosis is a degenerative disease of the medium and large arteries. The intima becomes thickened through the deposition of fibrofatty and fibrous plaques. The plaques are composed of excess cholesterol, other lipids, smooth muscle cells, connective tissue, calcium, fibrin, and specialized cells. Atherosclerosis may be primary or associated with hyperthyroidism, insulin-dependent diabetes, hepatic or renal disease, alcoholism, infection, hypertension, and other disorders.

Incidence

An estimated 5 million Americans have atherosclerosis, which renders it the second most prevalent cardiovascular disease.

Etiologic Risk Factors in Primary Atherosclerosis

Etiological risk factors with nutritional implications include obesity; high intake of fat (especially saturated fat), cholesterol, refined sugars, alcohol, and sodium; and low intake of fiber and polyunsaturated fats (see List of Etiologic Risk Factors in Cardiovascular Disease).

Drug Therapy

Medications are added to treatment in the same progressive steps used in hypertension treatment if hypertension is the precipitating factor. Other medications presently prescribed are listed in Table 3-11.

Diet Therapy

Goals

- Reduce low-density lipoproteins (LDL)* and cholesterol blood levels by limiting exogenous sources of saturated fats and cholesterol and increasing intakes of polyunsaturated fats (PUFA) such as vegetable oils and mucilaginous fibers (*e.g.*, guar and pectin; Table 3-12)
- Increase high-density lipoprotein (HDL) blood levels by encouraging body-weight reduction, which is facilitated by increased energy expenditures, when recommended by the physician; additionally, encourage client to abstain from cigarette smoking
- Reduce triglyceride (fats formed from 3 fatty acids attached to 1 glycerol molecule) and very-low-density lipoprotein (VLDL) blood levels by limiting exogenous sources of total fat, refined sugars, and alcohol (limiting these foods also decreases caloric intake, which enhances endogenous triglyceride reduction)
- Adapt dietary restrictions to attain a nutritionally balanced diet that will maintain optimal nutritional status, including ideal body weight for height and body build (strict lipid restrictions adjust lipid levels but also decrease the ingestion and utilization of other essential nutrients such as protein, calcium, iron, vitamin B complex, and fat-soluble vitamins)
- Lower blood pressure levels by reducing sodium and calorie intake and increasing potassium intake (see Table 3-7)
- Encourage lifelong compliance with dietary modifications by adapting adjustments to client's lifestyle

---

* Protein density is used as a guide for diagnosing and classifying hyperlipidemia because lipids are not water soluble. Consequently, for lipids to be transported in the blood, they must be enveloped by a protein molecule (lipoprotein) since blood is 90% water, and water and fat, like vinegar and oil, do not mix.

The four major lipoprotein classifications (Table 3-13) are:

1. *Chylomicrons*, which predominately transport exogenous triglycerides from the small intestines to the cells
2. *Very-low-density lipoproteins (VLDLs)*, which predominately transport endogenous triglycerides
3. *Low-density lipoproteins (LDLs)*, which predominately transport cholesterol to the cells, including blood vessel cells
4. *High-density lipoproteins (HDLs)*, which predominately transport cholesterol from the cells, including blood vessel cells, back to the liver where it can be excreted in the form of bile

Table 3–12
Cholesterol Content of Some Common Foods

Food Source	Cholesterol Content (mg)
Beef, lean, 1 oz	25
Lamb, lean, 1 oz	28
Veal, lean, 1 oz	28
Cheese, cheddar, 1 oz	29
Liver, calves', 1 oz	122
Egg, medium, 1	252
Fish, halibut, 1 oz	18
Shrimp, 1 oz	42
Bacon, 1 strip	3
Butter, 1 tsp	12
Whole milk, 1 cup	32
Skim milk (<1% fat), 1 cup	4
Ice cream, 3½ oz	40
Peanuts, ½ oz*	0
Chocolate sauce, 1 oz	0
Margarine, 1 tsp	0
Soybean oil, 1 tsp	0

* Cholesterol is a fatty alcohol (sterol) found in all animal tissues but *not* in plant tissues
(Pemberton CM, Gastineau CF (eds): Mayo Clinic Diet Manual. Philadelphia, WB Saunders, 1981)

Nutritional Care Plan

- Factors in Developing a Nutritional Care Plan for Atherosclerosis
  1. Interview Chart (Components With Special Significance)
     a. Sex. Higher incidence in males than in females
     b. Age. Lipid levels increase with age (Table 3-14)
     c. Diagnosis, etiology (primary or secondary hyperlipidemia). Influences dietary restrictions (Tables 3-15 and 3-16)
     d. Medications. Dietary restrictions less severe when medications are used
     e. History of modified diets. Helps nurse to judge client's knowledge of present dietary restrictions and degree of compliance
  2. Nutritional Assessment (Data With Special Significance)
     a. Diet history. Intakes of saturated animal fats, vegetable fats, refined sugars, alcohol, and total calories
     b. Vital signs, blood pressure, hypertension. May cause or enhance atherosclerotic progression
     c. Anthropometric measurements. Height and weight determine need for and extent of caloric restriction

d. Laboratory data
   (1) Blood
      (a) Simple assessment. Triglyceride and cholesterol plasma levels determine nutrient restriction needed. American Heart Association recommended levels for adults: triglycerides, 150 mg/dl; cholesterol, 130 mg/dl–190 mg/dl
      (b) Advanced assessment. Plasma lipoprotein density ranges by ultracentrifuge and electrophoretic migration; determine detailed levels of dietary modifications needed (Table 3-13)
e. Clinical evaluations
   (1) Extent of obesity. Determines caloric restrictions
   (2) Other clinical presentations (see Table 3-15)

Consult Chapter 2 for details on developing a nutritional care plan. Consult Chapter 1 for details on how to evaluate nutritional assessment data.

- Nutritional Care Plan Alterations for Primary Hyperlipoproteinemia (atherosclerosis)
  1. General nutritional care plan, a prudent diet (Tables 3-17 and 3-18)
  2. Specific nutritional care plan (Table 3-16)
- Nutritional Care Plan Alterations for Secondary Hyperlipoproteinemia
  1. Same as for primary hyperlipoproteinemia
  2. Primary disease may call for additional dietary alterations

Cerebrovascular Accident (CVA, Stroke)

Description

Cerebrovascular accident is a symptom complex resulting from an impairment of the blood supply to a portion of the brain. It is caused by a vascular lesion in the brain, which may be the result of a brain hemorrhage, related to hypertension, or of a thrombosis or embolism of the cerebral vessels, related to atherosclerosis.

Cerebral infarction occurs when the brain is deprived of blood.

Incidence

- 10% of all fatalities are secondary to stroke
- 20 million disabled

Etiologic Risk Factors

See List of Etiologic Risk Factors in Cardiovascular Disease.

Drug Therapy

Antihypertensives (Table 3-3), antihyperlipidemics (Table 3-11), or anticoagulants (Table 3-11) may be prescribed.

Diet Therapy

Goals

- See goals of diet therapy for hypertension and atherosclerosis.
- Reach and maintain optimal nutritional status by adapting dietary modifications (*e.g.*, food texture and others) to the client's impaired neuromuscular system.

Nutritional Care Plan

- Factors in Developing a Nutritional Care Plan
  See factors considered for hypertension and atherosclerosis.
- Other Factors
  1. Extent, if any, of dysphagia (difficulty in swallowing). Individuals with this condition have impaired control over the muscles needed for mastication, deglutition (swallowing), and movement of the tongue. This creates problems with moving food from the front to the back of the mouth and channeling food into the esophagus. The symptoms include drooling, choking, coughing (during or after meals), squirreling of food in cheeks, inability to gag, aspiration of food or saliva, chronic upper respiratory infections, weight loss, and anorexia.
  2. Sensory-perceptual alterations (*e.g.*, decreased visual field or diminished tactile sensation). These conditions may augment swallowing difficulties since the sight, smell, and texture of food enhance the swallowing act. Additionally, the presence of communication impairments affects the client's ability to express food preferences.
  3. Neuromuscular difficulties (*e.g.*, paralysis or spasticity of head, neck, and limbs) that impair the ability to feed oneself.
  4. Ill-fitting dentures. Twisting of the mouth may render dentures ill-fitting, which will interfere with the mastication and swallowing of food.
- Nutritional Care Plan Alterations for Cerebrovascular Accident
  1. Acute Stage
     a. Parenteral solutions for severely ill patients. Consult Chapter 2 for details on the composition and administration of parenteral solutions.

    b. Nasogastric feedings are contraindicated in many patients for a tube in the esophagus may cause dysphagia or aspiration and interfere with speech therapy. If tolerated, as client recovers, use only between meals so that he will be encouraged to try to ingest oral feedings.

2. Rehabilitative Stage

    a. Caloric alterations. Caloric restrictions only with extreme obesity. Most CVA patients have trouble meeting caloric and nutrient requirements (see dysphagia diet, Table 3-19).

    b. Sodium alterations. Mild sodium restriction, use 2000-mg sodium diet.

    c. Sodium–potassium ratio alterations. Foods high in sodium are restricted; high-potassium foods are encouraged; and potassium supplements may be necessary if diuretics are prescribed.

    d. Fat alterations. Cholesterol and saturated fats are limited with atherosclerosis.

    e. Consistency alterations. Pureed and chopped foods are encouraged; clear liquids and fibrous foods are limited when the client has difficulty in swallowing or chewing (Table 3-19).

- Techniques to Assist Food Ingestion by Dysphagic Clients

1. Provide mechanical devices customized to minimize feeding difficulties; prepare foods before serving (*e.g.*, blenderize, chop, and cut)

2. Stimulate saliva production by serving attractive foods with desired consistency, smell, and taste; if excess mucus is formed or drooling prevalent, limit milk products, chocolate, sweet foods, and citrus fruits

3. Consult family members on food preferences when communication is impaired

4. Promote mouth opening by applying light pressure to the chin, stroking digastric muscle beneath the chin, or touching lips with a spoon; if lips cannot be opened, use long straw and thick liquids

5. Remove distractions so that client's concentration can be directed toward using utensils, chewing, and swallowing; remind client to pick up fork, chew, and swallow

6. Place food tray on unafflicted side, within visual field

7. Help client perform oral hygiene techniques after each meal

- Techniques to Assist Swallowing by Dysphagic Clients

1. Position individual properly: sit him upright with hips flexed at 90° angle, back straight, feet flat on the floor, neck slightly forward, and arms flexed on arm rests; keep this position for 15–30 minutes to prevent aspiration

2. Increase head control by placing your hand on his forehead; additionally, teach client to flex his neck when swallowing

3. Stimulate lip closure by stroking lips with your fingers, or place his lips between your two fingers and apply pressure on upper lip

4. Minimize tongue thrust by applying pressure under mandible

5. Teach client to place and chew food on unaffected side of the mouth

6. Serve foods of suitable consistency such as foods that form a bolus in the mouth (*e.g.*, meat loaf with gravy; without gravy, foods may be too dry and sticky) or foods that do not break apart (*e.g.*, casseroles; small pieces of food cause choking, squirreling of food, and coughing)

7. Never rush

Nurses' Responsibilities in the Nutritional Care of the Client With Cardiovascular Disease

Dietary adaptations may be a part of the client's *lifelong* treatment. The modifications may control the progression of the disease or enhance rehabilitation but only if the client applies them on a day-to-day basis.

- Initiate Good Care

    1. Procure trained professional instruction immediately following prescription. Accurate instruction after diagnosis will enhance understanding and compliance.

    2. Initiate public educational programs that explain cardiovascular risk factors; participate in screening programs such as community blood pressure readings.

- Participate in Care

    1. Enhance client compliance: provide emotional support (for example, try the client's diet yourself for one day [*e.g.*, limit salt]; record palatability of food, your emotions related to the food, and so on—this will increase empathy); help client make food choices that will enhance palatability; emphasize the positive side of this treatment (*e.g.*, lack of side-effects, often not true of drug therapy).

    2. Enhance the quality of a stroke client's life: assist him at meals (position before meals, cut meat, and so on) but do not feed client if he is capable. Self-feeding relieves feeling of dependence and poor self-image.

    3. Watch for signs of dysphagia.

- Coordinate Care

    1. Organize information and contribute to health-team conferences.

    2. Obtain the following information and report data that will influence compliance such as economic and cultural background; family background (*e.g.*, the person who prepares meals must

understand the cooking and food modifications needed); lifestyle (*e.g.*, number of restaurant meals); indications of noncompliance, such as having food brought in from home; other information that indicates compliance or noncompliance such as weight changes, blood pressure changes, and symptoms of hypokalemia or hyperkalemia (see text).

3. Collect necessary data (*e.g.*, 24-hour urine samples) and report findings.

- Reinforce and Follow Up Care

1. Assure the client that he is not alone.

2. Obtain a working knowledge of how these dietary adaptations can control his disease progression and how the modifications can be adjusted to his lifestyle. Obtain this knowledge by attending dietary conferences and nutrition workshops, acquiring and studying the diet manual and your local American Heart Association booklets, and reading supermarket and medication labels.

3. Compliment compliance by relating reduced blood pressure, lipid levels, and edema to dietary adherence, namely, modifying intake of calories, fat, sodium, and potassium.

4. Consult Chapter 2 for more details on how to obtain dietary compliance.

Table 3-1
Progressive Nutritional Care Plan for a Coronary-Care Unit

Time	Foods Allowed	Nutrients Procured
Day 1	Nothing by mouth (NPO) or sips of cool water (not ice water) Parenteral solutions, 1–2 liters of 5%–10% dextrose solutions	170–680 kcal Carbohydrate Water
After medical treatment on Day 1 or Day 2	Fluids, fruit juices, skim milk, regular or salt-free (SF) broth, ginger ale; tea and coffee, which are stimulants, may be limited to lessen vagal responses Serve liquids at room temperature	500–800 kcal Carbohydrate Limited protein and fat Sodium, potassium Water (1–1.5 liters) Vitamin and mineral supplements may be needed
Days 2–5	Bland, soft, low-roughage foods served in small portions, frequently Tender cooked meat and vegetables, canned fruits, plain breads, and desserts	1000–1200 kcal Carbohydrate, 50%–58% of kcal Protein, 12%–20% of kcal Fat, 25%–30% of kcal (limit saturated fat) Sodium, 1–2 g or less Fluid, 1–1.5 liters Vitamin and mineral supplements may be needed
Day 5 (nutritional care plan based on client's clinical status)	Foods allowed usually low in calories, saturated fat, cholesterol, and sodium Fluids sometimes limited Foods high in potassium advised	Calories are adjusted to weight (*e.g.,* 1200–1800 kcal) Carbohydrate, 50%–58% of kcal Protein, 12%–20% of kcal Fat, 25%–30% of kcal Cholesterol, 300 mg Sodium, 2 g Potassium, 2 g or more Fluids are adjusted to calorie intake in a 1:1 ratio. That is, 1 ml of fluid is given per kcal (*e.g.,* 1800 ml/1800 kcal)

Table 3–3 111

Table 3–3
Medications Used to Treat Hypertension and Cardiac Dysfunctions

Medication Category	Mechanism of Action	Adverse Side-Effects With Nutritional Implications	Dietary Adaptations
Step I Diuretics Potassium-wasting diuretics Thiazides and thiazide derivatives (*e.g.*, hydrochlorothiazide [HydroDiuril], chlorothiazide [Diuril], methyclothiazide [Enduron])	*In general*, diuretics ↳→ CO ↓ TPR ↓ PV ↑ PRA Add to or potentiate the action of other antihypertensive drugs *Specifically*, thiazides affect renal tubular mechanism of electrolyte (*e.g.*, sodium and potassium and chlorine) reabsorption; consequently, excretion enhanced	*In general*, diuretics induce Dry mouth and thirst Salt craving *Hypokalemia* (thiazide and thiazidelike) Low potassium may precipitate digitalis toxicity Hypochloremic alkalosis	Suck ice chips or hard candies if calories are not restricted Limit sodium intake to 2 g/day (see Tables 3-6, 3-7, and 3-8) Use herbs at the table and in cooking Increase intake of plain fruits, vegetables, and fruit juices (see Conversion Table for Sodium-Restricted Diets and List of Signs and Treatment of Hypokalemia and Hyperkalemia) Avoid licorice; it enhances hypokalemia Give potassium chloride supplements Acid ash diet may be indicated (rare)

(continued)

Table 3–3
Medications Used to Treat Hypertension and Cardiac Dysfunctions *(continued)*

Medication Category	Mechanism of Action	Adverse Side-Effects With Nutritional Implications	Dietary Adaptations
Step I (continued)			
		Hyperglycemia	Adjust intake of refined carbohydrates, hyperglycemic oral agents, and insulin according to individual hyperglycemia
		Hyperuricemia	Limit meat and meat extracts that contain purines, which metabolize to uric acid (see Chap. 9 on low purine diets for gout)
		Hypercalcemia (thiazides)	Limit dairy products Avoid vitamin D supplements
		Elevated LDLs	Limit foods that contain saturated fat and cholesterol (*e.g.*, animal fats)
		May precipitate increased excretion of zinc, magnesium, and water-soluble vitamins, especially riboflavin	A well-balanced, nutrient-dense diet is advocated Dietary supplements of these nutrients may be necessary
		Dilutional hyponatremia	Restrict fluid; do not increase salt intake
		Dehydration may occur with excessive dosage	Monitor weight and BUN levels frequently

(continued)

Table 3–3 113

Table 3–3
Medications Used to Treat Hypertension and Cardiac Dysfunctions (continued)

Medication Category	Mechanism of Action	Adverse Side-Effects With Nutritional Implications	Dietary Adaptations
Step I (continued)			
		Anorexia, nausea, vomiting, abdominal pain	Individualize diet to symptoms Give small frequent bland meals Limit fluids to between meals to decrease volume (see Tables 4-6 and 7-3)
		Diarrhea	Give low-residue foods until diarrhea subsides (see Table 7-5) Increase fluids; monitor electrolytes
		Constipation	Increase intake of fibrous foods; increase fluids
		Increased alcohol sensitivity	Abstain from or limit alcohol intake Taking these drugs with meals may alleviate or lessen GI adverse effects Administer with breakfast
Thiazidelike diuretics (*e.g.*, chlorthalidone [Hygroton])	Cause extensive diuresis with greatly increased excretion of sodium and chlorine Site of action appears to be ascending limb of Henle's loop of nephron	Same as thiazide diuretics	Same as thiazide diuretics

(continued)

Table 3–3
Medications Used to Treat Hypertension and Cardiac Dysfunctions (continued)

Medication Category	Mechanism of Action	Adverse Side-Effects With Nutritional Implications	Dietary Adaptations
Step I *(continued)*			
Loop diuretics (*e.g.,* furosemide [Lasix], ethacrynic acid [Edecrin])	Act on the ascending limb of the loop of Henle and in proximal and distal tubules of kidney; consequently, supress water and electrolyte reabsorption and enhance excretion	Same as thiazide diuretics	Same as thiazide diuretics
Potassium-sparing diuretics Triamterene (Dyrenium)	Inhibit the reabsorption of sodium ions in exchange for potassium and hydrogen ions at the segment of the distal tubule under the control of adrenal mineralocorticoids	Nutritional adverse effects similar to those of potassium-wasting diuretics except hypokalemia and hypochloremic alkalosis are prevented	Dietary adaptations are the same as with thiazide diuretics except high-dietary intakes of potassium and dietary supplements (*e.g.,* K-Lor) are not necessary
	Consequently, blocks sodium–potassium exchange in kidney, leading to sodium excretion and potassium retention	Dyrenium may be a folic-acid antagonist; consequently, megaloblastic anemia may develop	Give foods high in folic acid (*e.g.,* green leafy vegetables; see Chap. 10 for other foods high in folic acid). Supplements may be needed
		Azotemia (nitrogen retention)	Limit intake of high-protein foods (*e.g.,* meat, fish, and dairy products)

(continued)

Table 3-3 115

Table 3-3
Medications Used to Treat Hypertension and Cardiac Dysfunctions (continued)

Medication Category	Mechanism of Action	Adverse Side-Effects With Nutritional Implications	Dietary Adaptations
Step I (continued)			
		Increases urinary excretion of calcium	Calcium supplements may be needed Give drug after meals or with meals to lessen adverse GI effects
Spironolactone (Aldactone)	Aldosterone antagonist; consequently, inhibits exchange of sodium for potassium in distal renal tubule and helps prevent potassium wasting	Nutritional adverse effects similar to those of other diuretics except does not appear to elevate serum uric acid or alter carbohydrate metabolism However, hyperchloremic acidosis may develop when excessive doses precipitate hyperkalemia	Dietary adaptations are the same as with other potassium-sparing diuretics except that purine intake may not have to be limited and carbohydrate and insulin adjustments may not be necessary If hyperkalemia develops, foods high in potassium may be limited Give drug after meals to lessen adverse GI effects
Amiloride HCl (Midamor)	Potassium-conserving diuretic that is not an aldosterone antagonist	Gastrointestinal adverse effects similar to thiazide diuretics Excessive dosage may elevate BUN and potassium blood levels over time	Same as thiazide and other potassium-sparing diuretics

(continued)

Table 3-3
Medications Used to Treat Hypertension and Cardiac Dysfunctions (continued)

Medication Category	Mechanism of Action	Adverse Side-Effects With Nutritional Implications	Dietary Adaptations
Step II			
Sympathetic depressants (adrenergic-inhibiting agents)	*In general*, sympathetic depressants $\leftarrow \rightarrow \downarrow$ CO $\leftarrow \rightarrow \downarrow$ TPR $\uparrow$ PV $\downarrow$ PRA	*In general*, sympathetic depressants induce Dry mouth Depression	Increase fluids, suck on ice cubes frequently, or hard candies if calories are not restricted. Monitor for weight gain and dental caries May suppress or increase appetite; adjust caloric intake to individual needs
Reserpine (Serpasil)	Used in agitated psychotic states (*e.g.*, schizophrenia), especially when individual also needs hypertensive medications	Water and sodium retention with resultant edema Weight gain may be result of edema or increased appetite	Low-sodium diet regimen may be indicated (see diuretic salt-craving dietary adaptations) Adjust caloric intake to individual gains
Methyldopa (Aldomet)	Causes a net reduction in tissue concentration of serotonin, dopamine, norepinephrine, and epinephrine Lowers plasma renin activity and blood pressure	Anemia, especially from methyldopa, which may precipitate hemolytic anemia Precipitates peptic ulcers, especially reserpine	High-dietary intake or dietary supplements of vitamin B_{12}, vitamin C, folate, and iron may be indicated Conservative or liberal bland diet may be indicated (see Table 7-3) *(continued)*

Table 3–3 117

Table 3–3
Medications Used to Treat Hypertension and Cardiac Dysfunctions (continued)

Medication Category	Mechanism of Action	Adverse Side-Effects With Nutritional Implications	Dietary Adaptations
Step II (continued)			
Clonidine (Catapres)	Inhibits sympathetic outflow from brain, which stimulates vessel dilatation	Anorexia, nausea, and vomiting	Give antacids between meals See diuretic dietary adaptations
		Diarrhea	See diuretic dietary adaptations
		Constipation	See diuretic dietary adaptations
		Increased alcohol sensitivity	Abstain from or limit alcohol intake
		Competes with amino acids for absorption, especially methyldopa	Avoid protein or amino acid supplements Administer with meals, food, or milk to lessen adverse GI effects
Beta blockers (Beta-adrenergic blocking agents)	*In general*, beta blockers ↓ CO ↑ TPR ← → PV ↓ PRA	*In general*, beta blockers induce Masked symptoms of hypoglycemia (*e.g.*, tachycardia) and may potentiate insulin-induced hypoglycemia	Diabetics' diet, including timing of meals and division of nutrients, especially carbohydrates, should be monitored closely
Propranolol (Inderal)	Decrease adverse sympathetic (epinephrine) and norepinephrine stimulation by blocking beta receptor sites Used for angina and arrhythmias	Edema	See diuretic salt-craving dietary adaptations
		Depression	See sympathetic depressant dietary adaptations

(continued)

Table 3–3
Medications Used to Treat Hypertension and Cardiac Dysfunctions (continued)

Medication Category	Mechanism of Action	Adverse Side-Effects With Nutritional Implications	Dietary Adaptations
Metoprolol (Lopressor), nadolol (Corgard), atenolol (Tenormin)	Thought to be competitive antagonists of catecholamines at peripheral (especially cardiac) adrenergic neuron sites, leading to decreased CO Believed to suppress renin activity	Nausea, epigastric pain, vomiting Diarrhea Constipation Increased alcohol sensitivity	See diuretic dietary adaptations See diuretic dietary adaptations See diuretic dietary adaptations Abstain from or limit alcohol intake Give these drugs with food to increase absorption
Step III Vasodilators	*In general,* vasodilators ↑ CO ↓ TPR ↑ PV ↑ PRA	*In general,* vasodilators induce Decreased absorption of pyridoxine (vitamin B_6)	Increase intake of animal foods, especially pork and glandular meats (*e.g.,* liver) Give vitamin B_6 supplements
Hydrallazine (Apresoline)	Relax smooth muscles of blood vessels	Paresthesia (tingling in the fingers), especially from hydralazine, which may be relieved by vitamin B_6 supplements Water and sodium retention with resultant edema, especially from minoxidil	
Prazosin (Minipress)	Reduce elevated systolic and diastolic blood pressure by decreasing peripheral vascular resistance	Nausea and vomiting Alcohol enhances hypotensive effect	See diuretic salt-craving dietary adaptations Diuretics are usually necessary See diuretic dietary adaptations Abstain from alcohol Give these drugs with food to increase absorption

(continued)

Table 3–3 119

Table 3–3
Medications Used to Treat Hypertension and Cardiac Dysfunctions (continued)

Medication Category	Mechanism of Action	Adverse Side-Effects With Nutritional Implications	Dietary Adaptations
Step IV			
Potent sympathetic depressants Guanethidine (Ismelin)	*In general*, potent sympathetic depressants $\longleftrightarrow \downarrow$ CO $\longleftrightarrow \downarrow$ TPR $\uparrow$ PV $\downarrow$ PRA Slow heart rate	*In general*, potent sympathetic depressants induce Irritable colon, especially diarrhea Dizziness, orthostatic hypotension, and weakness	See diuretic dietary adaptations Symptoms may impair ability to procure and prepare foods Check weight often but keep in mind that maintained or gained weight may be water weight not dry weight
Minoxidil (Loniten)	Peripheral vasodilator that reduces elevated systolic and diastolic blood pressure by decreasing peripheral vascular resistance $\downarrow$ TPR	Nausea and vomiting Salt and water retention diuretics must be used concomitantly Does not produce orthostatic hypotension	See diuretic dietary adaptations See diuretic salt-craving dietary adaptations
Angiotensin Blocker			
Captopril (Capoten) May be used as a step II, III, or IV agent in clients resistant to other therapy or because of intolerable	Competitive inhibitor of angiotensin I–converting enzyme (ACE), which converts angiotensin I to angiotensin II In addition, captopril elevates	*In general*, captopril induces Dysgeusia (loss of taste), which may be enhanced by captopril's ability to bind with the zinc contained in ACE	Zinc supplements may be indicated (see Table 4-6 for dietary adaptations recommended for clients with dysgeusia)

(continued)

Table 3–3
Medications Used to Treat Hypertension and Cardiac Dysfunctions (continued)

Medication Category	Mechanism of Action	Adverse Side-Effects With Nutritional Implications	Dietary Adaptations
side-effects from other medications	the activity of the kallikrein–kinin and prostaglandin systems, which reduces blood pressure		See diuretic dietary adaptations
	In general, captopril $\leftrightarrow \uparrow$ CO $\leftrightarrow \rightarrow \uparrow$ TPR $\uparrow$ Renal blood flow $\downarrow$ PV $\uparrow$ PRA	Anorexia, abdominal pain, nausea, diarrhea, or constipation	Protein intake may need to be increased
		Proteinuria—protein in the urine may exceed 1 g/day, and edema may develop as a result	Sodium intake may be limited to lessen edema
			See diuretic salt-craving dietary adaptations
		Hyperkalemia may develop Potassium-sparing diuretics are not advised	Foods high in potassium should be limited (see potassium-sparing diuretic dietary adaptations and Tables 3-6 and 3-7)
			Administer 1 hr before meals to enhance drug effectiveness
Calcium Channel Blockers			
Verapamil* (Isoptin) (Calan) Diltiazem HCl (Cardizem) Nifedipine (Procardia)	*In general,* calcium blockers Inhibit the calcium ion influx through slow channels into conductile and contractile myocardial cells and vascular smooth muscle cells	*In general,* calcium blockers induce Nausea, vomiting, abdominal discomfort, diarrhea, or constipation	See diuretic dietary adaptations
	Increase coronary blood flow by	May interfere with the release of pituitary hormones and in-	Refined carbohydrate intakes may have to be limited

(continued)

Table 3–3 121

Table 3–3
Medications Used to Treat Hypertension and Cardiac Dysfunctions (continued)

Medication Category	Mechanism of Action	Adverse Side-Effects With Nutritional Implications	Dietary Adaptations
	relaxing coronary artery smooth muscle; this relaxation reduces coronary vascular resistance, resulting in improved myocardial oxygen supply Decrease peripheral resistance and increase blood flow Approved for treatment of angina pectoris and cardiac arrhythmias May be approved for treatment of cardiomyopathy and hypertension	sulin; subsequently, glucose metabolism may be impaired	Diabetics may need additional monitoring *Note.* These drugs are still under investigation; at present, physicians recommend diet therapy, moderate exercise programs and smoking abstinence in addition to drug therapy
Cardiac Drugs			
Cardiac glycosides Digitalis Digitoxin (Crystodigin) Digoxin (Lanoxin)	*In general,* cardiac glycosides ↑ myocardial contractility ↓ heart rate ↑ CO	*In general,* cardiac glycosides induce increased calcium, magnesium, and thiamine excretion in some individuals	Foods high in calcium (*e.g.,* dairy products), magnesium (*e.g.,* unsalted nuts), and thiamine (*e.g.,* pork products) should be increased Dietary supplements of these nutrients may be necessary Calcium supplementation must be monitored

(continued)

Table 3–3
Medications Used to Treat Hypertension and Cardiac Dysfunctions (continued)

Medication Category	Mechanism of Action	Adverse Side-Effects With Nutritional Implications	Dietary Adaptations
Cardiac Drugs *(continued)*		Decrease carbohydrate absorption	Monitor diabetics on insulin levels closely
			Avoid excessive intake of fiber (*e.g.*, bran); it inhibits drug absorption
		Toxicity when hypokalemia is a complication	Increase potassium intake
			See thiazide diuretic dietary adaptations (supplements of potassium may be necessary)
		Toxicity when hypercalcemia is a complication	Avoid megadoses of vitamin D
		Few GI adverse effects unless dosage is excessive, then nausea and vomiting may be induced	A nutritionally balanced diet advised unless nausea or vomiting occur; then consult diuretic dietary adaptations
			Absorption delayed or reduced when taken with food
			See diuretic dietary adaptations
Nitroglycerin (Nitrostat), isosorbide dinitrate (Isordil)	*In general,* nitroglycerin and related drugs relax smooth muscles, which produces a vasodilatory effect that relieves angina pectoris episodes	*In general,* nitroglycerin and related drugs induce	*In general,* dietary adaptations are made to augment the drug's effectiveness or decrease the need for it (*e.g.*, caloric adjustments to augment weight loss and reduced alcohol intake is advised)
		Dry mouth	
		Nausea and vomiting	

(continued)

Table 3–3 123

Table 3–3
Medications Used to Treat Hypertension and Cardiac Dysfunctions (continued)

Medication Category	Mechanism of Action	Adverse Side-Effects With Nutritional Implications	Dietary Adaptations
Potassium Chloride Supplements (*e.g.,* Kay Ciel, K-Lor, Slow-K)	*In general,* potassium chloride supplements replace potassium wasted or lost during diuretic therapy	*In general,* potassium chloride supplements induce Nausea and abdominal cramps Diarrhea Decreased vitamin B_{12} absorption Aftertaste	See diuretic dietary adaptations See diuretic dietary adaptations Increase animal foods or give vitamin B_{12} supplements GI distress and aftertaste will be minimized if supplement is dissolved and diluted well in cold juice or water and a straw is used to limit aftertaste Do not administer with milk or milk products Take with or after meals: food delays absorption but reduces adverse GI effects

↤→ little or no change or effect; ↓ decreased; ↑ increased; CO, cardiac output; TPR, total peripheral resistance; PV, plasma volume; PRA, plasma renin activity
* Intravenous preparation approved for supraventricular tachycardia. Intravenous nifedipine and diltiazem HCl are still under investigation, as are oral medications.

Table 3–4
Increased Mortality for Insured Men and Women With Rise in Blood Pressure

| Pressure (mm Hg) | Chance of Death Compared to Normal (%) | | | |
| | Men | | Women | |
	1959 Build and Blood Pressure Study*	1979 Build and Blood Pressure Study*	1959 Build and Blood Pressure Study*	1979 Build and Blood Pressure Study*
Systolic				
138–147	55	36	22	22
148–157	94	68	40	35
158–167	144	110	130	67
168–177	†	124	†	†
178–192	†	132	†	†
Diastolic				
88–92	50	38	22	33
93–97	88	71	68	63
98–102	134	104	118	83
103–108	162	164	†	†

* The 1959 Build and Blood Pressure Study reflects the mortality experience among insured lives covering the years 1935 through 1954, and the 1979 Build and Blood Pressure Study reflects provisional experience among insured lives covering the years 1954 through 1972.
† Too few cases for analysis
(Ad Hoc Committee of the New Build and Blood Pressure Study, Association of Life Insurance Medical Directors of America and Society of Actuaries, 1979)

Table 3-6 125

Table 3-6
Daily Meal Plan High in Calories, High in Sodium, Low in Potassium*

Foods	Amount	Calories	Sodium (mg)	Potassium (mg)
Breakfast				
Apple Danish (Sara Lee, frozen)	1 roll	360	408	163
Coffee, freeze-dried	1 tbsp	3	0	83
Sugar, granulated	1 tsp	16	0	0
Total		379	408	246
Lunch				
Split pea soup, (canned)	1 cup	172	912	37
Corned beef on rye bread sandwich	1	296	1214	140
Mustard, prepared, brown	1 tsp	4	65	7
Cucumber dill pickle	1 large	11	1428	200
Fresca	12 oz	4	65	0
Total		487	3684	384
Dinner				
Big Mac (McDonalds)	1 serving	541	963	387
French fries	1	211	112	567
Salt	1 tsp	0	1955	0
Catsup	1 tbsp	16	156	55
Apple pie	1 slice	295	408	38
Coca Cola	12 oz	144	1	4
Total		1207	3595	1051
Daily Total		2073	7687	1681

Tsp = teaspoon, tbsp = tablespoon
* Meal plans can be used as teaching tools
(Pennington JAT, Church HN: Bowes and Church's Food Values of Portions Commonly Used, 13th ed.
Philadelphia, JB Lippincott, 1980)

Table 3–7
Daily Meal Plan Low in Calories, Low in Sodium, High in Potassium*

Foods	Amount	Calories	Sodium (mg)	Potassium (mg)
Breakfast				
Orange juice, diluted	⅔ cup	45	1	186
Shredded Wheat cereal	1 biscuit	89	1	87
Skim milk	½ cup	45	64	204
Sanka, instant	1 cup	5	0	87
Sugar, granulated	1 tsp	16	0	0
Total		200	66	564
Lunch				
Sliced chicken (dark)	3½ oz	176	86	321
Whole wheat bread	2 slices	112	242	126
Mayonnaise	1 tbsp	61	82	1
Grapes, American	22 med	69	3	158
Iced tea	1 glass	12	4	255
Total		430	417	861
Dinner				
Hamburger, lean	1 pattie	140	41	480
Hamburger roll	1	89	152	28
Catsup	1 tbsp	16	156	55
Cole slaw with mayonnaise	1 cup	119	149	230
Strawberries, whole	10	37	4	164
Skim milk	1 cup	89	128	408
Total		490	630	1365
Daily total		1120	1113	2790

Tsp = teaspoon, tbsp = tablespoon
* Meal plans can be used as teaching tools
(Pennington JAT, Church HN: Bowes and Church's Food Values of Portions Commonly Used, 13th ed.
Philadelphia, JB Lippincott, 1980)

Table 3-8 127

Table 3-8
Sodium Alteration Classifications and Dietary Intake Adaptations

Sodium Alteration Classifications	Dietary Intake Adaptations
Normal Daily Dietary Intake Sodium, 100–300 mEq 2300–6900 mg Salt, 6–16 g	Salt addition at the table allowed Salt addition in food preparation allowed Processed foods allowed Very salty foods allowed (See Table 3–6 and Conversion Table for Sodium-Restricted Diets)
Mild Sodium Restriction Sodium, 87–197 mEq 2000–4500 mg Salt, 5–11.44 g	Salt addition at the table not allowed Salt addition in food preparation allowed only at upper limits (3000–4500 mg) Processed foods with large quantities of sodium not allowed (read labels) Low-sodium processed foods in limited amounts may be substituted, such as Del Monte Low-Sodium green beans or peas (<10 mg sodium per ½ cup) and Stop and Shop's Low-Sodium Bread with Flavor Very salty foods not allowed (see Table 3–6 and Conversion Table for Sodium-Restricted Diets)
Moderate Sodium Restriction Sodium, 44 mEq 1000 mg Salt, 2.5 g (see Conversion Table for Sodium-Restricted Diets) Salt substitutes may be used with physician's permission (Table 3–9)	Salt restrictions same as for mild sodium-restricted diet Foods naturally high in sodium are controlled (*e.g.,* bread, butter, milk)

(continued)

Table 3-8
Sodium Alteration Classifications and Dietary Intake Adaptations (*continued*)

Sodium Alteration Classifications	Dietary Intake Adaptations
Strict Sodium Restriction Sodium, 22 mEq 500 mg Salt, 1.3 g	Salt restrictions the same as for moderate sodium-restricted diet Foods naturally high in sodium further restricted (*e.g.*, low-sodium breads and cereals are used; regular milk is restricted to 2 cups; meat is restricted to 5–6 oz daily)
Severe Sodium Restriction* Sodium, 11 mEq 250 mg Salt, 0.65 g	Salt and natural sodium restrictions the same as for strict sodium-restricted diet Low-sodium milk (Lonolac) used instead of regular, and eggs restricted

* Restrictions lower than this, or use of low-sodium diets for long periods of time, especially if diuretics are prescribed, may precipitate symptoms of hyponatremia: muscle cramps, vomiting, hypotension, hypovolemia, and oliguria

(American Dietetic Association: Handbook of Clinical Dietetics. New Haven, Yale University Press, 1981; and American Heart Association booklets [see References])

Table 3-10 129

Table 3-10
Calorie, Sodium, and Potassium Content of Common Foods in the Basic Five Food Guide*

Food Group and Foods	Amount	Calories	Sodium (mg)	Potassium (mg)
Milk				
Whole milk	1 cup	150	120	370
Ice cream (16% fat)	1 cup	349	108	221
Blue cheese	1 oz	103	390	72
Cottage cheese (1% fat)	½ cup	81	459	97
Meat				
Beef pot roast	2 slices	302	57	438
Cod fish, broiled	4 ounces	162	105	386
Crab, canned	½ cup	86	850	94
Egg, boiled	1	78	59	62
Soy beans, cooked	½ cup	130	2	540
Fruit and Vegetable				
Banana	1 small	85	1	370
Apple	1 small	58	1	110
Potato	1 medium	76	3	407
Artichoke	1 bud	44	30	301
Peas, fresh, shelled	¾ cup	86	2	316
Peas, canned and drained	¾ cup	88	236	96

(continued)

Table 3–10
Calorie, Sodium, and Potassium Content of common foods in the Basic Five Food Guide*

Food Group and Foods	Amount	Calories	Sodium (mg)	Potassium (mg)
Bread and Cereal				
White bread, enriched	1 slice		62	117
Rice, long-grain, parboiled, cooked	1 cup		159	538
Macaroni, cooked	1 cup		151	1
Corn flakes, Kellogg's	1 cup		84	216
Sweets and Fats				
Sugar, granulated	1 tsp		16	0
Butter	1 tsp		36	41
Margarine	1 tsp		36	49

* Consult Daily Meal Plans for other common foods.
(Pennington JAT, Church HN: Bowes and Church's Food Values of Portions Commonly Used, 13th ed. Philadelphia, JB Lippincott, 1980)

Table 3–11 131

Table 3–11
Medications Used to Treat Atherosclerosis

Medication Category	Mechanism of Action	Adverse Side-Effects With Nutritional Implications	Dietary Adaptations
Antihyperlipidemics Cholestyramine (Questran) Colestipol (Colestid)	Bile acid sequestrants (bind bile acids in the intestines) Consequently, less cholesterol absorbed, liver uptake of LDL-c increased, and more cholesterol excreted May also bind warfarin (an anticoagulant) and digoxin (a cardiac medication) Absorption of thiazides (antihypertensive medications) also decreased	Impair absorption of fats, carotene, iron, carbohydrate (xylose), calcium, vitamins A, D, E, K, B_{12}, and folic acid Enhance constipation since bile salts are bound Alter taste	A nutritionally balanced diet is advocated in order to ensure adequate intake of these nutrients. Supplements of vitamins and minerals may be necessary if medication is used over an extended time. Increase the fiber content of the diet by increasing intake of whole-grain products, raw fruits, vegetables with skins, and adding bran to foods, gradually. Individualize food intake to taste. Granules have limited palatability and suspend in water and other liquids; therefore, they should be ground and mixed with food at mealtime.

(continued)

Table 3–11
Medications Used to Treat Atherosclerosis (continued)

Medication Category	Mechanism of Action	Adverse Side-Effects With Nutritional Implications	Dietary Adaptations
Antihyperlipidemics *(continued)*			
Clofibrate (Atromid)	Lowers triglyceride levels by increasing catabolism of VLDLs to LDLs and probably by decreasing hepatic secretion of VLDLs; however, LDLs may rise if extensive decrease in VLDLs	Enhances risk of gallstones	Limit total fat and cholesterol intakes.
		Induces nausea, vomiting, and abdominal distress	Individualize diet to symptoms. Give small bland meals frequently. Limit fluids to between meals to decrease volume (see Tables 4-6 and 7-3).
		Enhances weight gain	Caloric intakes should be adjusted to individual weights.
		Alters taste	Individualize food intake to taste.
		Decreases absorption of carotene, vitamin B_{12}, iron, and glucose	Foods with high contents of these nutrients should be increased. Dietary supplements of these nutrients may be necessary.
		May decrease disaccharidase enzymatic activity in small intestines	Limit refined sugar and dairy product (*e.g.*, milk) intake.
Nicotinic acid (Nicolar)	Inhibits VLDL secretion In large doses, gradually causes reduction in serum lipids	Causes flushing of skin Decreases glucose tolerance	Carbohydrate intake may have to be adjusted.

(continued)

Table 3–11 133

Table 3–11
Medications Used to Treat Atherosclerosis (continued)

Medication Category	Mechanism of Action	Adverse Side-Effects With Nutritional Implications	Dietary Adaptations
	Increase dosage gradually	Induces hyperuricemia	Limit meat and meat extracts, which contain purines that metabolize to uric acid (see Chap. 9 for low-purine diets used in gout).
			See clofibrate dietary adaptations.
		Induces epigastric distress, nausea, and vomiting	Conservative or liberal bland diet may be indicated (see Table 7-3).
		Activates peptic ulcers	Antacids are given between meals.
		Alcohol may enhance drug's adverse effects	Limit alcohol intake.
Probucol (Lorelco)	Inhibits early stages of cholesterol synthesis and dietary absorption	Induces diarrhea and flatulence	Give with meals to minimize GI distress.
			Give low-residue foods until diarrhea subsides (see Tables 7-5 and 7-7).
	Increases excretion of fecal bile acids	Induces nausea and vomiting	Increase fluids (see Table 7-4).
			See clofibrate dietary adaptations.

(continued)

Table 3–11
Medications Used to Treat Atherosclerosis *(continued)*

Medication Category	Mechanism of Action	Adverse Side-Effects With Nutritional Implications	Dietary Adaptations
			Give with meals to increase absorption (if client follows a low-cholesterol, low-saturated fat diet, drug dosage may be decreased).
Anticoagulants Warfarin sodium (Coumadin)	Sequential depression of blood clotting factors VII, IX, X, and II Degree of depression dependent upon dosage administered	Induces hemorrhage in extensive doses	Avoid high-fat meals, which increase prothrombin activity. Limit intake of foods high in vitamin K (*e.g.*, leafy green vegetables, beef liver, brussel sprouts, alfalfa sprouts, and green tea), which may inhibit the hypoprothrombinemic effect of the drug. However, if hemorrhage occurs, increase above intake and give vitamin K supplements. Avoid megadoses of vitamin E and vitamin C, which alter drug effects.
		Induces abdominal cramps and nausea	See clofibrate dietary adaptations. *(continued)*

Table 3-11 135

Table 3-11
Medications Used to Treat Atherosclerosis *(continued)*

Medication Category	Mechanism of Action	Adverse Side-Effects With Nutritional Implications	Dietary Adaptations
Anticoagulants *(continued)*			See probucol dietary adaptations. Avoid alcohol; it interferes with drug action. Administer with meals to increase absorption.
Salicylates (*e.g.*, aspirin)	Decrease aggregation of blood platelets	Decrease uptake of vitamin C by leukocytes	Increase intake of foods high in vitamin C (*e.g.*, orange juice and tangerines). Give vitamin C dietary supplements if necessary. See nicotinic acid dietary adaptations.
		Activates peptic ulcers	See warfarin sodium dietary adaptations. Give with meals to limit GI distress.
		Induces hemorrhage in extensive doses (see Table 9-1 for other adverse effects of aspirin)	

Table 3–13
Classification and Properties of the Major Human Plasma Lipoproteins

Property	Chylomicrons	Very-Low-Density Lipoproteins	Low-Density Lipoproteins	High-Density Lipoproteins
Density ranges (g/ml) ultracentrifuge	<0.95	0.95–1.006	1.006–1.063	1.063–1.21
Electrophoretic migration	Origin	Preβ	β	α
Average composition (%)				
Protein	2	8	21	50
Cholesterol	7	20	45	22
Triglyceride	84	51	11	4
Phospholipid	7	19	22	24
Apolipoproteins				
Major	ApoB ApoC-I, II, III ApoA-I	ApoB ApoC-I, II, III ApoE	ApoB	ApoA-I, ApoA-II
Minor	ApoA-II, ApoE (PRP—prolinerich)	ApoA-I, II, ApoD	ApoC-I, II, III	ApoC-I, II, III, ApoD, ApoE
Origin	Intestine	Intestine, liver	Metabolic product of VLDL	Intestine, liver
Function	Transport dietary triglycerides	Transport hepatic triglycerides	Regulate cellular cholesterol metabolism	Transport cholesterol from peripheral cells to liver

(Reprinted with permission. Bond JT, Filler, LJ, Leveille GA et al: Infant and Child Feeding, p 286. New York, Academic Press, 1981)

Table 3–14 137

Table 3–14
**Age Variations of "Normal" Limits of
Plasma Lipid and Lipoprotein Cholesterol Concentrations***

Age of Subjects (yr)	Plasma Cholesterol (mg/dl)	Very-Low-Density Lipoproteins (mg/dl)	Low-Density Lipoproteins (mg/dl)	High-Density Lipoproteins (mg/dl)		Plasma Triglycerides (mg/dl)
				M	*F*	
Newborn "cord blood"	50–95	0–15	20–45	30–55	30–55	10–65
1–9	120–230	5–25	50–170	30–65	30–65	10–140
10–19	120–230	5–25	50–170	30–65	30–70	10–140
20–29	120–240	5–25	60–170	35–70	35–75	10–140
30–39	140–270	5–35	70–190	30–65	35–80	10–150
40–49	150–310	5–35	80–190	30–65	40–85	10–160
50–59	160–330	10–40	80–210	30–65	35–85	10–190

* "Normal" limits as used here are not necessarily "safe" or acceptable limits. The normal limits listed in this table are based on a Washington area population sample. They do not necessarily hold for other countries or even for other regions of the United States.
(Adapted from Stanbury JB, Wyngaarden JB, Fredrickson DS (eds): The Metabolic Basis of Inherited Disease, 3rd ed, p 547. New York, McGraw Hill, 1972)

Table 3–15
Five Types of Primary Hyperlipoproteinemia*

Type	Incidence	Origin: Possible Mechanism	Age of Detection	Appearance of Plasma (after storage at 4°C)
I	Very rare	Genetic recessive; deficiency in lipo- protein lipase	Early child- hood	Cream layer over clear infranatant fluid on standing
IIa	Common	When genetic, dominant, spo- radic; decreased catabolism of beta-lipoprotein	Early child- hood (in severe cases)	Clear
IIb or III	Relatively uncommon	When genetic, re- cessive; sporadic?	Adulthood (over age 20)	Clear, cloudy or milky
IV	Common	When genetic, dominant, spo- radic; excessive endogenous glyc- eride synthesis or deficient glycer- ide clearance?	Adulthood	Slightly turbid to cloudy, unchanged with standing
V	Uncommon	Probably genetic, dominant, spo- radic	Early adulthood	Cream layer over turbid infranatant on standing

* LDL = low-density lipoproteins; VLDL = very-low-density lipoproteins; ILDL = intermediate low-density lipoproteins

Table 3-15 139

Cholesterol	Triglyceride	Lipoprotein Family	Clinical Presentation	Conditions to Be Excluded[†]
Normal or elevated	Markedly elevated	Elevated chylomicrons	Lipemia retinalis, eruptive xanthomas, hepatosplenomegaly, abdominal pain	Dysgammaglobulinemia, insulinopenic diabetes
Elevated	Normal or slightly elevated	Increased LDL	Xanthelasma, tendon and tuberous xanthomas, juvenilis corneal arcus, accelerated atherosclerosis	Dietary cholesterol excess, porphyria, myxedema, myeloma, nephrosis, obstructive liver disease
Elevated	Usually elevated	IIb Increased LDL and VLDL III Increased ILDL	Xanthoma planum; tuberoeruptive and tendon xanthomas; accelerated atherosclerosis of coronary and peripheral vessels	Myxedema, dysgammaglobulinemia
Normal or elevated	Elevated	Increased VLDL	Accelerated coronary vessel disease, abnormal glucose tolerance, hyperuricemia	Diabetes, glycogen storage disease, nephrotic syndrome, pregnancy, Werner's syndrome
Elevated or normal	Elevated to markedly elevated	Increased chylomicrons and VLDL	Lipemia retinalis, eruptive xanthomas, hepatosplenomegaly, abdominal pain, hyperglycemia, hyperuricemia	Myeloma, dysproteinemias, diabetic acidosis, nephrosis, alcoholism, pancreatitis

† Secondary hyperlipoproteinemias
(Adapted from Anderson L et al: Nutrition in Health and Disease, 17th ed. Philadelphia, JB Lippincott, 1982)

Table 3–16
**Recommended Nutrient and Dietary Adaptations
for the Five Types of Hyperlipoproteinemia**

Type	Diet Prescription	Kilocalories	Protein
I	Low fat, 25–35 g	Not restricted	Total protein intake is not limited
IIa	Low cholesterol Polyunsaturated fat increased	Not restricted	Total protein intake is not limited
IIb and III	Low cholesterol Approximately: 20% kcal, protein 40% kcal, fat 40% kcal, CHO	Achieve and maintain ideal weight, *i.e.*, reduction diet if necessary	High protein
IV	Controlled CHO Approximately 45% kcal Moderately restricted cholesterol	Achieve and maintain ideal weight, *i.e.*, reduction diet if necessary	Not limited other than control of patient's weight
V	Restricted fat, 30% kcal Controlled CHO, 50% kcal Moderately restricted cholesterol	Achieve and maintain ideal weight, *i.e.* reduction diet if necessary	High protein

(Adapted from Frederickson DS, Levy RI, Jones E, et al: The Dietary Management of Hyperlipoproteinemia: A Handbook for Physicians and Dietitians. Washington, DC, DHEW Publication No. [NIH 73-110])

Table 3–16 141

Fat	Carbohydrate	Cholesterol	Alcohol
Restricted to 25-35 g Type of fat not important	Not limited	Not restricted	Not recommended
Saturated fat intake limited Polyunsaturated fat intake increased	Not limited	As low as possible; the only source of cholesterol is the meat in the diet	May be used with discretion
Controlled to 40% kcal (polyunsaturated fats recommended in preference to saturated fats)	Controlled—concentrated sweets are restricted	Less than 300 mg—the only source of cholesterol is the meat in the diet	Limited to 2 servings (substituted for carbohydrate)
Not limited other than control of patient's weight (polyunsaturated fats recommended in preference to saturated fats)	Controlled—concentrated sweets are restricted	Moderately restricted to 300-500 mg	Limited to 2 servings (substituted for carbohydrate)
Restricted to 30% kcal (polyunsaturated fats recommended in preference to saturated fats)	Controlled—concentrated sweets are restricted	Moderately restricted to 300–500 mg	Not recommended

Table 3–17
Comparison of the Current American Diet, the American Heart Association Prudent Diet, and United States Dietary Goals

Nutrient	Current American Diet	Prudent Diet	U.S. Dietary Goals
Total Calories	Excessive	Reduce to achieve and maintain ideal body weight	Same as prudent diet
Total Fat % of Calories	40%–42%	30%–35%	30%
Saturated	16%	10%	10%
Monosaturated	19%	10%–15%	10%
Polyunsaturated	5%–7%	10%	10%
P:S Ratio	0.3–0.4: 1	1–1.5: 1	1: 1
Cholesterol	500–700 mg	300 mg	300 mg
Carbohydrate % of Calories	40%–46%	45%–55%	58%
Complex, starch	22%	Increase	48% complex starch and natural sugars
Simple sugars			
Natural	6%	Decrease sugars	
Refined	18%		Refined 10%
Protein % of Calories	12%	12%–15%	12%
Sodium	100–300 mEq	130 mEq	87 mEq
	2300 mg–6999 mg	3000 mg	2000 mg

(US Department of Agriculture, Agricultural Research Service, 1974; American Heart Association: Diet and Coronary Heart Disease, New York, AHA, 1973; Dietary Goals for the United States. Washington, DC. US Government Printing Office, Stock No 052-070-04376-8, 1977)

Table 3-18 143

Table 3-18
**Comparison of the Basic Five Food Guide for
Adults and the Prudent Diet Food Recommendations**

Basic Five	Prudent Diet
Milk Group	
2 servings of whole milk, cheese, or yogurt	2 servings of skim milk, cheese, or yogurt
Meat Group	
2 (3-oz) servings of meat (beef, lamb, pork), poultry, or fish Eggs (1–2), dry beans, or peas (¼ cup for 1 oz of meat)	Limit beef, lamb, and pork; consume more fish, poultry, and dry beans or peas Limit eggs (4/wk) and shellfish
Vegetable and Fruit Group	
4 servings or more per day with at least one citrus fruit	Use generous amounts in meal planning—high in vitamins and minerals, low in calories and fat, free of cholesterol
Bread and Cereal Group	
4 servings per day, including rice, pasta, bread, and cereals	4 servings per day—low in fat and cholesterol Use whole-wheat products instead of refined white products Use only unsweetened cereals
Sugar and Fats	
Add to diet to meet caloric needs	Limit empty calorie foods: sodas, desserts, candy Use vegetable oils and soft margarines instead of animal fats—high in polyunsaturated fat, low in saturated fat

Table 3–19
Progressive Dysphagia Diet

Food Consistency in Ascending Order*	Foods Allowed	Foods Not Allowed
Thick Liquids and Purees Foods combined in a blender; liquid added to consistency of thick soup	Ice cream, thinned yogurt, pureed soft-cooked egg, cheese melted into other foods, refined cooked cereals, pureed fruits and vegetables; nectar, sherbet, ice cream, custard, thick soups, Carnation Instant Breakfast, thinned cream of wheat	All others
Ground Food Foods put through food grinder to break down fiber and connective tissue content so that food requires little or no chewing	All ground meats, bite-size vegetables, junior baby foods, soft canned fruits, custards, moist cake, soups with chunks of meat or vegetables; all foods in previous categories	Fibrous vegetables such as celery, asparagus, and so on; fruits with pits, skins, or connective tissue such as oranges; bagels, bran cereals, and others
Finely Chopped Food Foods chopped smaller than ¼ inch, including meats, starches, vegetables; some chewing required; consistency of uncooked hamburger	All foods listed previously except they need not be ground	Same as listed for ground foods
Chopped Food Foods chopped in ¼-inch chunks including meats, vegetables, and fruits; re-	All meats, chopped as indicated, flaked fish, bite-size vegetables, soft canned	Fibrous stringy vegetables, berries, cherries, figs, dates, and raisins

(continued)

Table 3–19 145

Table 3–19
Progressive Dysphagia Diet (continued)

Food Consistency in Ascending Order*	Foods Allowed	Foods Not Allowed
quires fair amount of chewing; good for those who need texture in their diet for palatability or elimination or who need chewing practice	fruits, fresh fruits (cut in small pieces without the skin or membranes), tuna or egg salad, pasta or noodles cut up, boiled potato cut in small pieces, soft-cooked eggs, small pieces of refined breads, hot cereals	

Cut Foods

Food is cut to ½-inch pieces of edible size

* Consistency categories based on manual dexterity and ability to chew and swallow
(Reprinted with permission. Lee KA: Dysphagia And Its Dietary Management: A Review for Dietitians. Personal Correspondence, 1981)

Bibliography

American Dietetic Association: Handbook of Clinical Dietetics. New Haven, Yale University Press, 1981

American Heart Association: Planning Fat Controlled Meals for 1200 and 1800 Calories. Dallas, American Heart Association, 1966

American Heart Association: Your 500 Milligram Sodium Diet. Dallas, American Heart Association, 1968

American Heart Association: Your Mild Sodium Restricted Diet. Dallas, American Heart Association, 1969

American Heart Association: Your 1000 Milligram Sodium Diet. Dallas, American Heart Association, 1969

Anderson L, Dibble MV, Turkk PR et al: Nutrition in Health and Disease, 17th ed. Philadelphia, JB Lippincott, 1982

Batterman B: Hypertension. Part I: Detection and evaluation. Cardiovascular Nursing 11:38, 1975

Beard TC, Cooke HM, Bray WR et al: Randomised controlled trial of a no-added-sodium diet for mild hypertension. Lancet 2:455, 1982

Bond JT, Filler LJ, Leveille GA et al: Infant and Child Feeding. New York, Academic Press, 1981

Frederickson DS, Levy RI, Jones E et al: The Dietary Management of Hyperlipoproteinemia: A Handbook for Physicians and Dietitians, rev. Bethesda, MD, National Heart and Lung Institute, 1973. DHEW Publication No (NIH 73-110)

Freis ED: Mild Hypertension. Postgrad Med 73:180, 1983

Friedewald WT: Current nutrition issues in hypertension. J Am Diet Assoc 80:17, 1982

Gaffney TW, Cambell RP: Feeding techniques for dysphagic patients. Am J Nurs 74:2194, 1974

Galli C, Agardi E, Petroni A et al: Dietary factors affecting prostaglandin formation in tissues. In Hegyeli RJ (ed): Prostaglandins and Cardiovascular Disease. New York, Raven Press, 1981

Green ML, Harry J: Nutrition. In Contemporary Nursing Practice. New York, John Wiley & Sons, 1981

Grundy SM, Bilheimer D, Blackburn H et al: Rationale of the diet-heart statement of the American Heart Association. Circulation 65:839A, 1982

Hemzacek KI: Dietary protocol for the patient who has suffered a myocardial infarction. J Am Diet Assoc 72:182, 1978

Heyden S, Williams RS: Cholesterol controversy: Where do we go from here? Cardiology 69:110, 1982

Hunt SM, Groff JL, Holbrook JM: Nutrition: Principles and Clinical Practice. New York, John Wiley & Sons, 1980

Jordan SC: A Synopsis of Cardiology, 2nd ed. Chicago, Year Book Medical Publishers, 1979

Kaplan NM: Newer anti-hypertensive agents. Postgrad Med 73:213, 1983

Kaplan NM: Therapy for mild hypertension. JAMA 249:365, 1983

Khaw KT, Simon T: Randomised double-blind cross-over trial of potassium on blood pressure in normal subjects. Lancet 2:1127, 1982

Krause MV, Mahan LK: Food, Nutrition, and Diet Therapy, 6th ed. Philadelphia, WB Saunders, 1979

Langford HG: Potassium in hypertension. Postgrad Med 73:227, 1983

Lee KA: Dysphagia and Its Dietary Management: A Review for Dietitians. Personal correspondence.

Lewis CM: Nutrition and Diet Therapy (Self-Instructional Units) Sodium and Potassium. Philadelphia, FA Davis Company, 1976

MacGregor GA, Smith SJ, Markandu ND et al: Moderate potassium supplementation in essential hypertension. Lancet 2:567, 1982

Moser M: Stepped-care treatment of hypertension. Postgrad Med 73:199, 1983

Multiple Risk Factor Intervention Trial Research Group: Multiple Risk Factor Intervention Trial: Risk factor changes and mortality results. JAMA 248:1465, 1982

Oliver MF: Diet and coronary heart disease. Human Nutrition: Clinical Nutrition 36C:413, 1982

Pemberton CM, Gastineau CF (eds): Mayo Clinic Diet Manual, 5th ed. Philadelphia, WB Saunders, 1981

Pennington J: Nutritional Diet Therapy. Palo Alto, CA, Bull Publishing, 1978

Pennington JAT, Church HN: Bowes and Church's Food Values of Portions Commonly Used, 13th ed. Philadelphia, JB Lippincott, 1980

Preliminary Findings of the 1979 Build and Blood Pressure Study. Chicago, IL, Association of Life Insurance Medical Directors and the Society of Actuaries, 1979

The Prudent Diet. New York, Bureau of Nutrition, Dept of Health, 1969

Puska P, Nissinen A, Vartiainen et al: Controlled, randomised trial of the effect of dietary fat on blood pressure. Lancet 3:1, 1983

Roe DA: Interactions between drugs and nutrients. Med Clin North Am 63:985, 1979

Roe DA: Clinical Nutrition for the Health Scientist. Boca Raton, FL, CRC Press, 1979

Rossi LP, Antman EM: Calcium channel blockers. Am J Nurs 83:382, 1983

Shank FR, Park YK, Harland BF et al: Perspective of Food and Drug Administration on dietary sodium. J Am Diet Assoc 80:29, 1982

Singh B, Cocco G, Haeusler G et al: Calcium antagonists today and tomorrow. Cardiology 69 (Suppl 1):237, 1982

Smith CH, Bidlack WR: Food and drug interactions. Food Technology 36:99, 1982

Songu-Mize E, Bealer SL, Caldwell RW: Effect of AV3V lesions on development of DOCA-salt hypertension and vascular Na^+K^+-Pump Activity. Hypertension (Suppl) 4:575, 1982

Stanbury JB, Wyngaarden JB, Fredrickson DS: The Metabolic Basis of Inherited Disease. New York, McGraw–Hill, 1972

Suitor CW, Hunter MF: Nutrition: Principles and Application in Health Promotion. Philadelphia, JB Lippincott, 1980

Tilton CN, Maloof M: Diagnosing the problems in stroke. Am J Nurs 82:596, 1982

Wenger NK: Guidelines for dietary management after myocardial infarction. Geriatrics 33:72, 1978

Suggested Readings

American Heart Association: American Heart Association Cookbook. New York, David McKay, 1975

American Heart Association Booklets: Fat Restricted Diets and Recipes— Sodium Restricted Diets and Recipes.

Dahl LK: Salt and hypertension. Am J Clin Nutr 25:231, 1972

Resin E, Abel R, Modan M et al: Effect of weight loss without salt restriction on the reduction of blood pressure in overweight hypertensive patients. New Engl J Med 298:1, 1978

chapter 4

Cancer

Description

Cancer is a general term that covers many malignant conditions. All cancers start from a single cell that is genetically different from the normal cells in the tissue from which it arises. The cancer cell transfers its genetic properties to its descendants, which are able to grow without regard to the homeostatic mechanisms that control normal tissue growth. Cancers can be subdivided into two general types: solid tumors and hematologic malignancies. Cancer, then, is a set of diseases, rather than a single disease, and must be treated accordingly.

Incidence

- National number 2 killer, 20% of all fatalities, 356,000 fatalities per year
- 1,000,000 or more persons under treatment
- 30% to 60% of all cancers in the United States may be related directly or indirectly to dietary components, dietary patterns, or food-processing technology.

Etiologic Risk Factors With Dietary Implications

High dietary intake of
Total dietary fat; alcohol, especially when augmented by cigarette smoking; smoked, fried, charcoal-cooked, or broiled meats; moldy

149

foods that contain aflatoxins (*e.g.*, grains and peanuts); foods that contain high nitrate concentrations (*e.g.*, beer and fried bacon); salt, especially salt-cured meats; fermented foods (*e.g.*, pickled foods); unrefrigerated perishable foods

Low dietary intake of
Foods that contain preformed (retinol) vitamin A (*e.g.*, dairy products) or provitamin A; carotene (*e.g.*, green leafy vegetables and deep yellow vegetables or fruits); fiber (*e.g.*, whole grains, fruits with skins, nuts, and leafy vegetables); nutrients that act as antioxidants (*e.g.*, vitamin C, vitamin E, and selenium). Supplements of these nutrients, however, are not recommended at the present time.

In the fall of 1982, the Committee on Diet, Nutrition, and Cancer of the National Research Council of the National Academy of Sciences recommended four dietary guidelines for Americans in order to help reduce their risk of cancer. These guidelines are as follows:

- Reduce the consumption of fat, both saturated (*e.g.*, animal fats) and unsaturated (*e.g.*, vegetable oils), to 30% of caloric intake.
- Eat fruits, vegetables, and whole-grain products every day, especially foods high in vitamin C and beta-carotene, such as citrus fruits and dark green and deep yellow vegetables; supplements of vitamin C and especially vitamin A are not recommended at this time.
- Minimize consumption of salt-cured, salted, pickled, or smoked foods such as smoked sausages, smoked fish, bacon, bologna, and hot dogs.
- Drink alcohol only in moderation (not defined) particularly if you also smoke cigarettes.

Drug Therapy

Drugs commonly used in chemotherapy and their nutritional implications are given in Table 4-1.*

Diet Therapy

Goals

In clients with cancer, the goals of diet therapy, as well as the nutritional care plans, differ with the prognosis. When the disease may be arrested or cured, food is used as part of the therapeutic care plan. When the disease is advanced or terminal, food is used as a source of pleasure or emotional support and is part of the palliative care plan. These two

---

* See tables at the end of this chapter.

treatments are often used concomitantly; however, for purposes of clarity, they are described separately here (Tables 4-2 to 4-4).

Therapeutic Care

- Maintain or improve optimal nutritional status by meeting the increased metabolic demands of the disease before, during, and after drug, surgical, or radiation treatment.
- Maximize the optimal chance for response to cancer treatment.
- Improve the client's quality of life (performance status) by alleviating or reducing the symptoms and complications related to tumorogenesis and treatment (see Table 4-1).
- Maintain normal weight and height patterns of children.

Palliative Care

- Meet the increased metabolic demands of the disease but not at the expense of individual control and acceptance.
- Use food as a means of pleasure and emotional support.
- Quality of life considerations are the same as in therapeutic care but should not be undertaken at the expense of individual control and acceptance.
- Use food as a means of pleasure, not as a body builder.

Nutritional Care Plan Alterations for Therapeutic and Palliative Care

- Oral Feedings
  1. A well-balanced, nutrient-dense, nutritional care plan is advised when tolerated by the client.
  2. Oral supplements may be added to increase nutrient density if tolerated.
  3. Alterations of this plan are based on present nutritional status, clinical symptoms, prognosis, and individual food preferences.

There are no set dietary adaptations that benefit each cancer client, however, so the following recommendations are only suggestions, they are not set rules.

  1. Dietary adaptations suggested for host metabolic alterations induced by tumorogenesis and antineoplastic treatment (Table 4-5)
  2. Dietary adaptations suggested for clinical symptoms induced by tumorogenesis and antineoplastic treatments (Table 4-6)
- Enteral Feedings
  1. Therapeutic Care
     a. Indications. Clients who will not eat, cannot eat, or cannot eat enough to prevent catabolism.
     b. Feedings may be used as a sole source of nourishment or as

supplements to oral foods. Factors to consider when selecting feedings are

(1) Client's tolerance to this method of feeding and presence or absence of food allergies or intolerance (*e.g.*, lactose intolerance)

(2) Availability of an enteral route

(3) Pathophysiological and psychological complications induced by tumorogenesis and treatment (see Tables 4-1, 4-5, and 4-6)

(4) Calorie and nutrient requirements

(5) Composition of the enteral product: natural *versus* predigested nutrients, osmolality, and fluid *versus* caloric content

(6) Cost

2. Palliative Care

a. Indications. Clients cannot eat or cannot eat enough to maintain desired performance status.

b. Feedings, as with therapeutic care, may be the sole source of nourishment or a supplement. The factors to consider when selecting feedings are the same as those considered when feedings are used for therapeutic care.

- Parenteral Solutions*

1. Therapeutic Care. Indications: Clients will not eat, cannot eat, or cannot eat enough to prevent catabolism but have a good prognosis (*i.e.*, there are realistic expectations that antineoplastic treatments may cure the disease or arrest its progression or that parenteral feedings will add to the client's comfort or improve the quality of life).

2. Palliative Care. Seldom indicated, sometimes helpful in adding to the client's comfort or improving the quality of life.

Nurses' Responsibilities in the Nutritional Care of the Client With Cancer

- Oral Nutritional Care Plans

1. Initiate Good Care. Procure instructions and dietary adaptation suggestions from the dietitian immediately following diagnosis. Instructions are especially important for clients receiving antineoplastic treatment as outpatients. These clients are less likely to understand that food is a part of their treatment and more likely

---

* Consult Chapter 2 for details on enteral and parenteral nutritional support.

to decrease food consumption when clinical symptoms make food unappealing and difficult to prepare.

2. Participate in Care

   a. Empathize; provide emotional support.

   b. Encourage client to eat but do not force him to eat. Instead, emphasize the importance of nutritional care in his overall treatment. Then, help client gain control over this treatment by assisting him with food choices and meal patterns.

   c. Enhance the quality of his life by making mealtime a pleasant experience: give medications that relieve pain before meals, help client wash his hands before meals, remove bedpans and other unpleasant objects, deliver foods at the desired temperature, and visit the client often during meals so that he does not feel abandoned. Encourage and help client practice good oral hygiene after meals.

3. Coordinate Care

   a. Organize and contribute to health-team conferences.

   b. Obtain and report the following information during these conferences:

      (1) Food preferences and aversions mentioned by the client so that these can be served or avoided

      (2) New lab data

      (3) New treatment plans

      (4) Other factors that may influence food consumption

4. Reinforce and Follow Up Care

   a. Assure client that he is not alone when disease or treatment make food unappealing, but do not reveal any additional information that will increase his anxiety or lead him to imagine food-related symptoms.

   b. Obtain a working knowledge of how tumorogenesis and treatment affect nutritional status (see Table 4-1) and how dietary adaptations may alleviate or relieve these symptoms (see Sample Nutritional Assessment Sheets [pp. 154–156] and Tables 4-5 and 4-6). Additional information is available from many sources (see Suggested Readings at the end of this chapter). Assist clients to acquire these booklets; most are free or inexpensive.

   c. Compliment clients who are willing to sacrifice comfort occasionally in order to augment their nutritional care.

• Enteral and Parenteral Care Plans

Nurses' responsibilities to cancer clients on specialized care plans are the same as those for any individual receiving these care plans. Consult Chapter 2 for details on responsibilities.

Memorial Sloan–Kettering Cancer Center Initial Nutrition Assessment Form

1. a. What is your usual weight? ____ pounds.
   b. What is your height?____ feet ____ inches.
   c. In the last 2 months, have you gained weight?
      No ____ Yes ____. If yes, how many pounds? ____
      Lost weight? No ____ Yes ____. If yes, how many pounds? ____.

2. Is your present appetite usual? ____ better? ____ or worse? ____ than normal.

3. a. Do you have a problem related to eating? No ____ Yes ____. If yes, check the appropriate reason(s): Sore mouth ____ Swallowing ____ Chewing ____ Choking ____ Salivation ____ Change in taste ____ Food aversion ____ Nausea ____ Vomiting ____ Diarrhea ____ Constipation ____ Other ____
   b. Do you need help eating? No ____ Yes ____.

4. Do you wear dentures? Upper ____ Lower ____ None ____.

5. a. Were you previously on a special diet? No ____ Yes ____. If yes, please check ____ Low sodium ( ), Low fat ( ), Low sugar ( ), Other ____
   b. Do you take vitamins or minerals? No ____ Yes ____.
   c. Do you have any personal or religious dietary restrictions? Kosher ____ Vegetarian ____ Other (specify):____.

6. Do you have any allergies or intolerances for food? No ____ Yes ____. If yes, please list:

7. Do you take any other special food regularly? No ____ Yes ____. If yes, please list:

8. Do you have any major food dislikes? No ____ Yes ____. If yes, please list:

DO NOT WRITE BELOW THIS LINE—FOR DIETITIAN'S USE ONLY

Date of initial visit: _____

1. Diagnosis: _____

2. Expected treatment plan: Surgery _____
   RT _____ Chemo _____ Other _____

3. Abnormal lab data (list): _____

4. Metabolic and other problems:
   Diabetes _____ Hyperlipidemia _____
   Other endocrine _____ Malabsorption _____
   Hypertension _____ Type _____
   Heart disease _____ GI obstruction _____
   Persistent fever _____ Partial _____
   Severe trauma/burns _____ Complete _____
   Alcohol/drug abuse _____ GI fistula _____
   Renal disease _____
   Liver disease _____

5. Present medications: _____

6. Ht: ____ cm Adm Wt: ____ kg Avg Std ____ kg
   Pre-illness Wt: ____ lbs ____ kg
   Percentage Wt Change (%): _____
   (pre-illness—Adm/Pre-illness X100)

7. Anticipated problems due to illness or
   treatment plan? No ____ Yes ____

8. Edema/Ascites: (Site) Degrees-0-4 +
   Ascites: ____ Sacral _____

9. Nutritional Care Plan:
   a) No apparent problem _____
   b) Diet Rx _____
   c) Supplements Rx _____
   d) Date to reevaluate _____
   e) Nutrition team consult _____

10. Discharge plan/comments: _____

DIETITIAN: _____

**Calvary Hospital Nutritional Support
and Assessment Sheet hx:** _____

ANTHROPOMETRIC DATA

Height _____in _____cm

Weight   ADM. _____ lbs _____ kg   TSF _____ mm
           USUAL _____ lbs _____ kg   MAC _____ cm
           IDEAL _____ lbs _____ kg   MAMC _____ cm

LAB DATA

FBS _____ (M71-114/F75-117 mg/dl)
Hematocrit _____ (M42-48/F42-48)
Creatinine _____ (MO.6-1.2/FO.5-1.0 mg/dl)
Lymphocytes _____(1500/mm^3)
Albumin _____(M4.2-5.4/F3.8-5.2 G/dl)
BUN _____ (M8-25/F7-27 mg/dl)
Edema and degree: (1-4) _____
Sites _____Ascites _____ _____ Other _____
                           Yes   No

DIET HISTORY

Present food likes
Present food dislikes
Food allergies
Appetite   (circle)   Good   Fair   Poor
DENTITIAN   (circle)   Natural   Dentures   Oral Problems
What factor(s) appear(s) to hinder eating?   (circle)
Nausea   Anorexia   Food Served
Pain   Chewing   Smell
Taste   Swallowing   Other: _____

PRESENT MEDICATIONS/INTERACTIONS

OTHER PERTINENT INFORMATION

Tube for feeding (site and status)?
Do you need help feeding yourself? Yes _____ No _____
Current bowel function?
Constipation   Diarrhea
Use of laxatives
Colostomy (site and status)

DIET ORDER

PROGNOSIS FOR TREATMENT

Recommended Caloric Intake _____

Table 4–1 157

Table 4–1
Factors That Affect Nutritional Status in Clients With Cancer

	Factors Related to the Neoplastic Process		Factors Related to Treatment		
Clinical Signs	**Tumor-Related Factors**	**Pain and Psychological Disturbances**	**Chemotherapy***	**Radiotherapy**	**Surgery**
Anorexia and other appetite disturbances	Changes in metabolism may cause increased production of lactic acid and urea. This leads to alterations in sense of taste, such as aversion to bitter taste and sensitivity to glucose and salt. Obstruction of the salivary glands by a tumor causes dry mouth, dental caries, and dysphagia. Metabolic and chemical imbalances induced by tumor secretions may cause nausea and vomiting.	Stress hormones reduce production of insulin (decreased insulin enhances lipolysis) and digestive secretions, and peristalsis. Stress hormones increase production of lactic acid and urea. Stress may stimulate the vomiting center of the brain. Pain may affect ability to swallow. Food aversions may develop when foods are associated with nausea and vomiting.	Doxorubicin (Adriamycin), methotrexate (Mexate), fluorouracil (Adrucil), cyclophosphamide (Cytoxan), and mechlorethamine (Mustargen) decrease appetite. Steroids may increase appetite (*e.g.,* prednisone). Vinblastine (Velban), bleomycin (Blenoxane), methotrexate (Mexate) and fluorouracil (Adrucil) may induce stomatitis, dry mouth, or dysphagia.	Radiation to the head and neck area decreases saliva production, causing dry mouth, dental caries, dysphagia, taste changes, stomatitis, and nausea and vomiting. All these conditions decrease the ingestion and digestion of food.	Nausea and vomiting after surgery decrease food ingestion. Resection of a tumor in the oropharyngeal area may decrease saliva production, leading to dysphagia, dental caries, and chewing difficulties. These conditions decrease food ingestion.

(continued)

Table 4–1
Factors That Affect Nutritional Status in Clients With Cancer (continued)

Clinical Signs	Factors Related to the Neoplastic Process		Factors Related to Treatment		
	Tumor-Related Factors	Pain and Psychological Disturbances	Chemotherapy*	Radiotherapy	Surgery
Early satiety (bloating, feeling of fullness, "heartburn")	Taste alterations lead to alterations in digestive secretions. Malnutrition decreases absorption area, which decreases digestion. Secretions produced by the tumor may alter function of the hypothalamus (hunger center). Tumor obstruction in the GI tract inhibits normal digestion and absorption	Decreased secretions of digestive juices and decreased peristalsis cause decreased digestion and early satiety.	Most anticancer drugs cause nausea and vomiting. Drugs that alter taste (e.g., mechlorethamine) lead to a decrease in digestive secretions. Drugs that cause malabsorption resulting in malnutrition (e.g., dactinomycin, Cosmegen, trade generic methotrexate) will creased absorption and early satiety. also cause decreased absorption and early satiety.	Altered taste, decreased absorption, and decreased digestion cause malnutrition.	Obstruction in the stomach decreases digestion. If the stomach is removed, the individual may develop the dumping syndrome (see Chap. 7). Obstruction in the small intestines decreases absorption.

(continued)

Table 4–1
Factors That Affect Nutritional Status in Clients With Cancer (continued)

	Factors Related to the Neoplastic Process		Factors Related to Treatment		
Clinical Signs	Tumor-Related Factors	Pain and Psychological Disturbances	Chemotherapy*	Radiotherapy	Surgery
Weight loss[†]	Basal metabolic rate (BMR) is increased by 10%–25%; body is unable to adapt to starvation. Catabolism of protein and adipose tissue is increased to enhance gluconeogenesis (tumors use carbohydrate almost exclusively for energy) but ketosis is only slightly increased. Weight loss may be masked by edema. See also Anorexia and Early Satiety, above.	Stress hormones alter food ingestion, absorption, and utilization (decrease tissue synthesis). Pain decreases food ingestion by affecting desire or ability to prepare food.	Almost all drugs used in cancer therapy cause weight loss due to side-effects (e.g., nausea, diarrhea). Steroids (e.g., estrogen, prednisone), however, may increase appetite or may mask weight loss by causing edema.	Radiation to the head and neck causes weight loss by decreasing food ingestion. Radiation to the abdominal area decreases synthesis of intestinal epithelial cells, causing decreased absorption of nutrients and clinical side-effects (e.g., diarrhea). Malnutrition is the result.	Resection of any area of the gastrointestinal tract will cause decreased absorption of nutrients. In addition, postsurgical complications such as fistulas, ulcer formation, and strictures may further decrease the absorption area and enhance diarrhea or steatorrhea. Malnutrition and weight loss may be the result.

(continued)

Table 4–1 159

Table 4–1
Factors That Affect Nutritional Status in Clients With Cancer (continued)

| Clinical Signs | Factors Related to the Neoplastic Process | | Factors Related to Treatment | | |
	Tumor-Related Factors	Pain and Psychological Disturbances	Chemotherapy*	Radiotherapy	Surgery
Anemia	Endogenous and exogenous sources of iron, protein, folic acid, vitamin B_{12}, and vitamin B_6 may be used by the tumor to the detriment of the host.	Stress hormones and pain may decrease ingestion of exogenous supplies of iron, protein, folic acid, vitamin B_{12}, and vitamin B_6.	Methotrexate may cause anemia by interrupting folate and vitamin B_{12} function. Steroids and fluorouracil may cause gastrointestinal bleeding.	Radiation that causes decreased ingestion or absorption of nutrients will lead to anemia.	Resection of the stomach or ileal section of the intestine will decrease vitamin B_{12} absorption.
Asthenia (weakness, loss of strength)	Malnutrition caused by all other symptoms of cachexia (poor intake, ineffective metabolism, and depletion of protein stores) reduces intestinal cell synthesis and the absorption area. This de-	Depression, stress, and pain decrease the ingestion, absorption, and utilization of nutrients.	All drugs used in cancer therapy create host alterations and side-effects that may weaken the client.	Any radiation that causes gastrointestinal dysfunction will weaken the client.	Any surgery that causes gastrointestinal dysfunction will weaken the client.

(continued)

Table 4-1 161

Table 4-1
Factors That Affect Nutritional Status in Clients With Cancer (continued)

	Factors Related to the Neoplastic Process		Factors Related to Treatment		
Clinical Signs	Tumor-Related Factors	Pain and Psychological Disturbances	Chemotherapy*	Radiotherapy	Surgery
	creases the quantity of nutrients available for tissue synthesis and repair. In addition, it may enhance clinical symptoms (diarrhea and others) that increase host depletion.				

* Drugs listed are commonly used in cancer therapy; not all anticancer drugs are listed.
† Cachexia (tissue-wasting leading to weakness and emaciation) occurs in one third to two thirds of all cancer clients.

Table 4-2
Major Differences and Similarities of Therapeutic and Palliative Nutritional Care Plans

Therapeutic Care	Palliative Care
Major Goal	
Nourish the body as well as the spirit.	Nourish the spirit first and the body second.
Caloric and Nutrient Intake	
Caloric and nutrient intakes must be maintained or increased in order to meet the pathophysiological and psychological alterations induced by tumorogenesis and treatment, enhance response to treatment, and prevent complications.	Dietary adaptations should be made only to meet psychological needs, maintain performance status, and relieve discomforts (*e.g.*, nausea) induced by the disease.
Palatability	
Palatability of food may have to be sacrificed occasionally. Client should be taught that dietary alterations are an important part of treatment. If enteral feedings are a part of treatment, client should be allowed to taste several and choose the one most palatable.	Palatability of food is *never* sacrificed for nutrient density. For example, if client desires a "hot dog," he is allowed to have it, provided it does not cause added discomfort. Even then, it should be given if he is willing to trade pleasure for discomfort.
Meal Patterns	
Meal patterns are adapted to encourage maximum nutrient consumption and pleasure. For example, a large breakfast may be served instead of a large dinner. Meals should be served when the client is least fatigued and when treatment side-effects are at a minimum.	Meal patterns are the same as for therapeutic care. In addition, family members may be willing to prepare foods at home and bring them to the client.

(continued)

Table 4–2 163

Table 4–2
Major Differences and Similarities of Therapeutic and Palliative Nutritional Care Plans (continued)

Therapeutic Care	Palliative Care
Dining Area	
Dining area may be adapted to encourage maximum nutrient consumption. Individual is encouraged to eat in a pleasant, odor-free atmosphere (*e.g.*, the solarium) with pleasant companions.	Dining area considerations are the same as for therapeutic care. If client is bedridden, family members should be encouraged to bring food and eat with him.
Client Participation	
Control over dietary intake by the client should be encouraged. He should be allowed to select foods that appeal to his particular preferences with some guidance from the dietitian and nurse. Food consumption will be enhanced if menus are handed out close to mealtime or when client is feeling at his best.	Control considerations are the same as for therapeutic care, except that food suggestions should be related to the individual's psychological, not pathophysiological, needs. The client controls his eating patterns and decides whether or not he wishes to eat. His wishes in this area are respected.
Pediatric Considerations	
Malnutrition must be prevented, so that growth patterns of children are not affected.	Mealtimes and foods should be made as pleasant as possible.

Table 4–3
Factors in Developing a Nutritional Care Plan— Interview Chart

Initial or Therapeutic Care	Advanced or Palliative Care
Age	
Most cancer treatments are more effective in the young who have rapidly multiplying cells (*e.g.*, leukemia). Consequently, nutritional care plans must be intense in order to prevent growth abnormalities after treatment.	The older adult client may not desire changes in his food habits at this stage of the disease.
Ethnic Background	
This often determines what foods will be tolerated during nutritional support therapy.	This often determines what foods will provide the most pleasure and emotional support.
Household	
Persons living alone may use more processed and already prepared feedings such as enteral feedings (*e.g.*, Meritene) during nutritional support therapy.	Hospitalized persons from families with established food habits may desire foods brought from home.
Diagnosis	
This may indicate prognosis of the disease and the effects of treatment on nutritional status.	This may indicate the progression of the disease. Often it indicates the quantity and quality of foods tolerated.
Medications	
This indicates which nutritionally significant side-effects (*e.g.*, vomiting) are likely. Alterations in the nutritional care plan are often directed toward alleviating or preventing unpleasant symptoms. Extent of nutrient deficiencies determines the need for vitamin and mineral supplements.	Medications are usually administered to advanced cancer clients for comfort, not for treatment. Therefore, they may augment, not interfere with, the nutritional care plan.

Table 4–4 165

Table 4–4
Nutritional Assessment

Initial Assessment* — Therapeutic Care	Advanced or Follow-up Assessment† — Palliative Care
Goals	Initial assessment goals plus
1. Identify individuals deemed at nutritional risk	1. Determine treatment and nutritional care plan effectiveness
2. Determine the etiology of the nutritional risk	2. Determine whether the therapeutic nutritional care plan should be terminated and a palliative care plan initiated
3. Identify individuals most likely to become nutritional risks during treatment	Information necessary for accomplishing these goals includes the following.
4. Determine the nutritional care plan that will maintain or improve the individual's nutritional status.	
Information necessary for accomplishing these goals includes the following.	
Diet History	
Personal interview, note changes in food ingestion (*e.g.,* loss of appetite, taste aversions); digestion (*e.g.,* early satiety); absorption; and utilization of nutrients. Any one of these changes will affect nutritional status.	Personal interview, follow-up diet histories may reveal that food habits have changed owing to the progression or treatment of the disease. New nutritional care plans may be needed.
Vital Signs	
Temperature may indicate how efficiently the immune system is functioning.	A rise or fall in temperature indicates effectiveness of treatment.
Anthropometrics	
Height and weight (present, usual, ideal) indicate the extent of adipose tissue catabolism.	Daily follow-up weight measurements may indicate effectiveness of treatment and nutritional care plans. Advanced anthropometric

(continued)

Table 4–4
Nutritional Assessment (continued)

Initial Assessment* — Therapeutic Care	Advanced or Follow-up Assessment† — Palliative Care
Anthropometrics *(continued)*	data that may reveal changes in total body composition (adipose tissue as well as muscle tissue catabolism) are triceps skinfold measures, mid-arm circumference measures, and mid-arm muscle circumference measures.
Laboratory Data	
Fasting blood sugar (FBS) indicates the extent of gluconeogenesis (protein and fat catabolism).	Reevaluations of fasting blood sugars may determine effectiveness of treatment and nutritional care plans.
White Blood Count (WBC)	
Emphasis on total lymphocyte count (TLC). Low lymphocyte counts ($<1500/mm^3$) may indicate malnutrition at the subclinical level, since lymphocytes are an indicator of visceral, not somatic, protein stores. Lymphocyte counts also indicate how efficiently the immune system is functioning.	Frequent examination of lymphocyte counts determines effectiveness of treatment and nutritional care plans. A more complete analysis of individual immunocompetence can be obtained by the skin antigen test.
Albumin	
Low serum levels (below 4.2 g/dll for males and 3.8 g/dll for females) indicate that malnutrition may exist.	Frequent examination of albumin serum levels indicates effectiveness of treatment and nutritional care plans over time, but it may not be a good indicator of present nutritional status. Present nutritional status can be evaluated by the transferrin test. The transferrin test also detects iron deficiencies.

(continued)

Table 4–4 167

Table 4–4
Nutritional Assessment (continued)

Initial Assessment* — Therapeutic Care	Advanced or Follow-up Assessment† — Palliative Care
Clinical Evaluations	
Edema may indicate that colloidal osmotic pressure (low levels of albumin) is not functioning properly. This will cause fluid imbalances. Danger is that edema may mask overt signs of malnutrition (*e.g.*, weight loss).	The sudden appearance of extensive edema may indicate that protein stores are low or that the kidney is malfunctioning. If the therapeutic plan and treatment have been unable to curtail this disease progression, it may be time to initiate palliative care. Advanced assessment determinations that can be examined to evaluate kidney function and visceral protein stores are serum albumin, transferrin, blood urea nitrogen, and creatinine levels.

* Consult Memorial Sloan–Kettering Cancer Center's Initial Nutrition Assessment Form for other individual data necessary to evaluate nutritional status. Consult Chapter 1 for details on how to obtain and evaluate nutritional assessment data.
† Consult Calvary Hospital's Nutritional Support and Assessment Sheet for other individual data necessary to evaluate the nutritional status of advanced cancer clients. Consult Chapter 1 for details on how to obtain and evaluate nutritional assessment data.

Table 4–5
**Dietary Adaptations Suggested for Metabolic Alterations
Induced by Tumorogenesis and Antineoplastic Treatments**

Metabolic Alterations	Dietary Adaptations
Caloric Alterations	
Elevated basal metabolic rate (BMR) that does not adapt to starvation. Higher caloric expenditures are due to inefficient tumor metabolism (*e.g.*, an increased need for glucose for energy by the tumor).	Caloric requirements are increased from 30–35 kcal/kg/day for an adult to 40–45 kcal/kg/day Food intakes should provide for increased requirements: add calorie-dense foods (such as butter, cream, cream cheese, honey, and whole-milk yogurt) to favorite recipes
Protein Alterations	
Increased gluconeogenesis, ureagenesis, and possibly nitrogen trapping (retention of nitrogen by tumor while rest of body is losing nitrogen at accelerated rate); decreased insulin secretion related to presence of stress hormones	Protein requirements increased from 0.8–1 g/kg/day for an adult to 1.5–2 g/kg/day. Food intakes should provide for increased requirements: add high-protein foods (such as skim-milk powder, cheeses, yogurt, and eggs) to favorite recipes
Other Nutrient Alterations	
Subclinical deficiencies of all nutrients (malnutrition; tumor uses nutrients to detriment of host)	Carbohydrate and fat requirements increased Food intake should provide for increased requirements. Client should eat a well-balanced variety of foods of high-caloric density and nutrient density Vitamin and mineral intake should meet recommended daily allowances; seldom possible with diet alone — supplements may be needed

Table 4–6 169

Table 4-6
**Dietary Adaptations Suggested for Clinical Symptoms
Induced by Tumorogenesis and Antineoplastic Treatments**

Clinical Symptoms	Dietary Adaptations
Alterations in senses of taste and smell	If client has a high threshold to sugar, add fruits, marinate meats in sweet sauces, add honey to toast.
	Advise client to suck hard candies if he experiences a metallic taste. Avoid sugars between meals, however, if dental caries may be enhanced.
	Salt thresholds may vary—add salt when needed for taste appeal—avoid when food tastes too salty.
	If client has a low threshold to bitter taste, avoid meat (especially beef); substitute bland chicken and fish, eggs, dairy products, and vegetable proteins (all of these may be well tolerated in casseroles).
	Avoid tart foods like pickles and vinegar-based salad dressings; substitute cream salad dressings.
	Avoid citrus juices, substitute nectars.
	Enhance appearance of food; avoid bland-colored foods, substitute colorful ones.
	Enhance taste; avoid hot foods, substitute cold if client prefers.
	Avoid institutional foods; substitute foods prepared at home, if possible.
	Avoid giving enjoyable foods right before treatment; substitute dry crackers if necessary.
	Help client avoid cooking odors if client finds them unpleasant; substitute sweet smells or keep cooking areas separated from client's area.
	Avoid giving client foods to which he is averse; zinc supplements may help alleviate food aversions.
	Encourage good oral hygiene to lessen the time unpleasant tastes remain in the mouth. This practice will also decrease dental caries.

(continued)

Table 4–6
**Dietary Adaptations Suggested for Clinical Symptoms
Induced by Tumorogenesis and Antineoplastic Treatments** (continued)

Clinical Symptoms	Dietary Adaptations
Xerostomia (dry mouth), dysphagia (difficulty swallowing), stomatitis (inflammation of oral cavity)	Promote saliva production: avoid dry foods, colorless foods, foods with no taste (but do not make too spicy because spicy flavors may irritate ulcerations); substitute foods that have more liquid (*e.g.*, meat with added gravy, foods in sauces, creamy foods); encourage client to suck on ice cubes, sugar-free candies, or Popsicles or chew sugar-free gum.
	Adapt meal patterns; avoid 3 large meals, substitute 6 small meals.
	Adapt temperature of food when mouth is inflamed. Substitute cold foods (*e.g.*, buttermilk or yogurt) for hot foods. They may numb inflamed area.
	Avoid large pieces of food, substitute small bite-size pieces.
	Avoid sweets between meals; substitute protein and complex carbohydrate foods. Consult Chapter 3 for details on dietary adaptations for clients with dysphagia.
	Avoid alcohol, tobacco, and spicy and acid foods; substitute tea or milk, bland foods, or fruit nectars. Lidocaine (Xylocaine) can be used to relieve pain before eating if stomatitis in present.
Early satiety (bloating, feeling of fullness, "heartburn")	Avoid fatty foods, carbonated beverages, dairy products, coffee, alcohol, spicy foods, gaseous foods, and liquids with meals; substitute protein and complex carbohydrate foods, and bland foods, and have client consume liquids between meals.
	Adapt meal patterns; avoid 3 large meals, substitute 6 small meals, but avoid meals at bedtime.
	Adapt lifestyle; avoid sedentary lifestyle; substitute moderate exercise before and after meals.
	Give antacids after meals and at bedtime if prescribed by physician.
	Adapt food preparation methods; avoid frying, substitute steaming or baking.

(continued)

Table 4-6 171

Table 4-6
**Dietary Adaptations Suggested for Clinical Symptoms
Induced by Tumorogenesis and Antineoplastic Treatments** (continued)

Clinical Symptoms	Dietary Adaptations
Nausea and vomiting	Avoid giving enjoyable foods before treatment; substitute dry crackers, ginger ale, cola drinks, soda water, broth, and fruit nectars before and after treatment. Gradually progress to bland meals.
	Adapt meal patterns; avoid 3 large meals, substitute 6 small meals. Some clients find a large breakfast more palatable than a large dinner.
	Avoid fats and refined sugars, substitute protein and complex carbohydrates.
	Give nutrient-dense liquids (*e.g.*, milkshakes).
	Adapt food preparation methods; avoid fried foods, substitute steamed and baked ones.
	Help client avoid cooking smells. If client finds them unpleasant, substitute desirable odors.
	Enhance food appeal and digestion; avoid foods that have an unpleasant appearance, give antiemetics (*e.g.*, Compazine), tranquilizers (*e.g.*, Valium), and drugs that enhance GI motility (*e.g.*, Reglan) before meals if prescribed by the physician.
	Encourage good oral hygiene to relieve adverse tastes and dental caries.
Diarrhea and steatorrhea	Avoid foods with high-fiber content, dairy products, gluten (*e.g.*, wheat and rye products) and fat; substitute bland low-residue foods: white breads, refined cereals (*e.g.*, corn or rice cereals), eggs, or, in severe cases, chemically defined feedings. (See Chap. 2.)

(continued)

Table 4-6
Dietary Adaptations Suggested for Clinical Symptoms Induced by Tumorogenesis and Antineoplastic Treatments (continued)

Clinical Symptoms	Dietary Adaptations
Diarrhea and Steatorrhea (continued)	Adapt meal patterns: avoid 3 large meals, substitute 6 small meals. Avoid raw foods; substitute cooked ones. Consult Chapter 7 for more details on dietary adaptations for clients with intestinal dysfunctions.
Constipation	Enhance elimination by increasing fluid intakes; increasing fibrous food intakes, such as raw fruits and vegetables and bran products; increasing moderate exercise; establishing routine bowel habits; giving stool softeners or mild laxatives when advised by the physician.

Bibliography

Carson JAS, Gomican A: Taste acuity and food attitudes of selected patients with cancer. J Am Diet Assoc 70:361, 1977

Committee on Diet, Nutrition, and Cancer Assembly of Life Sciences National Research Council: Diet, nutrition, and cancer. Nutr Today 17:20, 1982

Diet and nutrition in cancer. Proc Am Cancer Soc NCI National Conference on Nutrition in Cancer, June 29–July 1, 1978. Cancer 43(Suppl):1955, 1979

Enig MG, Munn RJ, Keeney M: Dietary fat and cancer trends—A critique. Fed Proc 37:2715, 1978

Frytak S, Mertel CG: Management of nausea and vomiting in the cancer patient. JAMA 245:393, 1981

Geltman RL, Paige RL: Symptom management in hospice care. Am J Nurs 83:78, 1983

Groer M, Pierce M: Anorexia-cachexia. Nursing, 81(11):39, 1981

Kritchevsky D, Fink DJ: Introduction to the workshop on fat and cancer. Cancer Res 41:3684, 1981

March DC: Handbook: Interactions of Selected Drugs with Nutritional Status in Man, 2nd ed. Chicago, American Dietetic Association, 1978

Margan S, Caan B (eds): Applied nutrition in clinical medicine. Med Clin North Am 63:1027, 1979

Morrison SD: Origins of anorexia in neoplastic disease. Am J Clin Nutr 31:1104, 1978

Munro HN: Tumor–host competition for nutrients in the cancer patient. J Am Diet Assoc 71:380, 1977

Neilan BA: Cancer chemotherapy: Current status, coming innovations. Postgrad Med 73:125, 1983

Newel GR, Ellison NM (eds): Nutrition and Cancer: Etiology and Treatment. New York, Raven Press, 1981

Shils ME: How to nourish the cancer patient. Nutr Today 16(3):4, 1981

Van Eys J: Nutrition and neoplasia. Nutr Rev 40:353, 1982

Weisburger JH, Horn C: Nutrition and cancer: Mechanisms of genotoxic and epigenetic carcinogens in nutritional carcinogenesis. Bull NY Acad Med 58:296, 1982

William SR: Nutrition and Diet Therapy, 4th ed. St Louis, CV Mosby, 1981

Winick M: Nutrition and Cancer. New York, John Wiley & Sons, 1977

Yancey RS: Vitamins and trace elements in the etiology and treatment of cancer. Cancer Bull 32:177, 1980

Suggested Readings

Chemotherapy and You. US Department of Health and Human Services, NIH Publication No 81-1136. Bethesda, MD, National Cancer Institute, 1980

Diet and Nutrition: A Resource for Parents of Children with Cancer. US Department of Health, and Human Services, NIH Publication No 80-2038. Bethesda, MD, National Cancer Institute, 1979

Eating Hints: Recipes and Tips for Better Nutrition During Cancer Treatment. US Department of Health and Human Services, NIH Publication No 81-2079. Office of Cancer Communications, Bethesda, MD, National Cancer Institute (Building 31, Room 10A18), 1981

Fairchild M, Corbin C (eds): Nutrition Concerns . . . for Troubled Eaters During Radiation Therapy to the Head and Neck Areas. New York, Memorial Sloan–Kettering Cancer Center Food Services Department (1275 York Avenue), 1981

Nutrition for Patients Receiving Chemotherapy and Radiation Treatment. New York, American Cancer Society (777 Third Avenue), 1974

chapter 5

Diabetes Mellitus

Description

Diabetes mellitus is a chronic disease characterized by hyperglycemia and glycosuria, involving abnormalities in the metabolism of carbohydrate, protein, and fat. These nutrient imbalances are related to hormonal alterations, namely, absent, deficient, or ineffective insulin; excess glucagon; and a disturbance in somatostatin balance.

Metabolic alterations create pathophysiological disturbances that can induce clinical signs and symptoms (Fig. 5-1).

Incidence

- National number 3 killer—mostly from complications (*e.g.*, heart disease and stroke)
- Estimated incidence of 10.7 million—1 out of every 20 Americans, with a 6% rise in incidence annually
- Insulin-dependent diabetics, 10%
- Noninsulin-dependent diabetics, 90%
  1. Diagnosed diabetics, 5.7 million
  2. Estimated undiagnosed diabetics, 5 million

Etiologic Risk Factors

- Heredity
  Genetic predisposition established, but mode of inheritance not well defined

175

Insulin Absent, Insulin Deficient, or Insulin Ineffective		
Protein Metabolism Altered	Carbohydrate Metabolism Impaired	Fat Metabolism Accelerated
Protein anabolism ↓	Glucose uptake by the cell ↓	Fat anabolism ↓
Protein catabolism ↑		Fat catabolism ↑ (lipolysis)
Protein tissue used to produce glucose (gluconeogenesis)	Clinical signs and symptoms, weight loss (due to starvation) or gain (hyperinsulinemia), and fatigue	FFA in blood ↑, used for energy
Clinical sign, weight loss		Clinical sign, weight loss
Protein tissue necrosis with ↑ N and K levels in blood	Plasma glucose (hyperglycemia) ↑, (FBS > 110 mg/dl)	Lipids (VLDLs and cholesterol) ↑ in blood (hyperlipidemia)
Clinical signs and symptoms, azotemia, hyperkalemia, poor wound healing, tissue wasting	Vascular changes develop, renal glucose threshold exceeded (blood glucose > 160 - 180 mg/dl), which induces osmotic diuresis and glycosuria	Clinical signs and symptoms, atherosclerosis
N and K release into urine ↑		Ketone bodies in blood (ketonemia) and urine (ketonuria) ↑
Clinical signs and symptoms, diuresis and hypokalemia	Clinical signs and symptoms, nocturia, polyuria, polydipsia	Clinical signs and symptoms, ↓ pH and ↓ CO_2 blood levels, acid breath, heavy breathing ("Kussmauling"), dehydration (water and electrolyte loss ↑), dry skin, vomiting, abdominal pain, drowsiness, leading to
Ultimate result, cellular dehydration, which leads to	Water and electrolyte (Na) loss ↑, which induces dehydration with resultant hypovolemia and ↓ renal blood flow	
	Clinical signs and symptoms, anuria and drowsiness, leading to	

↓ HHNK (NIDDM) or DKA coma (IDDM), death.

Fig. 5–1.   Pathophysiology and clinical signs and symptoms of diabetes mellitus, in increasing severity, from top to bottom.
Abbreviations. ↓ decreased, ↑ increased, N = nitrogen, K = potassium, Na = sodium, FBS = fasting blood sugar, FFA = free fatty acids, VLDLs = very low density lipoproteins, HHNK = hyperglycemic hyperosmolar nonketotic coma, DKA = diabetic ketoacidosis, NIDDM = noninsulin-dependent diabetes mellitus, IDDM = insulin-dependent diabetes mellitus. (After Mitchell HS, Rynbergen HJ, Anderson L et al: Cooper's Nutrition in Health and Disease, 15th ed. Philadelphia, JB Lippincott, 1968)

- Age
  Incidence of insulin-dependent diabetes mellitus (IDDM) peaks during second decade, is low after age 30; incidence of noninsulin-dependent diabetes mellitus (NIDDM) increases with age and peaks after age 65
- Obesity
- Sedentary lifestyle
- Stress
  Physiological stress (*e.g.*, accidents, pregnancy)
  Psychological stress (increased amounts of stress hormones result in decreased secretion or sensitivity of insulin)
- Viral infections (*e.g.*, mumps, viral hepatitis, influenza)
- Low intake or impaired utilization of nutrients (*e.g.*, zinc and chromium)

Classifications* and Characteristics

- Primary Diabetes
  1. Insulin-Dependent Diabetes Mellitus (IDDM)
     Also referred to as juvenile-onset, youth-onset, Type I, and ketosis-prone diabetes
     a. Client usually, but not always, under age 40
     b. Symptoms begin abruptly
     c. Symptoms severe
     d. Symptoms progress rapidly (if not controlled) to ketoacidosis and coma (see Fig. 5-1)
     e. Client usually underweight
     f. Islet cell antibodies, 50% to 80% positive at diagnosis
     g. Human leukocyte antigens (HLA) high (B8, B15, Dw3/DR3, Dw4/DR4)
     h. Vascular complications
     i. Fasting plasma glucose (FPG) over 140 mg/dl
     j. Insulin low or absent

---

* These classifications of diabetes and related disorders of glucose tolerance were developed in 1979 by the National Diabetes Data Group of the National Institutes of Health and are approved by the American Diabetes Association and the International Diabetes Federation. (Details of classifications and characteristics are outlined in National Diabetes Data Group: Classification and diagnosis of diabetes mellitus and other categories of glucose intolerance. Diabetes 28:1039, 1979)

      k. Insulin needed along with dietary adaptations for control

      l. Adequate kilocalories needed to maintain weight and promote growth

  2. Noninsulin-Dependent Diabetes Mellitus (NIDDM). Also referred to as maturity-onset, adult-onset, Type II, and ketosis-resistant diabetes

      a. Client usually mature, over 40

      b. Symptoms may remain latent or occur gradually

      c. Symptoms usually milder

      d. Symptoms progress slowly: hyperosmolar coma may occur in severe cases, but diabetic ketoacidosis is rare except with severe stress or infection

      e. Most clients (60%–90%) are overweight

      f. Islet cell antibodies, 5% positive at diagnosis

      g. Human leukocyte antigens at normal levels

      h. Vascular complications

      i. Fasting plasma glucose (FPG) over 140 mg/dl

      j. Insulin may be deficient, delayed, ineffective, or high (hyperinsulinemia) but not absent

      k. Diet and exercise adaptations or hypoglycemic agents may be all that is needed for control; if hyperglycemia persists, however, insulin may be used for better control

      l. Kilocalories usually restricted to promote weight loss

- Impaired Glucose Tolerance (IGT). Plasma glucose (PG) levels between those considered normal and those considered diabetic
- Gestational Diabetes (GDM). Glucose intolerance that develops or is discovered in a woman during her pregnancy
- Previous Abnormality of Glucose Tolerance (PrevAGT). Normal glucose tolerance but a history of diabetic hyperglycemia or IGT that occurred either spontaneously or in response to an identifiable stimulus. Formerly called latent diabetes
- Potential Abnormality of Glucose Tolerance (PotAGT). No glucose intolerance but at greater risk than the general population for developing diabetes for a variety of reasons. Formerly called potential diabetes and prediabetes
- Secondary Diabetes. Diabetes mellitus caused by pancreatic disease, hormonal disorders, drugs (*e.g.*, corticosteroids), and chemical agents, viral infections, hemochromatosis, and others

  1. Similar to primary insulin-dependent diabetes or primary non-insulin-dependent diabetes, depending upon type and origin of disorder and severity of the condition

  2. Meal plans may be further adjusted to decrease adverse symptoms induced by primary disease

Table 5–2
Oral Hypoglycemic Preparations

Generic Name	Trade Name	Approximate Duration of Action (hr)
Sulfonylureas		
Tolbutamide	Orinase	6–10
Chlorpropamide	Diabinese	36–60
Acetohexamide	Dymelor	10–20
Tolazamide	Tolinase	12–24

(After Shuman CR: Pharmacological data on the Sulfonylureas. Medical Times 108:79, 1980)

Drug Therapy

Nutritional implications of drugs used in treatment of diabetes are given in Tables 5-1 and 5-2.*

Interactions Among Antihyperglycemic Agents, Nutrients, and Nutritional Status

- Insulin
  1. Indications
     a. Insulin-dependent diabetics
     b. Noninsulin-dependent diabetics with unstable blood sugar levels or unsatisfactory dietary compliance
  2. Definition
     A hormone secreted by the beta cells of the islets of Langerhans in the pancreas
  3. Composition
     a. A protein composed of two polypeptide chains, A and B, containing 21 and 30 amino acid molecules, respectively
     b. Clinical significance
        Insulin, like any other protein, digested by digestive enzymes into its component amino acids, if taken by mouth; therefore, must be injected directly into the bloodstream to be effective (insulin administration by pump is under research)
  4. Mode of Action
     a. Facilitates transport of glucose through cell membrane where it can be used for energy
     b. Enhances conversion of glucose to glycogen so glucose can be stored

---

* See tables at the end of this chapter.

    c. Enhances protein and fat synthesis and inhibits protein and fat catabolism

    d. Enhances glucose oxidation to pyruvate (aids glucose phosphorylation)

5. Insulin Preparations Commercially Available in the United States and Their Duration of Action (see Table 5-1)

    a. Composition

        1. Traditional commercial insulins prepared in amorphous or crystalline form from beef, pork, and sheep pancreas; consequently, amino acid pattern may not be same as in human insulin; in addition, some other pancreatic hormones (*e.g.*, proinsulin) or pancreatic polypeptides may remain, and antibodies may develop in the human host

        2. Research Insulin

        Human insulin now being prepared in *Escherichia coli* by using recombinant DNA technology

6. Dosage

    A normal individual secretes approximately 40 to 60 units of insulin/day (A standardized U-100 of insulin means that each milliliter contains 100 units of insulin.)

    Diabetic persons may not secrete any insulin, or the insulin they secrete may be delayed or have decreased sensitivity at the cell site. Consequently, the dosage of insulin administered must be individualized according to blood glucose levels, stage of growth, nutritional care plans, and lifestyle (*e.g.*, physical activity). It may be one type of insulin given in a single dosage, or it may be a multiple component "split-and-mixed" insulin regimen given in two or three injections/day.

7. Relation to Diet

    a. Traditional Insulin-Dependent Diabetics

        (1) Size of meals adjusted to insulin

        (2) Time of meals adjusted to peak of insulin action

        (3) Caloric and nutrient content of meals adjusted to insulin dosage

    b. Modified Traditional Insulin-Dependent Diabetics*

    Insulin adjusted to blood sugar levels and client's lifestyle (*e.g.*, exercise patterns); therefore, size, nutrient content (*e.g.*, carbohydrate), and time of meals may be more flexible. Insulin adjustment accomplished by multiple daily subcutaneous injections using a variety of delivery schedules or by continuous subcutaneous insulin infusion systems (CSII). The latter

---

* Adjusting insulin to blood sugar levels and lifestyle is still in the research stage and should not be undertaken unless the client and the health team are highly motivated and have specific training in monitoring blood sugar levels. Information on this subject is available from Diabetes Research and Training Center, Albert Einstein College of Medicine, Montefiore Hospital and Medical Center, 1825 Eastchester Road, Bronx, NY.

is accomplished by mechanical devices (*e.g.*, pumps) designed to simulate normal pancreatic insulin secretion.

8. Side-Effects in Relation to Diet
    a. *Hypoglycemia* when dosage too great; when normal dosage taken but food (glucose) not available; when normal dosage taken but exercise increased
    b. *Hyperglycemia* when dosage too low; when normal dosage taken but food (glucose) intake excessive; when insulin and food intake are the same but client is under stress (insulin not as effective when stress hormones are excessive)
    c. Allergies to insulin

- Oral Hypoglycemic Agents (see Table 5-2)
    1. Indications
       Noninsulin-dependent diabetics with unstable blood sugar levels or unsatisfactory dietary compliance
    2. Definition
       Synthetic chemical compounds
    3. Composition
        a. Sulfonylurea drugs have common core component, $-SO_2$ $-NH-CO-NH-$, responsible for their action
        b. Clinical significance
           Oral hypoglycemic agents *do not* contain amino acids; consequently, they will not be digested by digestive enzymes if taken by mouth; thus they will still be available for antihyperglycemic action
    4. Mode of Action
        a. Stimulate beta cells of the pancreas to secrete available insulin (some insulin must be available in order for these agents to have any antihyperglycemic action)
        b. Potentiate insulin action at the postreceptor level, possibly by modifying some aspect of intracellular metabolism
        c. Enhance insulin secretion in response to rising blood glucose concentrations
    5. Oral Hypoglycemic Agents Available in the United States and Their Duration of Action (see Table 5-2)
       Composition. Commercial hypoglycemic agents are synthetic chemical compounds
    6. Dosage
        a. Individualized according to blood glucose levels, nutritional care plan, and lifestyle
        b. Dosage also based on the drug's duration of action
        c. Dosage ranges from two to three doses/day for short half-life agents, (*e.g.*, tolbutamide [Orinase]) to one dose/day (usually before breakfast) for long-life agents (*e.g.*, chlorpropamide [Diabinese])

7. Relation to Diet
   a. Noninsulin-Dependent Diabetics
      (1) Size of meals and time of meals not strictly adjusted; agents only enhance available insulin action, do not lower blood sugar directly
      (2) Altering caloric and nutrient content of diet still advisable, since available insulin seems to be more effective when adipose cell is smaller
   b. Modified Traditional Insulin-Dependent Diabetics
      Agents used to augment insulin action for they may increase sensitivity
8. Side-Effects in Relation to Diet
   a. *Hypoglycemia* when dosage is too great; when normal dosage is taken but food (glucose) is not available; when normal dosage is taken but alcohol intake is excessive
   b. Additional dietary alterations may be required if coronary heart disease is evident, because according to the controversial University Group Diabetes Program (UGDP) study, diabetics on oral agents have greater incidence of vascular and coronary heart disease than those treated by diet alone or insulin

Diagnosis and Monitoring Control

- Urinary Analysis
  1. Volume
     Normal, 700 to 2000 ml/day
     Diabetic, increased volume, body attempts to dilute glucose
  2. Specific Gravity
     Normal, 1.008 to 1.030
     Diabetic, 1.030 or higher, increased glucose concentration
  3. Glucose
     a. Number and time of tests
        Double-voided urine tested four times daily, before meals and at bedtime
     b. Methodology of testing
        Concentration of glucose, in percentages (*e.g.*, ¼% = 250 mg/dl) read colorometrically by*

---

* At the recommendation of the American Diabetes Association, the plus (+) system formerly used for reporting glucose concentrations in urine has been removed from most products that are used in the home to reduce the possibility of confusion by persons who may use products of more than one manufacturer.

(1) Indicator paper strip (*e.g.*, Tes-Tape)

(2) Paper stick or reagent strips (*e.g.*, Diastix)

(3) Adding a reagent tablet to urine (*e.g.*, Clinitest)

4. Ketone bodies (incompletely oxidized fatty acids)
Concentration of ketones in mg/dl read colorometrically by

a. Paper strip or reagent strips, ketone bodies alone (*e.g.*, Ketostix)

b. Paper strip or reagent strip, ketone bodies plus glucose (*e.g.*, Keto-Diastix)

- Blood Analysis

  1. Purpose: Measurement of blood glucose levels

  2. Number and Time of Tests
  Home monitoring of blood glucose tested at least four to seven times per day before and 1 hour after meals and at bedtime or when symptoms of hyperglycemia or hypoglycemia occur. In addition, records are kept to analyze reasons for blood glucose changes (*e.g.*, lack of dietary compliance). Glycosylated hemoglobin (HbA_{1c}) measured every 4 to 8 weeks.

  3. Methodology of Testing

     a. In-home monitoring,* capillary or venous blood tested semi-quantitatively by reagent strips (*e.g.*, Visidex, Chemstrips bG) that contain oxidase; capillary blood readily obtained by pricking fingertip with an "Autolet" or a small 25- to 26-gauge disposable needle; results compared visually with a color chart; color changes with alterations in blood glucose levels.

     b. Capillary or venous blood tested semiquantitatively by a reflectance photometer (Glucometer, Glucochex)

     c. Glycosylated hemoglobin (HbA_{1c}) tested in laboratory; higher concentrations of this compound (10%–28% *vs.* 7% normal) have been found in blood samples of diabetics. Frequent measurement then can indicate the degree of blood glucose control.

  4. Oral Glucose Tolerance Test (OGTT)

     a. Methodology of Testing (Dietary Adaptations)

        (1) 150-g carbohydrate diet consumed for 3 days prior to test

        (2) Client fasts night before test but not more than 16 hours; no caffeine or nicotine allowed for 12 hours prior to test; additionally some medications may have to be eliminated prior to the test for they may influence results (*e.g.*, phenytoin, thiazide diuretics, glucocorticoids, oral contraceptives, and ascorbic acid)

---

* Specific training is necessary for both the health team and the client before home blood monitoring can become part of the diabetic's health care.

(3) The morning of the fourth day, the nonpregnant adult is given 75 g of glucose (calculated for children as 1.75 g/kg/IBW up to a maximum of 75 g); glucose load given as an oral glucose drink (glucose, water, and lemon flavoring) or in a glucola drink (hydrolysated cornstarch plus carbonated water and cola flavoring)

b. Diagnostic Procedures

(1) Blood sugar read before glucose preparation served; this determines fasting blood sugar levels

(2) Client continues to fast after the glucose load, and blood sugar read again at ½ hour, 1 hour, 2 hours, and 3 hours after consumption of glucose preparation

(3) Urine analyzed for determination of sugar percentage

(4) Blood sugar concentrations plotted against time and resulting curve compared with a normal curve (normal postprandial levels: 1 hour, 140 mg/dl; 2 hours, 120 mg/dl; 3 hours, 85–100 mg/dl [see Fig. 5-2])

(5) Diagnosis based upon two different test determinations since stress, drugs, and inactivity may affect results

5. Other Glucose Tests*

a. Intravenous glucose tolerance test

b. Cortisone and prednisone glucose tolerance test

c. Oral and intravenous tolbutamide tolerance tests

Diet Therapy

- Goals for Insulin-Dependent and Noninsulin-Dependent Diabetics

1. Improve the overall health of the client by attaining and maintaining optimal nutrition

2. Attain or maintain an ideal body weight

3. Provide for normal physical growth in the child; provide adequate nutrition for the pregnant woman and, hence, for her fetus; provide adequate nutrition for lactation needs if she chooses to breast feed

4. Maintain plasma glucose as near the normal physiological range as possible (see Fig. 5–2)

5. Prevent or delay the development or progression of cardiovascular, renal, retinal, neurologic, and other complications associated with diabetes, insofar as these are related to metabolic control

6. Modify the diet as necessary for complications of diabetes and for associated diseases

---

* Procedures used in these tests are beyond the scope of this book

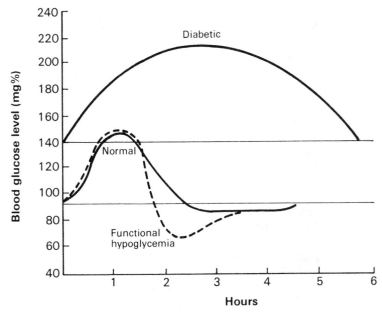

Figure 5-2. Glucose tolerance curve in the normal person, in the diabetic, and in the person with functional hypoglycemia. (Hunt SM, Groff JL, Holbrook JM: Nutrition: Principles and Clinical Practice, New York, John Wiley & Sons, 1980)

7. Make the diet prescription as attractive and realistic as possible by providing each patient with an individualized educational and follow-up program; repeat visits serve to extend and clarify the instruction, to provide assurance, and to check progress

Nutritional Care Plan

- Factors in Developing a Nutritional Care Plan for Insulin-Dependent and Noninsulin-Dependent Diabetics
  1. Interview Chart (Components With Special Significance)
     a. Age. Child, usually insulin-dependent; adult, noninsulin-dependent if clinical symptoms are recent
     b. Sex. Pregnant woman may have gestational diabetes; pregnant women with history of diabetes may need additional insulin and dietary adaptations
     c. Ethnic background. Diabetics need lifelong compliance; dietary adaptations should be directed toward an individual's beliefs, mores, cultural background (*e.g.*, traditional foods) and internalization of self-motivation toward prescribed behavior

    d. Occupation. Working in the evening may call for additional adjustments in the time insulin and meals dispensed

    e. Household. Family members, as well as clients, may need support and dietary instructions (family members can be a natural support system or hinder dietary compliance); clients living alone may need help adjusting their dietary adaptations to restaurant menus

    f. Diagnosis and Medical History. Newly diagnosed diabetics need extensive dietary instruction and assurance that their lifestyles need not be completely changed; complications may require additional dietary adjustments

    g. Medications. Consult list of Interactions Among Antihyperglycemic Agents, Nutrients, and Nutritional Status

    h. Allergies. Food aversions and allergies must be considered before recommending a nutritional care plan

    i. Special Diet. Often indicates client's knowledge of present dietary prescription and compliance; client may know diet prescription well or have many misconceptions; also, clients vary widely in their readiness to comprehend and integrate new information into an adjusted life pattern

2. Nutritional Assessment (Data With Special Significance)

    a. Diet History. Personal interview with special emphasis on amounts and types of nutrients consumed (carbohydrates, refined or complex; fats, saturated or polyunsaturated); total caloric content; frequency and time of meals; location of meal consumption (home, office, restaurant)

    b. Vital Signs

        (1) Blood Pressure. Diabetics have higher incidence of hypertension; additional dietary alterations will be required

        (2) Temperature. Insulin and glucose intake needs to be adjusted during stress (*e.g.*, infection) when insulin is less effective

    c. Anthropometric Measurements

        (1) Height, Weight* (Present, Usual, and Ideal), and Body Frame. Single most important dietary objective in treatment of all diabetics is to attain ideal body weight.

            (a) Insulin-Dependent Diabetics. Caloric needs increased; client usually malnourished when diagnosed

            (b) Noninsulin-Dependent Diabetics. Calories restricted; client usually overweight when diagnosed

---

* Keep in mind that limbs have weight (leg $=18\%$ of body weight, 9% below the knee). Amputees may appear to be at ideal body weight.

d. Laboratory Data

(1) Blood

(a) Plasma Glucose Levels. Determine need for and type of medication and severity of dietary modifications

(b) Cholesterol and Triglycerides. Diabetics have higher incidence of atherosclerosis and Type IV hyperlipoproteinemia. (↑VLDLs); high levels of cholesterol or triglycerides warrant additional dietary adjustments

(c) Albumin. Insulin-dependent diabetics may be severely malnourished

(d) Potassium. Determines extent of protein catabolism; BUN and creatinine increases may indicate impending nephropathy

(2) Urine

Glucose and Acetone Levels. Determine disease's severity and classification (noninsulin-dependent diabetics seldom spill ketones)

e. Clinical Evaluation

Extent of obesity or malnutrition determines caloric alterations. Consult Chapter 2 for details on developing a nutritional care plan; consult Chapter 1 for details on simple and advanced nutritional assessment data

• Nutritional Care Plan Alterations and Dietary Intake Adaptations for Insulin-Dependent and Noninsulin-Dependent (Obese) Diabetics

1. General Nutritional Care Plan for All Diabetics

a. Consume variety of nutrient-dense foods daily to maintain or obtain optimal nutritional status

b. Reduce or increase caloric content of diet to achieve and maintain ideal body weight

c. Apply nutrient distribution pattern for kilocalorie consumption recommended in Table 5-3 to daily meal plans*

d. See Table 5-4, Comparison of Insulin-Dependent and Noninsulin-Dependent (Overweight) Nutritional Care Plans

2. Specific Nutritional Care Plans for Individual Diabetics

Individual nutritional care plans are based on the diet prescription (includes modifications for special conditions); need for, dosage of, and type of medication; exercise patterns; individual food preferences calculated in exchanges (Tables 5-5 to 5-8)

a. Diet prescription to lower, control, or prevent fluctuations in blood sugar levels

---

* Note this distribution pattern is very similar to the pattern recommended for all Americans (U.S. Dietary Goals), except that refined sugars are restricted.

(1) Caloric Alterations for Insulin-Dependent Diabetics

    (a) Determine ideal body weight for adults; compare client's weight and height with average weight and height charts (see Appendix I) or estimate ideal body weight (females: allow 100 lbs for first 5 feet; males: 110 lb; add 5 lb for each additional inch, subtract 10% for small frame, add 10% for large frame)

    (b) Determine individual calories needed for basal metabolic rate and activity (see Chap. 6, Determination of Caloric Alteration Level chart, and Table 6-9). Caloric intake for most newly diagnosed, underweight, insulin-dependent diabetics needs to be *increased* from 30 to 35 kcal/kg/day to 40 to 45 kcal/kg/day

    (c) Determine ideal body weight for children; compare client's weight to average weights listed in the Recommended Daily Dietary Allowances (see Appendix IV); caloric intake for children should be sufficient to obtain ideal body weight, maintain growth development, and maintain activity level

    (d) Dietary adaptations: add calorie-dense foods, listed in the exchange lists (for example, margarine, cream, and yogurt) to favorite recipes (see Appendix V)

(2) Caloric Alterations for Noninsulin-Dependent Diabetics

    (a) See (a) under Insulin-Dependent Diabetics, above

    (b) Kilocalorie needs are determined as for insulin-dependent diabetics; caloric intake, however, for most newly diagnosed, noninsulin-dependent diabetics will need to be *reduced*

    (c) Dietary adaptations: consult Chapter 6 for ways to adjust body weight by caloric adjustments, behavioral modifications, and exercise alterations

(3) Protein Alterations for All Diabetics

    (a) 12% to 24% of total kilocalories. Upper limits for growing children, pregnant women, and lactating women

    (b) Dietary adaptations: limit animal protein (high in saturated fat and cholesterol); substitute vegetable proteins (soybeans and others) frequently

(4) Carbohydrate Alterations for Insulin-Dependent Diabetics*

    (a) 45% to 55% of total daily kilocalories

---

* The carbohydrate content of the diabetic diet has increased within recent years because high-fiber intake improves glucose metabolism, which in turn decreases the need for or dosage of insulin; when carbohydrate intake was low, fat was substituted to obtain total daily kilocalorie requirements, and diet became atherogenic.

(b) Complex carbohydrates, 30% to 45% of total carbohydrate kilocalories

(c) Natural sugars, 5% to 15% of total carbohydrate kilocalories

(d) Refined processed sugars, 0% of total carbohydrate kilocalories

(e) Dietary adaptations: Increase intake of foods containing complex carbohydrates such as foods containing starch (pasta or corn) and foods containing fiber (skins and seeds of raw fruits and vegetables, whole-grain and bran cereals, and leguminous plants [*e.g.*, lentils, dried beans, and dried peas]); limit intake of foods containing natural sugars such as peeled fruits and vegetables, natural fruit juices, and milk; restrict intake of foods containing refined processed sugars such as table sugar, honey, candies, and desserts; sugar substitutes such as aspartame and saccharin (not Sweet 'n Low, which contains lactose [milk sugar]) may be used, with discretion, instead of refined sugars, but pregnant women and children should be especially prudent in their use (see Chap. 6); restrict or limit alcohol, never consumed without physician's permission

(5) Carbohydrate Alterations for Noninsulin-Dependent Diabetics

(a) Same as insulin-dependent, above

(b) Same as insulin-dependent, above

(c) Natural sugars not as limited as in insulin-dependent nutritional care plan

(d) Same as for insulin-dependent diabetics, above; two exceptions: sorbitol and fructose are sometimes acceptable in certain individual nutritional care plans, as they produce a lessened postprandial hyperglycemia

(e) Dietary adaptations: Same as for insulin-dependent diabetics, except that use of alcohol, with a physician's permission, may be more liberal; if allowed, it must be taken as an exchange substitute, not in addition to allowed kilocalories (for example, 1 oz of alcohol = 1½ bread exchanges or 2 fat exchanges [approximately 90 kcal]

(6) Fat Alterations for All Diabetics*

(a) 25% to 35% of total daily kilocalories

---

* The total fat content of the diabetic diet has been decreased in recent years in order to try to prevent or control the complications and degenerative diseases (*e.g.*, atherosclerosis) related to diabetes.

(b) Saturated fats, 12% to 18% of total fat kilocalories (some sources state 10%)

(c) Monounsaturated and polyunsaturated fat, 12% to 18% of total fat kilocalories (some sources state 10% mono unsaturated and 10% saturated)

(d) Cholesterol, 300 g/day if atherosclerosis is a complication

(e) Dietary adaptations: limit intake of foods containing saturated fats and cholesterol such as animal fats (cheese, whole milk, butter and meats); limit intake of foods containing monounsaturated fats such as peanut oil and olive oil; increase intake of polyunsaturated fats such as soybean oils and soft margarines made of vegetable oils; however, increases should not be so extensive that total fat content of the diet is increased

(7) Vitamin and Mineral Alterations for All Diabetics

(a) Vitamin and mineral requirements (two thirds of the Recommended Dietary Allowances daily), as for any healthy adult (see Appendix IV)

(b) 100% of the allowances or supplements may be needed if client is malnourished or has complications

(c) Dietary adaptations: Intake of adequate amounts of calories and consumption of a variety of nutrient-dense foods daily should meet requirements

b. Meal Patterns
Altered to lower, control, or prevent fluctuations in blood sugar levels

(1) Insulin-Dependent Diabetic

(a) Meal Size. Determined by the diet prescription (establishes the kilocalories and grams of glucose-containing nutrients available daily) and type of insulin administered (establishes how much glucose can be metabolized after each meal); kilocalories available depend upon the individual's weight, activity level, age, and so on

(b) Time of Meals. Determined by type of insulin administered (establishes start of action, peak of action, and duration of action [see Table 5-1]); meals and insulin must be taken at specified times each day for effective control of blood sugar levels (clinical significance: insulin without glucose =hypoglycemia; glucose without insulin=hyperglycemia)

(c) Number of Meals and Snacks (Meal Division). Determined by diet prescription (establishes the kilocalories and grams of glucose-containing nutrients that can be

converted into foods daily); the type of insulin administered (establish the amount of food [glucose] that must
be available at any given time to prevent fluctuations in
blood sugar levels); and exercise patterns (establishes
insulin sensitivity—sensitivity is increased during and
after exercise, so more glucose must be available)

(i) Generalized Meal and Snack Division (see Tables
5-5 to 5-7)

Kilocalorie division. Each meal, 30% to 40% of total calories; snacks, 10% of total calories

Carbohydrate division. Each meal, 30% to 40% of
total carbohydrate kilocalories; snacks, 10% of total
carbohydrate kilocalories

Other nutrients. Equal division not usually necessary

(ii) General Criteria for Meal Size. Smallest meal when
insulin action is at its lowest point (usually breakfast), largest meal when insulin action is at its peak
(usually lunch or dinner)

(iii) General Criteria for Snack Size and Nutrient Composition

Snack at bedtime. Evening snack should provide a
simple sugar (quickly available source of glucose),
complex carbohydrate (intermediately available
source of glucose), and a protein or fat (slowly
available or prolonged source of glucose: 58% of
the protein molecule breaks down to glucose; 10%
of the fat molecule breaks down to glucose); this
regimen is recommended to prevent hypoglycemia
during the night or early morning hours

Example, apple, cheese and crackers

Snack for vigorous exercise (tennis, jogging, and so
on). Snack should provide simple sugar (quickly
available source of glucose); snacks with this nutrient composition should be consumed before, during, and sometimes after exercise

Example, natural fruit juices, lemonade, or even
sodas

Snack for moderate, prolonged exercise (golf, walking, housework, and so on). Snack should provide
complex carbohydrate and a protein or fat (see
bedtime snack) in order to provide extra glucose
over a period of time

Example, peanut butter and crackers plus a glass
of milk

(iv) General Recommendations for Exercise and Snack
Patterns. Perform same amount of exercise at ap-

proximately the same time each day. Carry a quick source of available glucose (candy, sugar cube) and complex carbohydrate (crackers) at all times so that hypoglycemia may be prevented, in case of unexpected activity

(d) Meal Plan. Conversion of the diet prescription into daily menus is accomplished by use of exchange lists for meal planning and food preferences

Specific exchange lists have been designed for diabetics; other lists are available for other disease conditions. Exchange lists for meal planning are substitute lists of foods with the same basic nutrients (carbohydrates, protein, fat, minerals, and vitamins) and calorie content. Foods within each group may be substituted for each other, but they *must not* be substituted for a food in another group (see Tables 5-5 to 5-8, and Appendix V)

(2) Noninsulin-Dependent Diabetics

(a) Meal Size. Determined the same way as for insulin-dependent diabetics; kilocalories available for meals usually less; client may have to reduce weight; glucose load during meals may still have to be controlled—even though exogenous insulin may not be needed—in order to prevent hyperglycemia because the endogenous source of insulin may be insufficient, delayed, or ineffective, even with the use of oral agents

(b) Time of Meals. Specific timing of meals is usually not necessary unless oral agents are being taken; clients are advised, however, not to skip meals, especially breakfast

(c) Number of Meals and Snacks (Meal Division). Strict division of kilocalories and carbohydrates between meals and snacks not usually necessary; client may be advised to eat only three meals a day in order to enhance weight reduction; snacks before exercise are only necessary when oral agents are used; noninsulin-dependent diabetics who require snacks before or during exercise are advised to use the same regimens recommended for insulin-dependent diabetics; moderate exercise for all noninsulin-dependent (obese) diabetics is encouraged as a means of augmenting weight reduction

(d) Meal Plan. Exchange lists for meal planning are advised, but other food plans may be followed; however, care should be taken that a variety of foods are consumed in order to provide adequate intake of macro- and micronutrients. Special foods (those containing sorbitol and others) are seldom needed if the individual chooses prudently the *amount* and *types* of foods eaten

   c. Enteral and Parenteral Nutritional Care Plans for All Diabetics
The same considerations are used when selecting an enteral feeding or parenteral solution for a diabetic as for any other individual (*e.g.*, which infusion route is available), except that the kilocalorie and nutrient content of the plan must be modified to meet the diabetic's individual diet prescription; insulin dosage may also have to be adjusted (consult Chap. 2 for details on enteral feedings and parenteral solutions)

Nutritional Care Plan and Drug Therapy Adjustments During Short-Term Complications of Diabetes Mellitus

Treating the short-term complications of diabetes requires the support of the complete medical team, especially the nurse. She must recognize when complications are imminent, recognize progressive symptoms, and institute treatment when necessary.

- Diabetic Ketoacidosis Coma
  1. Etiology. Undiagnosed diabetes, deliberate or accidental insulin omission, overeating without increasing insulin dosage, infection, vomiting, emergency surgery and others
  2. Progressive symptoms. Hyperglycemia (blood sugar levels of 400–800 mg/dl); others listed in Table 5-9
  3. Treatment
     a. Blood tested to estimate the severity of the emergency
     b. Insulin administered subcutaneously, or intravenously, depending on the client's needs
     c. Fluids and electrolytes replaced to relieve dehydration (4–8 liters of fluid plus electrolytes [K, Na, and P, especially] may be given, IV, the first 24 hr)
     d. Glucose (5%) given, IV, if hyperglycemia and glycosuria are diminished
     e. Oral feedings given as vomiting and nausea diminish: Usual progression is clear liquids (*e.g.*, broth, tea, and water); full liquids (*e.g.*, fruit juices and skim milk); soft diet in small feedings (usually given within 48 hr); regular meals within the patient's dietary prescription, with prescribed insulin; in some cases, to prevent future emergencies, the diet prescription and insulin dosage may have to be adjusted
- Hyperosmolar Nonketotic Coma
  1. Etiology. Undiagnosed noninsulin-dependent diabetes; noninsulin-dependent diabetes in client who is an older adult or experiencing extreme stress (*e.g.*, acute pancreatitis, myocardial infarc-

tion); may also occur in nondiabetic individuals receiving high intake of glucose (*e.g.*, TPN) or medications that reduce glucose tolerance

2. Progressive symptoms. Hyperglycemia (blood sugar levels of 600–3000 mg/dl), osmotic diuresis with accompanying dehydration; others listed in Table 5-9

3. Treatment. Same treatment progression used for ketoacidosis coma except that fluid replacement (hypotonic saline solutions) and insulin become the major priorities rather than diet; accurate fluid intake and output records are extremely important

- Hypoglycemia

    1. Characteristics. A symptom of a derangement in carbohydrate metabolism, usually defined as a blood glucose level of below 50 mg/dl (see Fig 5-2)

    2. General Symptoms. Sweating, weakness, hunger, tachycardia, inward trembling, unusual behavior, headache (see Table 5-9)

    3. Types

        a. Fasting Hypoglycemia

            (1) Etiology. Starvation, not eating enough but taking usual dosage of insulin, overadministration of insulin or oral agents, hypersecretion of insulin as a result of organic disorders in the pancreas or liver

            (2) Time Symptoms Usually Occur. Symptoms occur in "fasting" state, *usually 8 hours after eating* (at night or in early morning); symptoms progress if glucose is not consumed

            (3) Medical Treatment. Treat organic disorder, decrease dosage of medication, administer glucagon, give glucose and electrolytes by IV if individual is unconscious

            (4) Dietary Treatment. Give 5 to 15 g of carbohydrate in the form of direct sugar (*e.g.*, orange juice, tea, and sugar, hard candies) and follow with complex carbohydrates and protein (*e.g.*, milk and bread) for long-acting results

        b. Reactive or Functional Hypoglycemia*

---

* Functional hypoglycemia is a poorly understood disorder, which the American Diabetes Association, the Endocrine Society, the American Medical Association, and the American Dietetic Association decided warranted a "position paper." This paper was released, in 1973, by the American Dietetic Association and states,

After young or middle-aged people ingest a high carbohydrate meal (75 grams of glucose), it is not uncommon that the blood sugar decreases to levels below normal without the occurrence of any hypoglycemic symptoms. Even when low blood sugar can be demonstrated under these circumstances, it does not require treatment unless symptoms of hypoglycemia occur on a day-to-day basis when the patient ingests his usual diet. If these recurring symptoms can be relieved by food and a diagnosis of one of the common kinds of reactive hypoglycemia is made, the treatment is usually dietary.

(1) Etiology. Inherited metabolic disorders, gastrojejunosto-my, dumping syndrome, excessive intake of alcohol or caf-feine, crash dieting, stress (functional hypoglycemia)

(2) Time Symptoms Usually Occur. In the "fed" state, usually 2 to 4 hours after eating, but not in the fasting state; often subside spontaneously in 15 to 30 minutes; severity of the symptoms not progressive; attacks are more frequent when client is anxious or under stress

(3) Medical Treatment. Treat organic disorder, decrease dos-age of medication, administer glucagon, give glucose and electrolytes by IV if individual is unconscious

(4) Dietary Treatment

   (a) Caloric intake based upon individual's need to obtain or maintain ideal body weight

   (b) Small meals, 5 to 6 a day, rather than 3 large

   (c) Complex carbohydrates (75–100 g), and proteins (70–130 g) divided evenly throughout the 6 meals; fat makes up the remainder of calories

   (d) Natural sugars limited

   (e) Refined sugars, alcohol, and caffeine restricted

- Surgery. Regulation of glucose and insulin intake during emergency and elective surgery is the responsibility of the physician in most hospitals
- Infection and Febrile Illnesses
  1. Etiology. Same as for any other individual; concern is increased when the individual has diabetes because hormones (*e.g.*, epi-nephrine) released by stress decrease insulin release and insulin-receptor sensitivity. (Insulin receptors are located on the mem-branes of insulin-sensitive cells, including adipocytes, muscle cells, and monocytes; stress decreases their sensitivity. Ultimate-ly, the intracellular metabolism of glucose is impaired and blood glucose is increased [hyperglycemia])
  2. Treatment
     a. Medical. Same as for any individual, except that dehydration may be more severe and insulin may have to be increased or decreased according to the caloric adjustment; *insulin must still be taken*
     b. Dietary
        (1) Decrease caloric intake about 20% if fever is present
        (2) Give liquids frequently, including broth and fruit juices (these will replace not only fluid losses but also potassium and sodium losses)
        (3) Give only easily digested foods to prevent further vomiting and diarrhea

(4) Use regular sweets and sugar during illness to increase the ease of obtaining calories; however, must be taken in small doses (see list of Food Substitutions)

(5) Only necessary to consume the carbohydrate portion of the dietary prescription, which means that only the milk, bread, and fruit exchanges may have to be substituted (see list of Food Substitutions)

(6) If complications persist, consult a physician

Food Substitutions During Illness

Substitutions for difficult-to-digest foods

Fruit juices or soft drinks in place of whole fruit

Cooked cereals diluted with milk allowance

Milk toast made from bread and milk allowance

Cream soup using potato and vegetables (bread and milk allowance)

Eggs or cottage cheese in place of meat

Puddings or custards (milk and meat allowance)

Noodles and macaroni either in broth or in combination dishes using appropriate exchanges

Substitutions for carbohydrate exchanges

Substitutions for one fruit exchange (10 g of carbohydrate)

½ cup unsweetened orange juice or other juice

¼ cup grape juice

½ cup gingerale

2 tsp sugar

2 tsp honey, jelly, or jam

¼ cup regular Jell-O

6 Lifesavers

¼ twin Popsicle

2 unsweetened canned peach or pear halves

½ cup unsweetened applesauce or fruit cocktail

⅓ cup unsweetened apple, pineapple, apricot, or peach nectar

Substitutions for one milk exchange (12 g of carbohydrate)

1 cup skim or low-fat milk (whole milk contains fat, which may not be tolerated during illness)

1 cup artificially sweetened eggnog or cocoa (¼ cup dry skim or whole milk powder may be added to milk or other foods to increase carbohydrates)

1 cup commercial asparagus, chicken, or other creamed soup (to reconstitute, add equal amount of milk to contents of 1 can, or ½ cup

of milk to third of can—if soup is only reconstituted with water, it will provide only 5 g of carbohydrate or 1 vegetable exchange)

½ commercial twin pop bar

¼ cup instant or regular plain vanilla pudding or custard

Substitutions for one bread exchange (15 g of carbohydrate)

⅓ cup cranberry juice cocktail

½ cup regular cola-type beverage

½ cup instant or regular cream of wheat or rice cereal

5 small crackers

½ cup instant or regular rice or potatoes

¼ cup plain sherbet

⅓ cup sweetened gelatin

½ cup plain ice cream or ice milk

5 small vanilla wafers

Nutritional Care Plan Adjustments During Long-Term Complications of Diabetes Mellitus

Treating, controlling, and preventing the long-term complications of diabetes mellitus takes the support of the complete medical team. The scope of this book does not permit discussion of the nutritional care plans recommended for all these complications (*e.g.*, neuropathy, nephropathy, and retinopathy). Nutritional care plans for other complications such as coronary heart disease, stroke, atherosclerosis, hypertension, and gestational diabetes are discussed in other chapters. Keep in mind that nutritional care plans may need to be modified for both the primary disease (diabetes) and the secondary disease.

Nurses' Responsibilities in the Nutritional Care of the Client with Diabetes Mellitus

- Oral Nutritional Care Plans
  1. Initiate Good Care
     Procure trained professional instructions and dietary adaptation suggestions immediately following diagnosis. Converting the diet prescription into exchange lists for meal planning is difficult for most individuals to understand. If understanding is not clear at the beginning of care, the client is apt to become discouraged and unresponsive toward diet as a means of treatment in the future.

2. Participate in Care

   a. Weigh client in the office or outclient clinic and upon admittance. Weigh frequently after diagnosis to check progress and compliance.

   b. Still the fears of the client that he will never be able to eat normal foods again—a good teaching tool to alleviate these feelings of apprehension is shown in Tables 5-7 and 5-8.

   c. Encourage client to eat all the food on his tray, especially carbohydrate foods, but not to overeat.

   d. Motivate this behavioral adaptation by comparing food's relation to the necessity of use and dosage of insulin.

   e. Watch carefully for noncompliance. Check food consumption of insulin-dependent diabetics, especially carbohydrate foods. Make up lack through the use of orange juice, crackers, and so on.

   f. Enhance acceptance of the new nutritional care plan by making sure foods are palatable. Serve hot foods hot, cold foods cold, and so on.

   g. Modify the nutritional care plan during short-term illnesses. Use the guide for food consumption during illness to modify the plan (see list of Food Substitutions).

3. Coordinate Care

The overall responsibility of the nurse to the diabetic client is to help him achieve and maintain dietary compliance.

   a. Organize and contribute to health-team conferences.

   b. Obtain and report information such as the client's usual eating and drinking habits (*e.g.*, place of eating, time of eating, "special" foods that he likes which he now feels are restricted). Additionally, relate any complaints, requests, hopes, and expectations he has about his nutritional care plan so that treatment can be focused on his needs.

   c. Obtain new laboratory data (*e.g.*, lower or higher blood or urine sugars); new treatment plans (*e.g.*, introduction of insulin); and other factors that may influence food consumption.

4. Reinforce and Follow Up Care

   a. Compliment the noninsulin-dependent client who has lost weight. Provide motivation for continued compliance by relating weight loss to possible delayed progression of complications (*e.g.*, atherosclerosis or hypertension).

   b. Obtain a working knowledge of how the diet prescription can be calculated into exchange lists for meal planning by studying the hospital diet manual, the diabetic exchange lists for meal planning (see Appendix V), and booklets published by the American Diabetic Association and the American Dietetic Association).

c. In the hospital, check the client's knowledge of these exchange lists by having him choose foods available on the menu that will fit into his meal plan and reviewing the amount of food he is allowed (in other words, does he know what an ounce of meat looks like, a half-cup of fruit, and so on?)

d. In the outclient clinic or doctor's office, continually check the client's knowledge of his individual plan and advance his knowledge by helping him select foods that fit into his cultural, social, economic, and lifestyle habits. Insulin-dependent diabetics, during outclient care, should have special reinforcement of the relation of insulin to food (not too much food or too much insulin at any one time), the relation of exercise to insulin (the importance of ready snacks), and what foods contain recognizable and hidden sources of natural and refined sugars.

• Enteral and Parenteral Care Plans
Nurses' responsibilities to diabetes mellitus clients on specialized care plans are the same as those for any individual receiving these care plans, except that composition of the feedings receives special emphasis so they fit into the client's particular diet prescription (consult Chap. 2 for details of responsibilities).

Table 5-1
Insulins Available in the United States and Their Selected Characteristic Actions on Circulating Glucose Concentration (listed by manufacturer)

Onset of Action	Lilly	Nordisk	Novo	Squibb	Peak Effect (hr)		Duration of Action (hr)	
					Initial Rx*	Chronic Rx*	Initial Rx*	Chronic Rx*
Rapid	Iletin Regular[1,2,3]	Quick (regular)[4]	Actrapid (regular)[4]	Regular[7]	2-3	5-6	6	16-17
	Iletin Semilente[3]		Semitard (Semilente)[4]	Semilente[8]	3-6		12	
Combined		Mixtard (30% regular,[4] 70% NPH)						
Intermediate	Iletin NPH[1,2,3]	Insulatard NPH[4]	Monotard (Lente)[4]	Isophane (NPH[7])	6-12	10-12	14-24	24-26
	Iletin Lente[1,2,3]		Lentard (Lente)[5]	Lente[8]	8-14	10-12	18-24	24-26
				Globin[7]	6-8		18	
Slow (long)	Iletin Ultralente[3]		Ultratard (Ultralente)[6]	Ultralente[8]	20-30		36	
	Iletin PZI[1,2,3]			PZI[7]	16-24		36	

(continued)

Table 5-1 201

Table 5-1
Insulins Available in the United States and Their Selected Characteristic Actions on Circulating Glucose Concentration (listed by manufacturer) (continued)

* Initial Rx refers to patients receiving their first insulin injections, and chronic Rx refers to patients receiving their insulin injections for longer than 2 years. This has to be confirmed for the purified insulin preparations.

† Neutral Protamine Hagedorn

‡ Protamine Zinc Insulin

1 Purified pork (<10 ppm)

2 Purified beef (<10 ppm)

3 Single peak beef-pork (<50 ppm)

4 Purified pork (<5 ppm)

5 Purified beef-pork (<5 ppm)

6 Purified beef (<5 ppm)

7 Beef-pork (<10,000 ppm)

8 Beef (<10,000 ppm)

(Garber AJ, Owen OE: Diabetes mellitus and related disorders of carbohydrate metabolism. In Stein JH (ed): Internal Medicine. Boston, Little, Brown & Co, 1983)

Table 5-3
Comparison of the Current American Diet, the Newer Diabetic Diet, and the United States Dietary Goals

Nutrient	Current American Diet (%)	Newer Diabetic Diet (%)	U.S. Dietary Goals (%)
Total Calories	Excessive	Reduce or increase to achieve and maintain ideal body weight	Same as Diabetic Diet
Total Protein (% of calories)	12	12–24	12
Total Carbohydrate (% of calories)	40–46	45–55	58
Complex (starch and fiber)	22	30–45	48 (complex and natural)
Natural sugars	6	5–15	
Refined sugars	18	None allowed	10
Total Fat (% of calories)	40–42	25–35	30
Saturated	16	12–18	10
Monounsaturated	19	12–18 (mono- and polyunsaturated)	10
Polyunsaturated	7		10

(Senate Committee on Nutritional and Human Needs: Dietary Goals for the United States, 2nd ed [Washington, DC, US Government Printing Office, 1977]; American Diabetes Association and American Dietetic Association: A Guide for Professionals: The Effective Application of "Exchange List for Meal Planning" [New York, American Diabetes Association, 1977])

Table 5-4 203

Table 5-4
**Comparison of Insulin-Dependent and
Noninsulin-Dependent (Overweight) Nutritional Care Plans**

Insulin-Dependent	Noninsulin-Dependent
1. Maintain nutritional status and feeling of well-being	1. Same as insulin-dependent
2. Increase calories to obtain ideal body weight or growth	2. Decrease calories to achieve and maintain ideal body weight
3. Consume the same amount of kilocalories, carbohydrate, protein, and fat every day	3. Caloric and nutrient intakes, on a day-to-day basis, are not as rigid as for insulin-dependent
4. Consume the same ratio of kilocalories, carbohydrate, protein, and fat in each meal, every day, to control blood sugar levels	4. Not necessary to divide caloric intake into distinct ratios of carbohydrate, protein, and fat in each meal, every day Caloric intake is restricted, however, to prevent weight gain
5. Control intake of total fat	5. Same as insulin-dependent
6. Time meals to type and dosage of insulin — *extremely* important	6. Skipping meals not recommended, but rigid timing of meals, unless oral agents are used, is not necessary
7. Increase number and frequency of meals to correlate with insulin action and prevent fluctuations in blood sugar	7. Increased numbers of meals discouraged in order to enhance weight reduction
8. Increase intake of food before exercise to treat, abort, or prevent hypoglycemia	8. Increasing food for exercise not necessary unless individual is taking oral agents
9. Use food lists for meal planning to calculate meal plans so that a variety of the same types of foods and nutrients will be consumed daily	9. Food lists for meal planning are recommended for calculating meal plans, but strict adherence is not necessary Refined sugar intake, however, should be limited
10. Individualize diet plan for ethnic and previous dietary habits — make as flexible as possible	10. Same as insulin-dependent
11. During illness, provide small frequent feedings of carbohydrates, or carbohydrate intravenously, to prevent diabetic ketoacidosis	11. Small frequent feedings during short-term illnesses are advisable but strict adherence is not necessary; individual usually ketosis-resistant
12. Follow-up care is necessary in order to clarify instructions, check progress, and provide encouragement	12. Same as for insulin-dependent

Table 5–5
Composition of Food Exchange Lists Used for Diabetic Meal Planning

List	Food	Measure	Carbohydrate (g)	Protein (g)	Fat (g)	Kilocalories
1	Milk, nonfat	0.24 L (1 c)	12	8		80
	Milk, 1% fat	0.24 L (1 c)	12	8	2.5	103
	Milk, 2% fat	0.24 L (1 c)	12	8	5	125
	Milk, whole	0.24 L (1 c)	12	8	10	170
2	Vegetable	0.12 L (½ c)	5	2		28
3	Fruit	Varies	10			40
4	Bread	Varies	15			68
5	Meat, lean	28 g (1 oz)		7	3	55
	Meat, medium fat	28 g (1 oz)		7	5.5	78
	Meat, high fat	28 g (1 oz)		7	8	100
6	Fat	Varies			5	45

(The exchange lists are based on material in the *Exchange Lists for Meal Planning* prepared by Committees of the American Diabetes Association, and the American Dietetic Association in cooperation with the National Institute of Arthritis, Metabolism and Digestive Diseases and the National Heart and Lung Institute, National Institutes of Health, Public Health Service, US Department of Health and Human Services)

Table 5–6 205

Table 5–6
Sample Division Into Meals and Snacks for Insulin-Dependent Diabetic Diet

Diet Prescription

Total kilocalories: 1800
Nutrient division: 20% protein (90 g); 50% carbohydrate (225 g); 30% fat (60 g)

Exchange Lists

Food	Total Exchanges per Day	Carbohydrate (g)	Protein (g)	Fat (g)
Milk, skim	2	24	16	
Vegetables	2	10	4	
Fruit	2	20		
Bread	11	165	22	
Meat (medium fat)*	7		49	35
Fat	5			25
Total distribution		219	91	60

Meals and Snacks†

Food	Breakfast	Lunch	Snack	Dinner	Snack
Milk, skim	½ cup		½ cup	½ cup	½ cup
Vegetables		1		1	
Fruit	1	1			
Bread	2	3	1	3	2

(continued)

Table 5-6
Sample Division Into Meals and Snacks for Insulin-Dependent Diabetic Diet (continued)

Food	Meals and Snacks†				
	Breakfast	Lunch	Snack	Dinner	Snack
Meat, medium fat	1	3		3	1
Fat		1	1	2	
Total CHO‡ (g)	46	60	21	56	36
Total kcal	261	536	153	581	249

* The fat content of protein foods has been calculated as medium fat for convenience—check exhange lists for meal planning for foods included in the lean-, medium-, and high-fat categories.
† This is only one of many variations for the division into meals and snacks of kilocalories, carbohydrates, and exchange lists for meal planning. In general, the division is determined by the number of kilocalories and carbohydrates available, type and dosage of insulin available, occupation, and food preferences. The insulin used in this variation would be an intermediate-acting or long-acting insulin. Breakfast, therefore, is very small since the onset of insulin action may take up to 2 hours.
‡ CHO = carbohydrate

Table 5–7 207

Table 5-7
**Conversion of an 1800-Kilocalorie Diet
Prescription Into a Typical American Meal Plan**

Food	Amount	Exchange	Protein (g)	S CHO (g)	C CHO (g)	S Fat (g)	PUFA (g)
Breakfast							
Orange juice	½ cup	1		10			
Farina	½ cup	1	2		15		
Whole-wheat toast	1 slice	1	2		15		
Corn oil margarine	1 tsp	1					5
Skim milk	½ cup	½	4	6			
Coffee or tea	unlimited						
Lunch							
Club sandwich							
Whole-wheat toast	3 slices	3	6		45		
Sliced turkey	3 ounces	3	21			15	
Lettuce and tomato	3 slices	1	2	5			
Mayonnaise	1 tsp	1					5
Apple	1 small	1		10			
Coffee or tea	unlimited						
Snack							
Popcorn (popped)	3 cups	1	2		15		
Corn oil margarine	1 tsp	1					5
Skim milk	½ cup	½	4	6			

(continued)

Table 5-7
**Conversion of an 1800-Kilocalorie Diet
Prescription Into a Typical American Meal Plan** (continued)

Food	Amount	Exchange	Protein (g)	S CHO (g)	C CHO (g)	S Fat (g)	PUFA (g)
Dinner							
Pot roast of beef	3 slices	3	21			15	
Baked potato	1 large	2	4		30		
Broccoli spears	½ cup	1	2	5			
Dinner roll	1 small	1	2		15		
Corn oil margarine	2 tsp	2					10
Skim milk	½ cup	½	4	6			
Coffee or tea	unlimited						
Snack							
Graham crackers	4	2	4		30		
Cottage cheese, creamed	¼ cup	1	7			5	
Skim milk	½ cup	½	4	6			

S CHO = simple carbohydrate, C CHO = complex carbohydrate, S Fat = saturated fat, PUFA = polyunsaturated fat.

Obtaining only 15% of carbohydrate kilocalories in the form of simple sugars is difficult. The only alternative would be to eat raw fruits and vegetables with skins and seeds. These foods contain cellulose and pectin, as well as natural sugars, so they may also be considered complex carbohydrates.

Table 5-8 209

Table 5-8
Conversion of an 1800-Kilocalorie Diet
Prescription Into an Ethnic (Italian) Meal Plan

Food	Amount	Exchange	Protein (g)	S CHO (g)	C CHO (g)	S Fat (g)	PUFA (g)
Breakfast							
Grapefruit	½	1		10			
Hard roll	1 large	2	4		30		
Corn oil margarine	1 tsp	1					5
Buttermilk, skim	½ cup	½	4	6			
Coffee	unlimited						
Lunch							
Italian grinder							
Italian bread	¼ loaf	3	6		45		
Italian cold cuts	2 slices	2	14			10	
Provolone cheese	1 slice	1	7			5	
Lettuce and tomato	3 slices	1	2	5			
Corn oil margarine	1 tsp	1					5
Sliced orange	1 small	1		10			
Coffee, espresso	unlimited						
Snack							
Italian bread	1 slice	1	2		15		
Corn oil margarine	1 tsp	1					5
Yogurt, skim milk	½ cup	½	4	6			

(continued)

Table 5–8
**Conversion of an 1800-Kilocalorie Diet
Prescription Into a Ethnic (Italian) Meal Plan** (continued)

Food	Amount	Exchange	Protein (g)	S CHO (g)	C CHO (g)	S Fat (g)	PUFA (g)
Dinner							
Meat balls and spaghetti							
Meat balls	3 medium	3	21			15	
Tomato sauce, no sugar	½ cup	1	2	5			
Spaghetti	1 cup	2	4		30		
Italian bread	1 slice	1	2		15		
Olive oil*	1 tsp	1					5
Corn oil margarine	1 tsp	1					5
Buttermilk, skim	½ cup	½	4	6			
Coffee, espresso	unlimited						
Snack							
Hard roll	1 large	2	4		30		
Ricotta, cheese	1 ounce	1	7			5	
Yogurt, skim	½ cup	½	4	6			

S CHO = simple carbohydrate, C CHO = complex carbohydrate, S Fat = saturated fat, PUFA = polyunsaturated fat
* Olive oil is actually a monounsaturated fat, not a polyunsaturated fat

Table 5-9 211

Table 5-9
Signs and Symptoms of Diabetic Ketoacidosis (DKA); Hyperglycemic, Hyperosmolar Nonketotic Coma (HHNK); and Hypoglycemia

Findings	DKA	HHNK	Hypoglycemia
Onset	Gradual — hours or days	Gradual — hours or days	Rapid — minutes
Urine			
Output	Copious	Copious	Normal variation
Test for sugar	Strongly positive	Strongly positive	Not diagnostic
Test for ketones	Strongly positive	Negative	Not diagnostic
Appearance	Flushed		Pale, cold sweat
Respiration	May be deep and rapid (Kussmahl respiration)		Normal
GI	Nausea, vomiting		Hunger, sometimes nausea
Hydration	Dehydrated	Dehydrated	Normal
Sensorium	Drowsiness progressing to unconsciousness	Drowsiness progressing to unconsciousness	Dizziness, nervousness, staggering gait, inappropriate behavior, drowsiness progressing to unconsciousness, convulsions
Other	Fruity or acetone odor of breath		Lack of "squint reflex" (no squinting response when strong flashlight is beamed over closed eyelids of sleeping individual)

(Suitor CW, Hunter MF: Nutrition: Principles and Application in Health Promotion. Philadelphia, JB Lippincott, 1980)

Bibliography

American Diabetes Association: Principles of nutrition and dietary recommendations for individuals with diabetes mellitus: 1979. Diabetes 28:1027, 1979

American Diabetes Association and American Dietetic Association: A Guide for Professionals: The Effective Application of "Exchange Lists for Meal Planning." New York, American Diabetes Association, 1977

American Dietetic Association: Handbook of Clinical Dietetics. New Haven, Yale University Press, 1981

Anastasio P: New ways to control and manage diabetes. Environmental Nutrition 5:1, 1982

Anderson L, Dibble M, Turkki PR et al: Nutrition in Health and Disease, 17th ed. Philadelphia, JB Lippincott, 1982

Clarke WL: Continuous subcutaneous insulin infusion systems: A new approach to management of type 1 diabetes. Postgrad Med 73:319, 1983

Davidson JK: Controlling diabetes mellitus with diet therapy. Postgrad Med 59:114, 1976

El–Beheri Burgess BRB: Rationale for changes in the dietary management of diabetes. J Am Diet Assoc 81:258, 1982

Guthrie D: Helping the diabetic manage his self care. Nursing 80 10:57, 1980

Hansen B, Lernmark A, Nielsen JH et al: New approaches to therapy and diagnosis of diabetes. Diabetologia 22:61, 1982

Hunt SM, Groff JL, Holbrook JM: Nutrition: Principles and Clinical Practice. New York, John Wiley & Sons, 1980

Jenkins DJA, Taylor RH, Wolever TMS: The diabetic diet, dietary carbohydrate and differences in digestibility. Diabetologia 23:477, 1982

National Diabetes Data Group: Classification and diagnosis of diabetes mellitus and other categories of glucose intolerance. Diabetes 28:1039, 1979

Ney D, Stubblefield N, Fischer C: A tool for assessing compliance with a diet for diabetes. J Am Diet Assoc 82:287, 1983

Olefsky JM, Crapo P: Fructose, xylitol, and sorbitol. Diabetes Care 3:390, 1980

Owen OE, Boden G, Shuman CR: Managing insulin-dependent diabetic patients. Postgrad Med 59:127, 1976

Poplin LE: Diabetes that first occurs in older people. Nutr Today 17:4, 1982

Prater B: Education guidelines for self-care living with diabetes. J Am Diet Assoc 82:283, 1983

Reaven GM: Therapeutic approaches to reducing insulin resistance in patients with noninsulin-dependent diabetes mellitus. Am J Med 74:109, 1983

Rosett JW: Development of new educational strategies for the person with diabetes. J Am Diet Assoc 81:243, 1982

Shuman, CR: Pharmacological data on the sulfonylureas. Medical Times 108:79, 1980

Special Report: Principles of nutrition and dietary recommendations for patients with diabetes mellitus: 1971. Diabetes 20:633, 1971

Suitor CW, Hunter MF: Nutrition: Principles and Application in Health Promotion. Philadelphia, JB Lippincott, 1980

Thiele VF: Clinical Nutrition, 2nd ed St Louis, CV Mosby, 1980

Whitehouse FW: Classification and pathogenesis of the diabetes syndrome: A historical perspective. J Am Diet Assoc 81:243, 1982

Suggested Readings

American Diabetes Association and American Dietetic Association: Exchange Lists for Meal Planning. New York, American Diabetes Association, (1 West 48th Street), 1976

American Diabetes Association and American Dietetic Association: Family Cookbook. Englewood Cliffs, Prentice-Hall, 1980

Covelli P: New hope for diabetics. New York Times Newspaper March 8:62, 1981

Dwyer LS, Fralin FG: Simplified meal planning for hard to teach patients. Am J Nurs 74:664, 1974

Labrenz JB: Planning meals for the backpacker with diabetes—Nutritional values of freeze-dried foods. J Am Diet Assoc 61:42, 1972

Senate Committee on Nutritional and Human Needs: Dietary Goals for the United States, 2nd ed. Washington, DC, US Government Printing Office, 1977 (Pub No 052-070-04376-8)

chapter 6

Obesity

Description

- Overweight. A condition 10% to 19% above ideal body weight (IBW) for sex and age
- Obesity. An abnormal accumulation of fat in body tissue, generally 20% or more above IBW for sex and age; in some people, especially athletes, however, excess weight may be lean, not adipose, tissue

Incidence

- Number 1 United States nutritional disorder
- Overall national incidence, 50–80 million Americans, depending on method of measurement
- United States Health and Nutrition Examination Survey (HANES), 1971–1974, skinfold thickness statistics
    18% of all men aged 20–74 are overweight
    14% of all men aged 20–74 are obese
    13% of all women aged 20–74 are overweight
    24% of all women aged 20–74 are obese

Etiologic Risk Factors

See Table 6-1.*

Classifications and Characteristics

See Table 6-2.

---

* See tables at the end of this chapter.

Medical Treatment

The best medical treatment is prevention. Educate parents to prevent developmental obesity; educate teenagers and others to prevent adult-onset obesity. Psychiatric treatment may be helpful in preventing reactive obesity.

Surgical Treatment

- Criteria for Initiating Surgical Treatment
    1. Surgical procedures are performed only when all other attempts to control weight have failed.
    2. Client is 100 to 300 pounds above IBW.
    3. Client has a chronic condition, in addition to his obesity, that may shorten his life span (*e.g.*, hypertension, diabetes).
    4. Client is not over 50 years of age.
    5. Client has no history of alcoholism, psychiatric disorders, or renal or liver dysfunction.
    6. Client is highly motivated and willing to commit himself to extensive follow-up care.
- Goals. Increase satiety so that food ingestion is decreased, or decrease absorption of energy-producing nutrients so that energy storage (fat) is decreased.
- Surgical and Other Procedures. Dental splinting (commonly called "wiring the jaw"), suctioning (a salt solution is injected into a patch of fat cells, which ruptures the cells, and the liquid fat is "vacuumed out"), truncal vagotomy, gastric partitioning or gastroplasty (commonly called "gastric stapling"), wrapping the stomach in a polypropylene mesh, gastric bypass, jejunoileal bypass, and others
- Possible Complications. Diarrhea; steatorrhea; vomiting; psychiatric disorders; liver, renal, and gallbladder disorders; mineral or vitamin deficiencies and imbalances; peripheral nerve damage (suctioning); and many others
- Complications Related to Obesity That May Be Lessened or Prevented by Surgery. Cancer, hypertension, atherosclerosis, respiratory disorders (*e.g.*, pickwickian syndrome), degenerative arthritis, gout, skin irritations, and a shortened life span

Drug Therapy

See Table 6-3.

Diet Therapy

Goals for Juvenile- and Adult-Onset Obesity

- Promote a gradual weight loss (1–2 lb/wk) by altering nutrient intake, eating habits, and exercise patterns
- Maintain weight loss by motivating, educating, guiding, and supporting the client's own control over his body weight
- Prevent or delay the complications related to obesity, such as hypertension and diabetes mellitus
- Promote palatability by individualizing the diet prescription and meal plans

Nutritional Care Plan

Factors in Developing a Nutritional Care Plan for Juvenile- or Adult-Onset Obesity

- Interview Chart (Components With Special Significance)
  1. Age. Childhood obesity is more severe and more difficult to treat than adult-onset obesity; nurse should find out how long an adult has considered himself obese
  2. Sex. Determines kilocalorie restrictions needed
  3. Ethnic and Religious Background. Determines what foods to include in the meal plan, whenever possible, and what foods to omit
  4. Diagnosis and Medical History. Additional nutritional alterations may be necessary if other disease conditions such as hypertension and diabetes mellitus exist
  5. Medications. Some medications promote weight gain (*e.g.*, progesterone, estrogen, oral contraceptives, and cortisone); however, a client's having tried appetite depressants may indicate a motivation to try to control body weight
  6. Allergies. Food aversions and allergies must be considered in meal plan
  7. Special Diets. Client's motivation to control his own body weight may be low if previous attempts to diet have failed; fasting under medical care may be beneficial to enhance motivation; a history of "fad diets" may indicate interest in weight or misconceptions about how fast weight should be lost
  8. Appetite. May indicate whether the client is really hungry or eats according to external cues; keep in mind that actual appetite may not be revealed
  9. Mental Status. If client is anxious or depressed over other disease conditions or personal problems, nutritional treatment may

best be curtailed until after these conditions have been alleviated; some individuals find nutritional alterations extremely frustrating and depressing

- Nutritional Assessment (Data With Special Significance)
  1. Diet History. During the interview, special emphasis is placed on what and how much the client eats (*e.g.*, sweets, fried foods, fatty foods, and alcohol); why he eats (*e.g.*, is he motivated by his emotional state?); when he eats (*e.g.*, does he indulge in excessive nighttime eating?); where he eats (*e.g.*, in a room other than the usual dining area; in restaurants); with whom he eats (*e.g.*, does he have pleasant or nagging company?); how often he eats (*e.g.*, does he skip meals or consume meals plus snacks?)
  2. Vital Signs
     a. Blood Pressure. Obesity may precipitate hypertension
     b. Respiration. Severe obesity may precipitate respiratory problems
  3. Anthropometric Measurements
     a. Height and Weight. Present, usual, weight at 25 (if applicable), ideal; the single most important goal of all treatments is to achieve IBW or desired weight (if IBW is unrealistic, desired weight may be a more reasonable goal)
     b. Total Body Weight. This measurement and the percent of weight that is adipose tissue determine the severity of the condition and form of treatment
        (1) Methodology Used to Measure Total Body Weight
            (a) Adults and children over 3 years of age. Weigh individual on a beam scale (consult Chap. 1 for details)
            (b) Children under 3 years of age. Measure recumbent length, head circumference, weight on gram scale (infants)
        (2) To Determine What Portion of Total Body Weight Is Adipose Tissue (Adults and Children)*
            (a) Measure triceps skinfold (to determine subcutaneous fat stores)
            (b) Measure mid-arm muscle circumference (MAMC; to determine lean body mass)
            (c) Measure weight by densitometry (measures body fat and body water by specific gravity)
            (d) Measure weight using dilution methods (such measures determine body water)

---

* Consult Chapter 1 for details on how these measurements are obtained and compared to percentiles.

(e) Measure weight by total body potassium estimation (these measures determine lean body weight)

4. Laboratory Data

   a. Blood Glucose Levels. Hyperinsulinemia may have caused weight gain; obesity may precipitate noninsulin-dependent diabetes mellitus; endogenous insulin may be insufficient or ineffective — exogenous insulin may be needed

   b. Cholesterol and Triglycerides. Obesity causes increased levels of cholesterol and triglycerides in many individuals; these high levels may precipitate atherosclerosis; losing weight usually lowers blood levels of cholesterol and triglycerides; strong motivating factor for most clients

   c. Factors to Monitor During Treatment of Obesity (especially during fasting)

      (1) Resting and exercise electrocardiogram (EKG). Rapid weight loss can cause electrolyte imbalances that are detected by an EKG

      (2) Uric acid. Levels will rise if weight loss is rapid; indicates lean tissue depletion, manifested clinically by signs of gout

      (3) Hypokalemia. Indicates lean tissue is being depleted

      (4) Hematocrit. High levels indicate excessive water loss (dehydration). Reduced plasma volume may cause postural hypotension

      (5) Ketones. High levels in the urine or blood indicate fatty tissue depletion (lipolysis)

      (6) Urinary nitrogen. High levels indicate lean tissue depletion, may level as weight loss continues; protein-sparing fasts reduce lean tissue depletion

5. Clinical Evaluation

   Looking at a client is still a reliable way to determine the degree of overweight. Also, observe for the presence of other oral habits, such as gum chewing, nail biting, and smoking. Observe any signs of emotional disturbances: depression, anxiety, frustration, and poor body image (may lead to anorexia nervosa).

Nutritional Care Plan Alterations in Juvenile- and Adult-Onset Obesity

Treatment of obesity should not be thought of merely as a matter of willpower, nor should it be treated merely by altering kilocalorie intake. Instead, the health team should take into account the multiple factors such as emotions, eating habits, and exercise patterns that influence caloric intake. After considering all these factors, members of the health team should then motivate, guide, and support the client in a nonthreatening, nonjudgmental manner while he is modifying or controlling his own condition.

- Fasting
    1. Purpose. To obtain quick weight loss when the condition is resistant to all other forms of treatment; fasting should never be instituted unless the client can be placed under proper medical guidance, preferably in a hospital setting
    2. Types
        a. Total fast
            (1) Total caloric intake is first cut to 2000 kcal/day, to test client's emotional stability under semifasting conditions
            (2) The kilocalorie intake is then established at 0 kcal; the only nutrients allowed are water and vitamin and mineral supplements (in some cases, tea and coffee also)
            (3) Following the fasting period, the kilocalorie intake is raised to 600 kcal until the client can tolerate more
        b. Protein-sparing fast
            (1) Same as (1) under Total Fast, above
            (2) Kilocalorie intake is established at 120 to 400 kcal; the only nutrients allowed are protein (40–100 g/day or 1.5 g/kg IBW), water, and vitamin and mineral supplements (in some cases, tea, coffee, lean meat, fish, skinless poultry, or shellfish allowed)
            (3) Following the fasting period, kilocalories are raised gradually (according to tolerance) until a desired kilocalorie rate is reached that will help continue or maintain weight loss
    3. Duration. Two to three weeks, followed by partial abstinence, 2 or 3 days a week, until desired weight is obtained
    4. Advantages. Promotes quick, extensive weight loss that motivates client to participate in more conventional obesity treatments and lessens or prevents complications related to obesity such as diabetes mellitus and hypertension; protein-sparing fast decreases loss of lean tissue mass
    5. Disadvantages. Promotes adverse side-effects such as light-headedness, weakness, constipation, fluid and electrolyte imbalances, gout, anemia, ketogenesis, hypotension, psychological disturbances (irritability and depression), vitamin and mineral deficiencies, and others; should not be used to treat children
- Balanced Low-Calorie Nutritional Care Plan
    1. Premise. Calories do count
        a. 3500 kcal or 14,700 kilojoules (KJ) = 1 lb
        b. Nutrients that contribute kilocalories are carbohydrates (1 g

= 4 kcal or 17 KJ); protein (1 g = 4 kcal or 17 KJ; fat (1 g = 9 kcal or 38 KJ)

  c. Alcohol contributes kilocalories (1 g = 7 kcal or 29 KJ)

  d. Vitamins and minerals do not contribute kilocalories; they provide only the "spark" necessary for heat or energy production

2. Diet Prescription. Individualized to induce a weight loss of 1 to 2 lb per week

  a. Caloric alterations are determined by

    (1) Establishing present weight (consult nutritional assessment measurements)

    (2) Establishing age at which obesity developed

    (3) Establishing individual's IBW

      (a) Compare individual's present weight to desired weights listed in the Metropolitan Life Insurance Height and Weight Charts (Appendix 1)

      (b) Estimate IBW (allow 100 lb for the first 5 feet for a female and 110 lb for a male; add 5 lb for each additional inch [or subtract 5 lb for each inch under 5 feet]; subtract 10% for a small frame or add 10% for a large frame; see Appendix I)

    (4) Establishing the individual's IBW in kilograms (1 lb = 2.2 kg)

    (5) Establishing the individual's daily basal caloric needs (*i.e.*, 1 kcal is needed for every kg of IBW/hr; see chart on Determination of Caloric Alteration Level)

    (6) Establishing the individual's daily activity needs (see chart on Caloric Alteration and Table 6-9)

  b. Protein alterations

    (1) 20% of total kcal (normal is 12% of kcal)

    (2) Percentage of total kcal increased to provide satiety and ensure adequate vitamin and mineral intake

  c. Carbohydrate alterations

    (1) 45% to 55% of total kcal

    (2) Complex carbohydrate, 45% of total carbohydrate kcal

    (3) Dietary adaptations

      (a) *Limit* refined sugars and alcohol

      (b) *Increase* complex carbohydrates (*e.g.*, whole-grain breads and cereals and raw fruits and vegetables, which provide fewer concentrated calories, more satiety, and higher levels of vitamins and minerals)

    (4) If caloric restrictions are extreme, maintain minimum intake of 50 to 100 g daily to prevent ketosis

Determination of Caloric Alteration Level

Example, Medium frame, 5-ft 4-in woman
Determine ideal body weight (IBW)

5 ft	=	100 lb
1 in	=	5 lb
4 in	=	20 lb
IBW	=	120 lb

Determine daily caloric needs

120 lb	÷	2.2	=	55 kg
55 kg	×	24 hr	=	1320 kcal BMR*
30%†	×	1320	=	396 kcal of activity
		Total	=	1700 kcal (rounded) daily

Determine kilocalorie restriction to lose 1 lb weekly

1 lb = 3500 kcal
3500 ÷ 7 days = 500 kcal per day

Determine kilocalorie alteration level daily

1700 kcal − 500 kcal = 1200 kcal daily

---

* Basal metabolic rate
† Use 30% for light to moderate activity, 20% for sedentary activity, 40% for vigorous activity, and 50% for strenuous activity (see Table 6-9)

---

    d. Fat alterations

      (1) Fat contributes the remainder of total kilocalories allowed, 30% or less, depending on level of caloric alteration

      (2) Some fat intake should be allowed to provide satiety

      (3) Dietary adaptations

         (a) Limit margarine, cooking oils, fried foods, and gravies

         (b) Limit saturated fats if atherosclerosis is evident

    e. Vitamin and Mineral Alterations

      (1) Vitamin and mineral requirements may not be obtained when caloric alteration is severe; kilocalories must be obtained from nutrient-dense foods such as unsweetened fruits and whole-wheat products

      (2) Vitamin and mineral supplements, especially iron and thiamine, may be needed

  3. Meal Pattern. Individualized to enhance compliance

    a. Meal Size. Determined by diet prescription; usually smaller than before treatment began

    b. Time of Meals. Three meals a day, well spaced, to eliminate excessive hunger; eating at approximately the same time each day advisable, but flexibility is allowed; skipping meals, eating all the kilocalories allowed daily only in the evening, and binge-ing are *not* allowed

c. Number of Meals. Three small meals a day preferred; snacking creates temptation to overeat

d. Meal Plan. Nutrition tools used to convert the diet prescription into daily meal plans and menus include

(1) Basic Four Food Groups. Consult Table 6-4 and Chapter 1 for suggestions on how to use the Basic Four Food Groups when calculating a meal plan and individual menus

(2) Exchange Lists for Meal Planning. Consult Tables 6-5 and 6-6, Appendix V, and Chapter 5 for suggestions on how to use the exchange list for meal planning when calculating a meal plan and individual menus

(3) Recommended Daily Allowances. Consult Appendix IV, and Chapter 1 for suggestions on how to use recommended daily allowances when calculating a meal plan and individual menus

(4) Food Preferences and Aversions. Individual food preferences and aversions must be considered when using any nutrition tool to calculate meal plans and menus, or compliance will be short lived

- Elimination and Substitution Low-Calorie Regimens

1. Description. Based on the same premises as a balanced low-calorie nutritional care plan except the client is not given a specific dietary prescription; motivation is essential

Table 6–4
Basic Four Food Guide as an Instrument in Meal Planning

Sample Diet Prescription, 1200-Calorie Diet

Food	Serving Size	Number of Servings	Approximate Kilocalories*
Milk (whole)	1 cup	2	320
Meats, fish, poultry	1 oz	4	280
Egg	large	1	80
Breads or Cold	1 slice	4	315
Cereals	¾ cup		
Fruits	½ cup	2	100
Vegetables	½ cup	2	110
Total			1205

* Figures are slightly higher than those in exchange lists; individuals may consume fruits with higher contents of sugar, or other variations in calorie content may be present. If fats were desired to provide satiety, skim milk could be substituted (80 calories per cup *vs.* 160 calories for whole milk); approximately 4 teaspoons of margarine or oil could then be consumed (1 teaspoon = 45 kcal).

2. Methodology
   a. Client taught what foods contain excess calories that can increase weight gain gradually (Tables 6-7 and 6-8)
   b. Client taught how to substitute low-calorie foods for high-calorie foods (see list of Eating Habit Changes and chart of low-calorie substitutions)

Eating Habit Changes That Eliminate 100 Calories per Serving

Broil or bake foods instead or frying or breading

Drink skim milk instead of whole milk

Eliminate one slice of bread and margarine a day

Eat skimmed cottage cheese instead of cream cheese

Eat a salad, instead of pasta, as a side dish

Do not add sour cream to a baked potato

Use skim milk instead of cream in white sauces

Use low-calorie salad dressings or vinegar and lemon instead of creamed dressings

Drink coffee black; 4 cups a day with sugar adds up to 80 calories (1 tsp = 20 kcal)

Drink iced tea or unsweetened tomato juice instead of sweet soda drinks

---

Substitution of a Low-Calorie Food for a High-Calorie Food

Frozen apple pie, 1 piece

carbohydrate, 60 g × 4 calories/g	=	240 calories
protein, 3 g × 4 calories/g	=	12 calories
fat, 20 g × 9 calories/g	=	180 calories
TOTAL		432 calories

Apple, 1 large

carbohydrate, 33 g × 4 calories/g	=	132 calories
protein, 1 g × 4 calories/g	=	4 calories
fat, 1 g × 9 calories/g	=	9 calories
TOTAL		145 calories

---

   c. Client taught what low-calorie sweeteners and other low-calorie products may be substituted for natural sweeteners to enhance palatability while reducing caloric intake. Low-calorie sweeteners and other low-calorie products that may be substituted for natural sweeteners are

(1) Aspartame (APM; tradename Nutra Sweet), a dipeptide composed of two amino acids, aspartic acid and phenylalanine. One teaspoon equals one tenth of 1 calorie. One teaspoon of table sugar (sucrose) equals 16 to 20 calories. Nutra Sweet is added to some powdered drink mixes, presweetened cold cereals, instant puddings, gelatins, dessert toppings, and chewing gum. Additionally, Nutra Sweet is added to Equal, a new low-calorie, table-top sweetener. Equal is sold in boxes of individual packets. One packet has the same sweetening power as 2 teaspoons of table sugar (sucrose) and contains only 4 calories. *Caution.* Not recommended for individuals with phenylketonuria and may be toxic to clients with liver disease.

(2) Saccharin is derived chemically from phthalic anhydride, an organic compound. Saccharin is approximately 300 to 500 times sweeter than sucrose; thus 60 mg of saccharin equals 30 g of sucrose in sweetening power. Saccharin is added to baked goods and sodas. Additionally, it is sold in tablet form to be used as a table-top sweetener. *Caution.* Has been determined to cause cancer in laboratory animals.

(3) Sweet 'n Low is a blend of lactose (milk sugar), 4% soluble saccharin, and cream of tartar. One package has the sweetening power of 2 teaspoons of table sugar. Sweet 'n Low is added to some baked products, but it is mostly used as a substitute table-top sweetener. *Caution.* Sweet 'n Low should not be used imprudently by individuals with diabetes mellitus since it contains lactose, a sugar that can be metabolized to glucose in the human body.

(4) Polydextrose is a polymer prepared from dextrose and small amounts of sorbitol and citric acid. It contains only 1 calorie/g *versus* 4 calories/g of sucrose; however, it is not as sweet as sucrose. Polydextrose is used as a bulking agent in frozen desserts, cakes, salad dressings, chewing gum, and candies with a possible decrease in calories of 33% to 50% in some products when it is substituted for sucrose.

d. Client's knowledge reviewed and enhanced over time by follow-up visits, which enhance weight loss and maintenance

(1) Duration. Regimen usually necessary for lifetime unless individual has reactive or secondary obesity

(2) Advantages. Involves a gradual weight loss, teaches new eating habits gradually that can be followed for long periods, teaches wise food selections that help client control weight

- Lifestyle Alterations That Augment Low-Calorie Nutritional Care Plans

  Altering eating behavior as a means of treating obesity is based on the premise that behavioral changes not only enhance weight loss but also enable the individual to maintain the weight loss. The following behavioral changes may augment and support weight loss.

  1. Alterations in Eating Habits (Behavior Modifications)

     a. Shop for food right after you have eaten. Take a list. Do not be influenced by external cues such as the power of advertising and supermarket gimmicks (candy bars being placed temptingly next to the takeout counter where you have to wait). Read labels, look for hidden sources of calories. Avoid the tempting purchase of non-nutritious items.

     b. Plan meals the night before. Serve meals that are difficult to prepare—easily prepared meals tempt you to make extra amounts. Have other members of the family prepare meals if you nibble in the kitchen. Prepare small portions; do not allow for seconds.

     c. Serve food on small plates (portions look larger) in the kitchen instead of bringing serving dishes to the table.

     d. Drink a glass of water or eat your salad before the meal.

     e. Wait until everyone starts to eat before consuming your food. *Eat slowly*; put your utensils down between bites; swallow each mouthful of food before adding more food to your fork.

     f. Eat only in one room. Do not engage in other activities while eating such as reading or watching TV. Set the table every time you eat; this avoids snacking.

     g. Leave the table as soon as you are through eating. Clear and wash the dishes immediately.

     h. After meals, engage in activities that include moderate exercise or relieve tension such as sewing, knitting, or reading. Watching television may not be the ideal activity if commercials tempt you to eat.

     i. Join self-help groups such as Weight Watchers, The Diet Workshop Inc., TOPS (Take Off Pounds Sensibly), and Overeaters Anonymous. Once eating habits are under control, join community clubs that meet in the evening, to prevent slipping back into old eating habits, but do not eat the refreshments.

     j. Keep a food diary for at least 3 days, including 1 weekend day. An accurately kept diary can reveal your eating habits. It will also reveal the external or internal cues that trigger eating. Often these cues can be controlled when you become aware that they exist (see sample diary entry).

     k. Set up a reward system. Each week that you lose 1 or 2

One Entry in a Daily Food Diary

Day Tuesday

Time of day	Time spent eating	Food	Amount	Mood	Where	With whom	Activity	Calories
10 PM	5 min	Ice cream	1 cup	Bored	In front of TV set	Alone	Watching TV	278

pounds, treat yourself to a movie or the theater and, when weight loss is substantial, new clothes. If this sounds expensive, calculate how much you are saving by not purchasing snack foods and other high-calorie items.

2. Alterations in Exercise Patterns. Altering exercise patterns in order to augment weight loss is based upon the following premises:

a. Statistics indicate that sedentary living enhances weight gain and that obese people are more sedentary and move more slowly than others do. When an obese person merely changes very sedentary behavior to light or moderately active behavior, weight loss is enhanced (Table 6-9). For example, walk around the house to answer the telephone (remove telephone extensions); park the car in a lot that is farther from your destination; walk to work, if feasible.

b. Increased exercise enhances energy expenditure. When more calories are being burned, energy intake alterations will not need to be as severe.

c. Increased exercise creates a feeling of well-being. Exercise relieves the tensions and anxieties often experienced when low-calorie dietary regimens are first instituted.

d. Exercise helps to mobilize fat. Obese individuals who exercise will deplete adipose (fatty) tissue more than lean tissue.

e. Moving a greater weight for a given distance takes more energy than moving a lesser weight the same distance. Obese individuals moving the same distance burn up more calories than thinner people do.

   Example, 150-lb male burns up 105 calories walking 30 min at 2 mph; 225-lb male burns up 159 calories walking 30 min at 2 mph

   Example, 150-lb male burns up 201 calories walking 30 min at 4½ mph; 225-lb male burns up 294 calories walking 30 min at 4½ mph

f. Extensive exercise facilitates appetite control by suppressing appetite (decreases blood supply in the gastrointestinal tract). Obese individuals who *gradually* increase their activity to vigorous patterns will be able to increase calorie intake without enhancing appetite and weight gain.

- Unbalanced Low-Calorie Nutritional Care Plans ("Fad Diets")
  1. Statements commonly heard about fad diets (Table 6-10)
     a. "Eat all you want and still lose weight."
     b. "Lose weight while you continue to eat your favorite foods."
     c. "Lose weight quickly—lose 9 pounds in 2 days." (Recall how many calories constitute a pound. Is this statement believable?)
     d. "Lose weight quickly and change your life." (Weight loss does not automatically result in a life without problems. Dieters with such expectations usually gain back more weight than they lost.)
     e. "Let us tell you what to eat, when, so that no decisions are necessary on your part." (In this case, the individual never changes his eating behavior or exercise patterns. Consequently, weight is regained rapidly when the regimen is discontinued.)
  2. Factors to be evaluated before a new dietary regimen is begun
     a. Is the diet realistic?
     b. Does it suggest a physician's supervision?
     c. Are foods used in conjunction with drugs?
     d. Does the diet meet nutritional needs for all nutrients?
     e. Are alterations in eating behavior and exercise recommended?
     f. Will diet reduce scale weight by more than 1 to 2 pounds weekly?
     g. Does it state how much food should be consumed?
     h. Is it recommended for a lifetime or just for a short period?
- Self-Inflicted Starvation Regimens: Anorexia Nervosa
  1. Description. A psychological disorder in which the individual intentionally loses 25% to 35% of her ideal or usual body weight for height, sex, and age, resulting in cachexia
  2. Incidence. Highest in adolescent girls
  3. Etiologic Hypotheses. Underlying psychological problems that may precipitate metabolic disorders, disturbed patterns of family interest, or a strong desire to exert control over some aspect of life
  4. Characteristics
     a. Voluntary restriction of food intake, sometimes followed by impulsive ingestion of large amounts of foods (binge-ing) and then self-induced vomiting (purging); excessive preoccupation with weight loss and food

   b. Tension, distorted body image, compulsive physical and intellectual activity, perfectionist behavior, depression, and excessive use of laxatives and enemas

   c. Symptoms induced by persistent fasting and vomiting include: dehydration, electrolyte imbalances, malnutrition, esophageal irritation, dental erosion and decay, and endocrine and metabolic changes including menstrual disturbances (amenorrhea) and lower basal metabolic rates

5. Diet Therapy

   a. Goals. Nutritional care plans must provide a caloric content to enhance rapid weight gain, without which death may be imminent; individual must be under observation at all times if this weight gain is to be achieved

   b. Methodology. High-calorie parenteral solutions → high-calorie enteral feedings as a sole means of nutritional support or as meal supplements → high-protein, high-caloric liquid drinks with some solid foods at mealtime → solid foods with high nutrient-to-calorie density (consult Chap. 2 for the composition and administration of parenteral solutions and enteral feedings)

   c. Behavioral Modifications. Individual is allowed certain privileges (*e.g.*, going to bathroom alone) only when she eats and gains weight; treatment must be individualized and used with discretion, preferably under the observation of a psychiatrist

      Note. Individuals with *bulimia*, which is characterized by episodic patterns of binge eating (rapid consumption of large amounts of food in a short period of time), manifest characteristics and symptoms similar to those with anorexia nervosa, especially self-induced vomiting after a binge. Additionally, they fear that they will not be able to stop eating voluntarily, and they become severely depressed after a binge.

Nurses' Responsibilities in the Nutritional Care of the Obese Client

- Initiate Good Care

   Procure trained professional instruction and dietary adaptation suggestions immediately following the client's or physician's request for treatment. Professional advice is necessary in the beginning to help the individual convert the diet prescription or low-calorie substitution suggestions into palatable meals. Without this understanding, the client becomes discouraged and unresponsive. Procuring a dietitian's expert advice, however, although desirable, may not always be economically feasible in the physician's office, public schools, or industrial plants. Consequently, the nurse must take the initiative to teach the public how to lose weight sensibly and maintain weight loss. Special emphasis should be placed on guiding pregnant women, mothers of small infants, and teenagers, who represent the next generation, which may be either thin or obese, depending on the health-team's guidance.

- Participate in Care
    1. Set a good example. Achieve and maintain your own ideal body weight. This practice will enhance your client's respect, your own well-being, and your professional ability. Nursing is a demanding profession; carrying around extra weight will augment fatigue.
    2. Weigh client in the office or outclient clinic during appointment or upon admittance. Weigh frequently to check progress.
    3. In the hospital, watch for noncompliance. Is food being brought in from home or is client buying food from the "goodie wagon?" Encourage adherence by including the family in the treatment. Emphasize relation of ideal body weight to overall health, feeling of well-being, and mortality.
    4. In the hospital, enhance adherence to the new nutritional care plan by making the tray attractive and the food palatable. Serve hot foods hot, cold foods cold.
    5. In the community, enhance compliance by starting group sessions such as teenage clubs in the public schools. Include family members in these clubs whenever feasible, especially those who do the cooking.

- Coordinate Care
    The nurse has a pivotal role in helping the client achieve and maintain his ideal or desired body weight. Her role is to organize health-team conferences and to obtain, observe, and report subjective as well as objective information relevant to nutritional care.
    1. Subjective information. Appetite, motivation. Does client want to lose weight or is someone else urging him to lose weight? Is client a yo-yo dieter—has he lost weight before and regained it quickly? What and how much does the client usually eat? When does he eat? Where does he eat? With whom does he eat? How often does he eat? and so on
    2. Objective information. Present weight and recent weight gain or loss; present and past skinfold measurements; respiration and blood pressure; blood levels of cholesterol, triglycerides, uric acid, and potassium; acetone and nitrogen levels in the urine
    3. Clinical signs to be observed and reported. Mental status (signs of anxiety or irritability); oral habits (smoking, nail-biting); skin changes (may be caused by vitamin, mineral, or protein deficiencies); fatigue; postural or orthostatic hypotension on rising; and other noticeable findings

Increased Mortality With Rise in Weight by Cause of Death for Insured Men and Women*

IF YOU ARE	20% Above Average Weight		30% Above Average Weight		40% Above Average Weight		50% Above Average Weight	
YOUR CHANCE OF DEATH COMPARED TO NORMAL IS . . .								
	Men	Women	Men	Women	Men	Women	Men	Women
Cerebral Hemorrhage	8% higher	13% higher	37% higher	†	56% higher	†	†	†
Coronary Disease	19% higher	28% higher	44% higher	34% higher	58% higher	63% higher	75% higher	†
Diabetes	150% higher	75% higher	400% higher	†	†	†	†	†
Digestive Diseases	23% higher	30% higher	50% higher	†	120% higher	†	†	†

Note: This figure reflects provisional experience among insured lives from the 1979 Build and Blood Pressure Study covering the years 1954 through 1972. See Appendix for average weights of men and women.

* Women's mortality rates are substantially lower than men's. Thus, a given percentage increase in women's changes of death may reflect a much smaller increase in actual death rates.

† Too few cases for analysis

(Ad Hoc Committee of the New Build and Blood Pressure Study, Association of Life Insurance Medical Directors of America and Society of Actuaries, 1979)

- Reinforce and Follow Up Care
    1. Compliment weight loss and weight maintenance. Motivate continued adherence by relating weight loss to client's feeling of well-being, reduced blood pressure, and other beneficial effects (see chart on Increased Mortality).
    2. Obtain a working knowledge of how the diet prescription and low-calorie food substitutions can be converted into menus by studying the hospital diet manual, the Exchange Lists for Meal Planning, the Basic Four Food Groups, and reliable books on weight control (consult professional recommended reading lists before purchasing any books; use Tables 6-4 to 6-8 and lists on Eating Habits to Eliminate 100 Calories and Low-Calorie Substitutions as teaching tools, whenever applicable).
    3. In the hospital, check the client's dietary understanding. Have him choose foods available on the menu that fit into his meal plan; check his knowledge of the amount of food he is allowed (e.g., does he recognize that the amount of meat may be less than he normally consumes?).
    4. In the community
        a. Reinforce knowledge of individual plans and help clients select foods that fit into cultural, social, economic, and lifestyle habits

b. Motivate clients to continue exercising and increase their exercise, gradually; point out that weight loss makes extensive exercise easier to perform

c. Stay up-to-date on the latest fad diets being advocated; this is especially important with teenagers

d. Evaluate fad diets for unrealistic claims and convey your findings to your clients

e. Obtain knowledge about hidden calories in foods—read labels to find out how many calories are in common snack foods, for example; convey this information to your clients when applicable

f. Observe teenage clients for signs of self-inflicted starvation regimens (these signs can often be recognized during medical and dental examinations); suggest and initiate immediate care. Death may occur if care is not forthcoming

Table 6-1
Multiple Etiologic Risk Factors in Obesity

Genetic	Physiological	Psychosocial	Environmental
Somatotype Endomorph (round and plump) Laurence-Moon-Biedl syndrome	*Cytology* Hyperplasia and hypertrophy of adipose tissue cells Deficient brown adipose tissue deposits	*Emotions* Anger, boredom, depression, or loneliness may lead to overeating Poor body image and low self-esteem	*Sedentary Living* Energy intake exceeds energy output *External Cues* Sight, smell, taste, and availability of food
Parental Obesity Children born to 2 nonobese parents have a 7% incidence of obesity; children born to 2 obese parents have an 80% incidence of obesity (both genetic and environmental factors may be involved)	*Enzymatic Factors* Depressed levels of the "sodium pump" enzyme, sodium-potassium adenosine-triphosphatase (ATPase); high levels of lipoprotein lipase (under research)	*Reactive Obesity* Overeating related to stress, such as death, divorce, menopause *Economics* A higher incidence of obesity in lower economic groups	*Developmental Obesity* Overfeeding in childhood, bottle *vs.* breast feeding, feeding solid foods too soon, feeding to provide love and security *Technology* Use of labor-saving devices
	Hormonal Factors Low levels of thyroxin, growth hormone, and cholecystokynin; high levels of estrogen and insulin	*Eating Patterns* Cultural or traditional emphasis on large meals	*Alcohol Abuse* Alcohol is an appetite stimulant until intake is excessive

(continued)

Table 6-1 233

Table 6-1
Multiple Etiologic Risk Factors in Obesity (continued)

Genetic	Physiological	Psychosocial	Environmental
	Endocrine Disorders Froehlich's syndrome, Pradar–Labhart–Willi syndrome, Cushing's syndrome, hypothyroidism Destruction or tumor in the lateral feeding center or ventromedial satiety center of the brain ***Aging*** Basal metabolic rate (BMR) decreases with each decade ***Appetite Abnormalities*** Impaired interactions between neuropeptides, monoamines, and nutrients (under research)		

Table 6–2
Classifications and Characteristics of Obesity

Classification	Characteristics
Juvenile-onset obesity (also called metabolic, constitutional, and developmental obesity)	A child or an adult who has been obese since childhood Occurs in girls twice as often as in boys Hyperplasia (increased number of fat cells) Hypertrophy (increased size of fat cells) Excessive weight gain before age 10 Meal patterns characterized by large meals and snacks Difficult to lose weight and maintain weight loss
Adult-onset obesity (also called regulatory and reactive obesity)	Usually an adult in middle years Occurs in women twice as often as in men Hypertrophy (increased size of fat cells) Weight gain slow throughout adult years, unless obesity is reactive (owing to a specific stress, such as divorce) Meal patterns characterized by skipping breakfast and lunch and then eating throughout the evening (night-eating syndrome) Less difficult to treat than juvenile-onset obesity; client can lose weight more easily and maintain weight loss for longer periods

Table 6-3 235

Table 6-3
Medications Used to Treat Obesity*

Generic Name	Trade Name	Mechanism of Action	Adverse Side-Effects
Prescription Medications			
Amphetamines		*In general,* amphetamines	Palpitation
Dextroamphetamine sulfate	Dexedrine	Suppress appetite, stimulate	Tachycardia
Amphetamine sulfate	Benzedrine	the central nervous system,	Elevated blood pressure
Dextroamphetamine and am-	Obetrol	and elevate blood pressure	Overstimulation
phetamine sulfate plus dex-		Drug effectiveness may sub-	Euphoria
troamphetamine saccharate		side within a few weeks be-	Insomnia
and amphetamine aspartate		cause the body appears to	Dry mouth
Methamphetamine hydro-	Desoxyn	develop a tolerance	Dizziness
chloride		Drug dependence may	Diarrhea
		develop	Nervousness
			Others
Nonamphetamine anorexiants		*In general,* nonamphetamine	*In general,* adverse side-effects
Clortermine hydrochloride	Voranil	preparations have same	are the same as those in-
Benzphetamine hydrochlo-	Didrex	mechanism of action as am-	duced by amphetamine
ride		phetamines, except for	preparations.
Phenmetrazine hydrochlo-	Preludin	fenfluramine hydrochloride,	
ride		which appears to depress	
Diethylpropion hydrochlo-	Tepanil	the central nervous system	
ride			
Mazindol	Sanorex		

(continued)

Table 6-3
Medications Used to Treat Obesity* (continued)

Generic Name	Trade Name	Mechanism of Action	Adverse Side-Effects
Prescription Medications *(continued)*			
Phendimetrazine tartrate	Bontril PDM, Trimtabs		
Phentermine hydrochloride	Apidex-P, Fastin, T-Diet		
	Ionamin (resin)		Drowsiness
Fenfluramine hydrochloride	Pondimin		Constipation
			Depression
Nonprescription (over the counter) Diet Aids			
Phenylpropanolamine hydro-chloride	Dexatrim, Dietac, others. Several of these products are available with and without caffeine.	*In general*, mechanism of action is similar to that of amphetamines.	*In general*, adverse side-effects are similar to those induced by amphetamines.
Benzocaine	Ayds candies	Acts as a local anesthetic, which dulls the taste	Few adverse effects
Research Drugs			
Hydroxy citrate		Inhibits the formation of fat cells Blocks production of fat Reduces appetite	Adverse effects unknown as of 1983
Substance that will form a Teflon-like coating in the intestines		Will prevent the absorption of macronutrients that produce calories	Adverse effects unknown as of 1983

(continued)

Table 6-3 237

Table 6-3
Medications Used to Treat Obesity* (continued)

Generic Name	Trade Name	Mechanism of Action	Adverse Side-Effects
Research Drugs *(continued)*			
Naloxone		Endogenous opioid peptide antagonist	Adverse effects unknown as of 1983

* Bulk agents (*e.g.*, methylcellulose), diuretics, laxatives, and thyroid hormones have been used to promote weight loss. These medications can be dangerous to the health and should be used only under the supervision of a physician.

Table 6–5
1200-Calorie Diet Prescription Converted Into Exchange Lists for Meal Planning

Food	Amount per Serving	Number of Servings	CHO per Serving (g)	Protein per Serving (g)	Fat per Serving (g)	Calories per Serving	Total Calories
Skim milk	1 cup	2	12	8		80	160
Vegetable	½ cup	3	5	2		25	75
Fruit	½ cup or 1 small	3	10			40	120
Bread	1 slice						
Cereal		5	15	2		70	350
Hot	½ cup						
Cold	¾ cup						
Meat, medium fat	1 oz	5		7	5	75	375
Fat	1 tsp*	3			5	45	135
Total calories per day							1215

CHO = carbohydrate, g = grams, tsp = teaspoon
* Higher intake of cream and some salad dressings may be allowed. See Appendix V, Exchange Lists for Meal Planning

Table 6-6 239

Table 6-6
Sample Menu for 1200-Calorie Diet Based on Exchange List

Food	Amount per Serving	Number of Exchanges
Breakfast		
Grapefruit	½	1
Oatmeal (hot)	½ cup	1
Skim milk	1 cup	1
Coffee, black	unlimited	
Lunch		
Sliced turkey sandwich		
Turkey	2 oz	2
Whole-wheat bread	2 slices	2
Tomato and lettuce	3 slices	1
Mayonnaise	1 tsp	1
Blueberries	½ cup	1
Iced tea with lemon, no sugar	unlimited	
Dinner		
Cod fish fillet	3 oz	3
Boiled new potatoes	2 small	1
Margarine	1 tsp	1
Broccoli spears	½ cup	1
Tossed salad	small	1
Oil and vinegar	1 tsp	1
Cantaloupe	¼ small	1
Coffee or tea, no cream or sugar	unlimited	
Snack		
Graham crackers	2 small	1
Skim milk	1 cup	1

Table 6–7
Foods That Contain About 100 "Extra" Calories*

Food or Drink	Amount	Calories
Cream cheese	2 tablespoons	99
Chocolate chip cookies	2 average	104
Doughnut, plain Hostess	1 average	111
Crisco shortening	1 tablespoon	124
Triscuit crackers, Nabisco	4 pieces	84
Lollipop	1 medium	108
Pork link sausage	1 link	94
Mixed nuts, shelled	8–12 nuts	94
Coca-Cola	8 oz	96
Whisky (80 proof)	1½ oz	104

* 100 kcal × 30 days = 3000 kcal per month = approximately 1 lb per month; 1 lb per month × 12 months = 12 lb per year (Pennington JAT, Church HN: Food Values of Portions Commonly Used, 13th ed. Philadelphia, JB Lippincott, 1980)

Table 6–8
Foods That Contain About 500 "Extra" Calories*

Food or Drink	Amount	Calories
Cheese cake, Sara Lee	2 pieces	510
Ice cream (12% fat)	2 cups	556
Apple pie, homemade	1 piece	432
Burger King french fries	1 large serving	428
McDonalds, Big Mac	1 average	541
Pizza Hut, cheese pizza	3 pieces	450
Submarine sandwich, ham, salami, etc.	1 average	582
Milk shake, Borden (6% fat)	1 average	450
Eggnog with alcohol	1 cup eggnog, 1½ oz alcohol	446
Dairy Queen banana split	1 serving	540

* 500 kcal × 7 days = 3500 kcal per week = approximately 1 lb per week; 1 lb per week × 52 weeks = 52 lb per year (Pennington JAT, Church HN: Food Values of Portions Commonly Used, 13th ed. Philadelphia, JB Lippincott, 1980)

Table 6-9 241

Table 6-9
Caloric Expenditure for Various Activity Levels

Level of Activity	Type of Activity	Calories Used per Hour
Sedentary	Activities done while sitting that require minimal arm movement; *examples,* reading, writing, eating, watching television or listening to the radio, sewing, playing cards, typing, miscellaneous office work	80–100
Light	Activities done while sitting that are more strenuous, such as rapid typing; activities done while standing that require some arm movement; *examples,* household duties such as preparing and cooking food, washing dishes, dusting, and ironing; walking slowly; personal care; miscellaneous office work	110–160
Moderate	Activities done while sitting that require more vigorous arm movement; activities done while standing that require moderate arm movement, such as making beds, mopping, sweeping, light polishing and waxing, light gardening or carpentry work, walking moderately fast	170–240
Vigorous	Activities such as heavy scrubbing and waxing, hanging out clothes, stripping beds, walking fast, bowling, golfing, gardening	250–350
Strenuous	Activities such as swimming, tennis, running, bicycling, dancing, skiing, football	350+

(After Page L, Raper N: Food and Your Weight. Home and Garden Bulletin No 74, p 4. Washington, DC, US Department of Agriculture, 1973)

Table 6–10
Unbalanced Low-Calorie Nutritional Care Plans

Nutritional Care Plan	Comments	Adverse Side-Effects
High-Carbohydrate,Low-Protein, Low-Fat Diets		
Beverly Hills Drinking Man's Zen-Macrobiotic Fruitarian Pritikin Carbohydrate Craver's (to be released) Powders with a high percent of carbohydrate (*e.g.*, Cambridge Diet, Slim'Fast) Starch blockers (Calorex, Amylex, S.L.P.C., A.A.I., and Amy-less)	Consumption of the same types of foods becomes boring, resulting in reduced caloric intake. High-carbohydrate foods have fewer calories/g than do foods with a high-fat content; therefore, more food can be consumed without increasing the caloric content of the diet. Excess sugar in the diet can cause osmotic diarrhea—water is lost, scale weight goes down.	Gas and diarrhea, anemia, kwashiorkor, malnutrition, vitamin (B_{12}) and mineral (zinc and calcium) deficiencies may develop over time High intake of refined sugars may precipitate noninsulin-dependent diabetes mellitus Care plan should not be instituted during pregnancy—fetal growth will be impaired
High-Fat, Moderate-Protein, Low-Carbohydrate Diet		
Atkins Bio-Diet	High-fat intake increases satiety; less food is consumed. Insulin release is decreased—lypolysis increases—excessive amounts of free fatty acids are released into the blood. Incomplete oxidation of these acids causes an increased concentration of ketone bodies in the blood. Kidneys attempt to maintain acid-base balance by excreting these ketone bodies. Ketone bodies, water, and salts are released in excess—diuresis develops.	Dizziness, fatigue, irritability, nausea, excessive thirst, ketoacidosis, dehydration Blood levels of cholesterol and low-density lipoprotein increase—atherosclerosis may develop in time Vitamin and mineral deficiencies may develop Individuals with liver, kidney, or heart conditions should be advised not to use these diets

(continued)

Table 6–10 243

Table 6–10
Unbalanced Low-Calorie Nutritional Care Plans (continued)

Nutritional Care Plan	Comments	Adverse Side-Effects
High-Fat, Moderate-Protein, Low-Carbohydrate Diet *(continued)*	Additionally, without carbohydrate and insulin, glucose no longer enhances water retention, further increasing diuresis. End result: scale weight goes down.	
High-Protein, Low-Carbohydrate, Moderate-Fat Diet Stillman Scarsdale Last Chance Protein-modified fasts and formulas	Diet regimens usually tell the client what to eat and when; client has no decision to make. Increased numbers of solutes are excreted through the kidneys when individuals are on high-protein diets. Kidneys attempt to dilute them, and water, sodium, and potassium are lost in excess, with the result that scale weight goes down. Additionally, insulin release is decreased; ketoacidosis and reduced glycogen storage add to diuresis.	Fatigue, thirst, bad taste, foul breath (urea buildup), nausea, vomiting, diarrhea, irritability, postural hypotension, and dehydration Blood levels of low-density lipoproteins, cholesterol, and uric acid increase—atherosclerosis or gout may develop Blood levels of potassium decrease—tachycardia and cardiac arrest may occur Eating behavior remains unchanged, and weight is usually regained

Bibliography

American Dietetic Association: Statement on diet protein products. J Am Diet Assoc 73:547, 1978

Anderson L, Dibble MV, Turkki PR, et al: Nutrition in Health and Disease, 17th ed. Philadelphia, JB Lippincott, 1982

Bondy PK: Metabolic Obesity? N Engl J Med 303:1057, 1980

Bray GA: "Brown" tissue and metabolic obesity. Nutrition Today 17:23, 1982

Ferguson JM: Learning to eat: Behavior modification for weight control. Palo Alto, CA, Bull Publishing, 1975

Green ML, Harry J: Nutrition in Contemporary Nursing Practice. New York, John Wiley & Sons, 1981

Korcok M: Gastroplasty may lead field but it's not a winner yet. JAMA 246:2420, 1981

Larosa JC, Fry AG, Muesing R et al: Effects of high-protein, low-carbohydrate dieting on plasma lipoproteins and body weight. J Am Diet Assoc 77:264, 1980

Levine AS, Morley JE: The shortening pathways to appetite control. Nutrition Today 18:6, 1983

Marable NL, Hinners ML, Hardison NW et al: Protein quality of supplements and meal replacements. J Am Diet Assoc 77:270, 1980

Millman D: When thin is not beautiful: Anorexia nervosa. Med Times 109:71, 1981

Morley JE, Levine AS: The central control of appetite. Lancet 1:398, 1983

National Dairy Council: Energy balance throughout the life cycle. Dairy Council Digest 51:19, 1980

Page L, Raper N: Food and your weight. Home and Garden Bulletin No 74. Washington, DC, US Department of Agriculture, 1973

Pennington JAT, Church HN: Food Values of Portions Commonly Used, 13th ed. Philadelphia, JB Lippincott, 1980

Pi-Sunyer FX: Dietary practices in obesity. Bull NY Acad Med 58:263, 1982

Simonson M: An overview: Advances in research and treatment of obesity. Food and Nutrition News 53:1, 198 2

Van Itallie TB, Yang M–U: Current concepts in nutrition: Diet and weight loss. N Engl J Med 297:1158, 1977

Suggested Readings

American Diabetes Association and American Dietetic Association: Exchange Lists for Meal Planning. Chicago, IL, American Dietetic Association (430 North Michigan Ave) 1976

Better Homes and Gardens, (eds): Eat and Stay Thin, 2nd ed. Des Moines, Meredith Corporation, 1980

Brownell KD, Stunkard AJ: Couples training, pharmacotherapy and behavior therapy in the treatment of obesity. Arch Gen Psychiatry 38:1124, 1981

Danowski TS: Sustained Weight Control, the Individual Approach. Philadelphia, FA Davis, 1973

Edelstein B: Changing teenage eating behavior. Conn Med 45:496, 1981

Ikeda J: Change Your Habits to Change Your Shape—For Teenagers Only. Palo Alto, CA, Bull Publishing, 1978

Levitz LS: Behavior therapy in treating obesity. J Am Diet Assoc 62:22, 1973

Rynearson EH: Americans love hogwash. Nutr Rev (Suppl) 32:1, 1974

Stunkard A: I Almost Feel Thin. Palo Alto, CA, Bull Publishing, 1977

chapter 7

Gastrointestinal Tract

Description

The gastrointestinal tract is a tube that begins at the posterior region of the mouth, continues through the stomach and intestine, and terminates at the anus.

Functions

- Provides the chemical secretions, including enzymes and hormones, necessary for chemical digestion of food molecules
- Provides the neuromuscular functions necessary for mechanical digestion, which propels food along the gastrointestinal tract
- Provides the absorptive area and the nutrient carriers that enable end products of digestion to enter the body's circulatory system, which then delivers them to the body cells, where they can be utilized for energy and tissue synthesis

Etiologic Risk Factors

Etiologic Risk Factors for Gastrointestinal Dysfunctions

Psychosocial Factors

Disposition—anxious, aggressive, perfectionistic, compulsive
Skipping meals, eating on the run
Time oriented

Environmental Factors

Smoking

Poor eating habits—overindulgence in rich foods, eating more refined foods than nutrient-dense foods, consuming stimulative foods (*e.g.*, coffee) or drugs (*e.g.*, alcohol) without solid foods

Poor sanitation—microbial invasions enhance infections and inflammations

Excessive drug use—alcohol, antacids, aspirin, laxatives, vitamins, and minerals

Improper bowel habits

Drug Therapy

Consult Table 7-1.*

General Principles of Diet Therapy

Goals

- Alleviate or reduce pain and undesirable symptoms (*e.g.*, nausea, vomiting, and diarrhea)
- Give the dysfunctioning organ a complete rest or enable the damaged organ to function as easily and as efficiently as possible with the least amount of effort
- Restore damaged tissues by providing adequate calories and nutrients
- Maintain maximum nutritional status, which is accomplished by changing food consistency, limiting or eliminating nutrients that cause added distress, changing meal patterns to avoid over-distention, individualizing the diet to enhance palatability and consumption
- Long-term goal is to modify eating habits so that dysfunctions do not recur

General Nutritional Care Plan

General Factors in Developing a Nutritional Care Plan for Gastrointestinal Dysfunctions

- Interview Chart (Components With Special Significance)
  1. Age. Determines calories and nutrients needed to maintain or restore nutritional status and body tissues
  2. Sex. Same as for age

---

* See tables at the end of this chapter.

3. Ethnic and Religious Background. Determines what foods should be included in the meal plan, whenever possible, and what ones should be omitted to enhance consumption

4. Diagnosis and Medical History. Recurrent illnesses are often more severe; therefore, dietary restrictions may be more stringent; clients facing surgical procedures may need to have their nutritional status enhanced before surgery

5. Medications. Some medications taken for chronic illnesses (*e.g.*, antacids) may inhibit nutrient absorption or utilization; these interactions could impair nutritional status over time (see Table 7-1)

6. Allergies. Food allergies and aversions must be considered in the meal plan; eliminating certain foods (*e.g.*, dairy products in clients sensitive to lactose) may alleviate symptoms or improve condition; itching may indicate pending secondary organ (liver) dysfunction

7. Mastication or Swallowing Difficulties. May be the primary reason for dysfunction or secondary to other dysfunctions; in either case, eating patterns and food consistency must be altered, or nutritional status will be impaired

8. Special Diet. May help nurse judge client's present knowledge of dietary restrictions and degree of compliance; client may also have misconceptions about dietary restrictions that may be difficult to change (for example, clients who have been on conservative nutritional care plans may be afraid to try more liberal plans)

9. Appetite. Determines what meal plans must be adopted (*e.g.*, parenteral solutions, enteral feedings, or oral feedings), in order to meet nutritional needs

10. Mental Status. Anxious individuals will have increased difficulty adjusting to new nutritional care plans and should be reassured frequently that dietary treatment will enhance other treatments and recovery

- Nutritional Assessment (Data With Special Significance)
  1. Diet History. Personal interview with special emphasis on what foods cause pain or distress (liquids, solids, fatty foods, alcohol, and so on); when pain or distress occurs (*e.g.*, before or soon after eating; is pain relieved by food?); where client eats (*e.g.*, at home or at a fast-food establishment); how long he spends eating (eating on the run often impairs digestion); how often he eats (does he skip meals?); what medications seem to impair or enhance digestion

  2. Vital Signs. Temperature. Poor food sanitation may precipitate microbial invasion and infections that cause fevers

  3. Anthropometric Measurements
     a. Height and Weight. Present, usual, and ideal; determine extent of weight loss or gain

  b. Triceps Skinfold Test. Determines if weight loss is due to fatty tissue depletion

  c. Mid-arm Muscle Circumference Test. Determines if weight loss is due to lean tissue catabolism

4. Laboratory Data

  a. Blood

   (1) Hemoglobin and Hematocrit. Anemia is prevalent in clients with gastrointestinal dysfunctions because the ingestion or absorption of iron, folic acid, vitamin B_{12}, vitamin B_6, or protein may be impaired; in addition, excessive bleeding may deplete nutrient stores and blood volume

   (2) White Blood Count (WBC). High counts may indicate food poisoning or infection; low counts may indicate malnutrition

   (3) Fasting Blood Sugar Levels. High levels may indicate dysfunction secondary to diabetes mellitus

   (4) Blood Levels of Na, K, Cl, Ca, and P. Vomiting and diarrhea may cause decreased ingestion, digestion, and absorption of these nutrients; in addition, their excretion may be enhanced or impaired in some dysfunctions, which will affect the client's hydration

   (5) Albumin. Low levels indicate malnutrition and lean tissue depletion or decreased production (*e.g.,* liver disease)

   (6) Creatinine, Urea Nitrogen, and Serum Enzyme Levels. High levels indicate gastrointestinal dysfunctions secondary to other organ dysfunctions such as hepatic or renal disorders (*e.g.,* lactic dehydrogenase [LDH]; aspartate aminotransferase [AST], formerly known as serum glutamic oxalacetic transaminase [SGOT]; and alanine aminotransferase [ALT], formerly serum glutamic pyruvic transaminase [SGPT]).

   (7) Serum Levels of Vitamins and Minerals. Low levels may indicate malabsorption disorders; low levels of vitamin K may impair partial thromboplastin time (PTT)

  b. Urine

   (1) Urinary Nitrogen. Indicates the extent of lean tissue catabolism and effectiveness of treatment

   (2) Schilling Test. To diagnose vitamin B_{12} insufficiency; also indicates whether the dysfunction is gastric or small intestinal in origin

   (3) Urine Levels of Vitamins and Minerals. High levels may indicate malabsorption disorders; low levels indicate ingestion disorders or excretion disorders

      (4) Color. Changes in urine color (*e.g.*, brown) may indicate secondary organ (liver) dysfunction

   c. Stool Examination. Often denotes the location of the disorder, the severity of the dysfunction, and what nutrients must be avoided or replaced (see Table 7-4)

   d. Radiologic Examination. Diagnoses the origin of the disorder

   e. Specialized Diagnostic Examinations. Sigmoidoscopy and others diagnose the origin of the disorder so that proper treatment can be instituted

5. Clinical Evaluations

   a. Weight Loss. Excessive weight loss indicates severe ingestion, digestion, or absorption dysfunctions

   b. Skin. Dry skin or decubitus ulcer indicates nutrient deficiencies, especially of B-complex vitamins, vitamin C, fat-soluble vitamins, and protein; jaundice (yellow discoloration of the skin) indicates gallbladder or liver dysfunction

   c. Mouth. Red or swollen tongue or glossitis indicates vitamin B-complex deficiencies

   d. Mental Status. Irritability or mental confusion may indicate that some nutrients are not available for central nervous system function

Factors in Specific Gastrointestinal Dysfunctions

In addition to the general factors noted above, the following points are considered:

- Location of the dysfunction
- Normal functions of the organ involved
- Etiologic and risk factors
- Characteristics, symptoms, and clinical signs of the disorder
- Treatment of the disorder (*e.g.*, drug therapy, drug–diet interactions)

Mouth

Functions

- Mastication of food
- Production of saliva, which moistens food and facilitates swallowing
- Swallowing of food (the tongue pushes the bolus of food upward and backward into the pharynx)

Common Dysfunctions

Dental Caries

- Description. Bacterial decay that involves the loss of tooth structure
- Etiology. Initiation of decay depends on the interaction of several factors:
  1. A susceptible host
  2. Cariogenic bacteria
  3. A suitable substrate
  4. A sufficient period of time for fermentation
- Characteristics of the Decay Sequence
  1. Cariogenic bacteria react with a suitable substrate (sucrose) to form a plaque (a transparent gelatinous material)
  2. Plaque traps strains of bacteria that produce organic acids (*e.g.*, lactic acid)
  3. The acids formed dissolve the enamel minerals
  4. Tooth enamel is destroyed; decay is evident
- Symptom. Pain
- Dental Care. Prevention very important; plaque should be removed frequently
- Drug Therapy. No drug presently available to remove plaque
- Diet Therapy
  1. Nutritional Care Plan
     a. Methodology. Oral feedings
     b. Nutrients Increased. Protein; fat; complex carbohydrates with fiber; vitamins, especially A and D (from foods, not supplements); and minerals, especially iron, fluoride, calcium, and phosphorus
     c. Nutrients Decreased. Refined carbohydrates, especially those containing sucrose
     d. Dietary Adaptations.
        (1) Eat foods that promote chewing, such as meats, raw fruits and vegetables, and whole-wheat breads with crust (promotes saliva production, which can neutralize or dilute the acids formed in the plaque)
        (2) Eat only protein- or fat-containing foods between meals, such as cheese and peanuts
        (3) Limit refined sugar intake such as candy, sodas, and desserts
     e. Meal Plan Modifications. Limit snacks, especially those that contain refined carbohydrates

2. Behavioral Modifications
   a. Time is needed to ferment sugars and produce organic acids; to prevent this fermentation
      (1) Brush teeth after each meal and snack with a fluoride toothpaste
      (2) If brushing is not feasible after snacks, consume liquid snacks (not sweet sodas) rather than solid foods because liquids remain in the mouth for a shorter period of time
   b. Floss teeth at least once a day to help remove plaque

Dysfunctions Related to Cancer and Its Treatment

Altered taste, xerostomia (dry mouth), *stomatitis* (inflammation of the oral cavity), and *dysphagia* (difficulty swallowing). Consult Chapter 4 and Table 4-6 for dietary recommendations that may assist individuals with altered taste, xerostomia, and stomatitis. Consult Chapter 3 and Table 3-19 for dietary recommendations and behavioral techniques that will augment swallowing.

Esophagus

Functions

- The esophagus is a low-pressure tube protected by high-pressure valves called *sphincters.*
- Food is propelled down the esophagus by peristaltic waves and gravity to the lower esophageal sphincter (LES); the bolus of food and the swallowing act cause the LES to relax, and the sphincter opens.
- Food enters the stomach, after which the sphincter closes again and pressure is increased, preventing reflux of the gastric contents back into the esophagus.

Common Dysfunctions

Esophagitis or Gastroesophageal Reflux Disease ("Heartburn")

- Description. A syndrome that occurs when gastric or intestinal bile or pancreatic juices reflux into the esophagus
- Etiology. Obesity, pregnancy, possibly the aging process, tight-fitting garments
- Characteristics. Reflux is caused by a decrease in basal LES pres-

sure, which inhibits closing of the sphincter between swallows; decreased pressure may be caused by

1. An abnormal LES response to change in the intra-abdominal pressure
2. A decrease in gastrin (normally gastrin increases pressure)
3. An increase in secretin or cholecystokinin (normally these hormones decrease pressure)
4. A slow release of stomach contents

- Symptoms. Heartburn, dyspepsia, regurgitation, dysphagia, chest pain or esophageal spasm, symptoms from aspiration of regurgitated material
- Drug Therapy. Antacids (1 hr and 3 hr after meals and before bedtime), cholinergics, histamine blockers (see Table 7-1)
- Diet Therapy
  1. Acute Phase
     a. Nutritional Care Plan
        (1) Methodology. Oral feedings
        (2) Dietary Adaptations
           (a) Liquid diet, which is less abrasive
           (b) Foods allowed in this diet listed in Table 2-3
        (3) Meal Plan Modifications
           (a) Consume 6 small meals rather than 3 large meals
           (b) Avoid consuming foods for 2 to 4 hours before bedtime
     b. Behavioral Modifications
        (1) Consume liquids slowly
        (2) Eat slowly in a relaxed atmosphere
        (3) Avoid garments such as girdles and belts
        (4) Avoid bending and excessive exercise right after meals
        (5) Remain upright after meals
        (6) Sleep in an elevated position (extra pillows or wood blocks under the bedposts work well)
        (7) Cease smoking
  2. Chronic Phase
     a. Nutritional Care Plan
        (1) Methodology. Oral feedings
        (2) Nutrients Increased. Proteins and complex carbohydrates that increase LES pressure; total caloric intake decreased if individual is obese
        (3) Nutrients Decreased. Fats and refined carbohydrates that decrease LES pressure

(4) Dietary Adaptations

    (a) Limit or avoid foods that decrease LES pressure such as chocolate, coffee, tea, alcohol, peppermint and spearmint oils, fried foods, and all other fatty foods (*e.g.*, butter and margarine)

    (b) Increase foods that increase LES pressure, such as lean meats, fish, skim milk, and cheeses; substitute skim milk for whole milk

    (c) Limit or avoid foods that irritate the esophageal lining, such as coffee, citrus juices, and tomato juice

    (d) Limit foods that are high in calories, such as refined sugars; substitute complex carbohydrate foods (breads and cereals)

    (e) Increase vitamin supplements, if necessary, especially vitamin C

    (f) Limit or avoid all foods that cause distress

(5) Meal Plan Modifications

    (a) Same as Acute Phase

    (b) Also drink fluids only between meals

b. Behavioral Modifications

  (1) Chew foods thoroughly

  (2) Other modifications same as Acute Phase

Hiatal Hernia

- Description. An outpouching of a portion of the stomach through the diaphragm into the thoracic cavity
- Etiology. Gastric surgery; others the same as with esophagitis
- Characteristics. In one form of outpouching, a hiatal hernia may slide. Here part of the stomach, but not the esophagus, herniates through the diaphragm into the thorax. In another form of outpouching, gastroesophageal, the lower esophagus and part of the stomach protrude through the diaphragm into the thorax
- Symptoms. Same as those for esophagitis
- Drug and Diet Therapy. Same as for esophagitis

Achalasia (Esophageal Dyssynergia)

- Description. A disorder of lower esophageal motility
- Etiology. A neural disturbance dilates the esophagus; emotions or heredity may precipitate the condition

- Characteristics. Aperistalsis, elevated resting LES pressure, failure of the LES to relax completely, and esophageal dilatation
- Symptoms. Dysphagia, substernal pain following eating, regurgitation, weight loss, halitosis
- Drug Therapy. Same as for esophagitis and dysphagia
- Diet Therapy. Same as for esophagitis and dysphagia (consult Chap. 3 and Table 3-19 for dietary recommendations and behavioral techniques that will augment swallowing)

Stomach

Functions

- Receives and stores food for short periods of time; foodstuffs leave the stomach in the following order: liquids first, refined carbohydrates, complex carbohydrates, protein, fat, and mixed foods last; stomach empties in 1 to 4 hours, depending on amount and kinds of food eaten
- Secretes gastric juice, which contains hydrochloric acid (HCl), inorganic salts, water, mucin, intrinsic factor, and the enzymes rennin, pepsin, and gastric lipase; HCl enhances absorption of calcium, iron, and protein; intrinsic factor is necessary for absorption of vitamin B_{12}; rennin and pepsin are necessary for breakdown and absorption of protein
- Churns food mass into a semiliquid called *chyme*, which it releases, at certain intervals, into the duodenum

Common Dysfunctions

Acute Gastritis

- Description. A common dysfunction of the stomach marked by inflammation of the gastric mucosa; it may be acute or chronic
- Etiology. Dietary indiscretions such as overeating or drinking, eating too fast, eating when overtired or emotionally upset, eating rich or highly seasoned foods; eating contaminated foods
- Symptoms. Anorexia, nausea, vomiting, epigastric discomfort, and fever
- Drug Therapy. Emetic drugs and laxatives to rid the body of irritating foodstuffs or poisons

- Diet Therapy
  1. Acute Phase
     a. Nutritional Care Plan*
        (1) Methodology
            (a) Parenteral saline solutions for 24 to 48 hours
            (b) Oral feedings after 24 to 48 hours
     b. Behavioral Modifications. Rest
  2. Chronic Phase*
     a. Nutritional Care Plan
        (1) Methodology. Oral feedings
        (2) Nutrients Increased. All but fats
        (3) Nutrients Decreased. Fats
        (4) Dietary Adaptations
            (a) Avoid clear liquids (broth and others) because they stimulate gastric acid secretion
            (b) Give full liquids such as milk and cream soups (limit juices)
            (c) Progress to soft diet as time and tolerance increase
            (d) Progress to regular diet, eliminating foods known to cause distress (consult Chap. 2 for which foods are allowed on these diets and which should be avoided)
        (5) Meal Plan Modifications
            (a) Consume 6 small meals, rather than 3 large ones
            (b) Eat at regular times each day
     b. Behavioral Modifications
        (1) Eat more slowly, in a relaxed atmosphere
        (2) Chew foods well before swallowing
        (3) Store and prepare foods in a sanitary manner

Peptic Ulcer

- Description. A lesion occurring in either the stomach (gastric ulcer) or the duodenum (duodenal ulcer)

---

* If condition becomes chronic, it may be secondary to other diseases such as carcinoma of the stomach, pernicious anemia, or gastric ulcer. In this case, the primary disease as well as the gastritis must be treated in order to alleviate distress. Additionally, a complete diet history must be obtained to determine what foods or eating habits are causing distress. The nutritional care plan developed should be individualized and the information obtained from the diet history taken into consideration.

- Etiologic Risk Factors. Heredity; faulty dietary habits such as eating on the run, skipping meals, drinking excessive amounts of caffeine-containing liquids or alcohol; obtaining inadequate rest; psychological stress
- Characteristics and Symptoms. See Table 7-2
- Drug Therapy. Antacids, anticholinergics, histamine blockers, protein binders. See Table 7-1
- Diet Therapy
  1. Acute Phase
     a. Traditional Nutritional Care Plan
        (1) Methodology. Parenteral solutions of glucose and saline given until 24 to 72 hours after hemorrhage stops; oral feedings given after parenteral feedings are discontinued
        (2) Nutrients Increased and Decreased. See Table 7-3
        (3) Dietary Adaptations. Sippy diet or modifications
           (a) 3 to 4 oz of milk and cream served every 1 to 2 hours during the day and night, if client is awake; antacids given between servings
           (b) As pain subsides, small servings of soft bland foods such as milk toast, refined cereals (cream of wheat or rice), boiled eggs, strained cream soups, custards, and so on served 6 times a day
           (c) As tolerance increases, small servings of foods not considered mechanically, chemically, or thermally irritating are served as tolerated (consult Chap. 2 for specific foods considered soft in consistency and Table 7-3 for foods considered mechanically, chemically, and thermally irritating)
        (4) Meal Plan Modifications. See Table 7-3
     b. Traditional Behavioral Modifications. See Table 7-3
     c. Liberal Nutritional Care Plan
        (1) Methodology. Oral soft feedings are given frequently even when the client is bleeding or as bleeding subsides, if tolerated and prescribed.
        (2) Nutrients Increased and Decreased. See Table 7-3
        (3) Dietary adaptations
           (a) Nutritional care plan is individualized to enhance recovery and health maintenance
           (b) Foods avoided or limited are listed in Table 7-3
        (4) Meal Plan Modifications. See Table 7-3
     d. Liberal Behavioral Modifications. See Table 7-3

2. Chronic Phase
   a. Traditional Nutritional Care Plan
      (1) Methodology. Oral feedings
      (2) For nutrients increased and decreased, dietary adaptations, meal plan modifications, behavioral modifications, see Table 7-3
   b. Liberal Nutritional Care Plan. Same as above

Dumping Syndrome

- Description. A syndrome that develops during or shortly after a meal, involving excessively rapid emptying of the gastric contents
- Etiology. Gastric surgery, such as subtotal gastric resection, and tube feedings that pass directly into the jejunum
- Characteristics
  1. Stage I (15–20 min after a meal). Rapid release of hyperosmolar nutrients (refined carbohydrates) into the jejunum and their subsequent hydrolysis lead to a hypertonic intestinal content. This hypertonic material is rapidly diluted by fluid drawn from the plasma and extracellular fluid in an attempt to achieve osmotic balance. The end result is a rapid drop in circulating blood volume and a decrease in cardiac output. In addition, hormones such as histamine and prostaglandins are released as a result of the hyperosmolarity. These hormones are believed to enhance intestinal motility, resulting in diarrhea.
  2. Stage II (1–2 hr after a meal). Rapid digestion and absorption of concentrated carbohydrate create hyperglycemia and the rapid release of insulin. The end result is a rapid decrease in blood glucose levels (hypoglycemia), 1 to 2 hours after a meal.
- Symptoms
  1. Stage I. Sweating, abdominal distention, tachycardia, tremors, nausea, and diarrhea
  2. Stage II. Dizziness, nausea, faintness, and nervousness. Over time, malnutrition, weight loss, and anemia may develop
- Drug Therapy. Anticholinergics, antidiarrheals, iron supplements, and parenteral injections of vitamin B_{12} (see Table 7-1)
- Diet Therapy
  1. Nutritional Care Plan
     a. Methodology. Oral feedings, unless enteral feedings are indicated
     b. Nutrients Increased. Protein (20% of total calories), which repairs tissues; fat (30%–40% of total calories), which delays passage of food from the stomach, and enhances weight gain; vitamins and minerals (supplements may be needed to pro-

mote wound healing and nutrient absorption and utilization); complex carbohydrates, such as pastas and potatoes, to provide calories and nutrients (however, fiber-containing carbohydrates, such as whole grains, may be limited); caloric intake increased to extent of tolerance to enhance weight gain

c. Nutrients Decreased. Refined carbohydrates, which reduce hyperosmolarity and insulin release

d. Dietary Adaptations
   (1) Avoid refined sugars such as sugar, candy, colas, rich desserts, and alcohol
   (2) Limit intake of natural sugars such as fruits, vegetables, and milk
   (3) Limit salt intake
   (4) Increase intake of eggs, meat, fish, and cheese
   (5) Increase intake of margarines, mayonnaise, and salad dressings without sugar
   (6) Consume starchy carbohydrates (pasta and potatoes) but limit whole grains

e. Meal Plan Modifications
   (1) Consume 6 small meals rather than 3 large ones daily; this regimen decreases the hyperosmolic and hypoglycemic effects of the dumping syndrome and increases calories
   (2) Drink liquids 1 hour before and after meals but not with foods, so that food will pass from the stomach more slowly
   (3) Use the diabetic exchange lists as a guide when calculating and dividing nutrient allowances into daily meal plans

2. Behavioral Modifications
   a. Lie down after eating; this position slows passage of food from the stomach; adequate rest decreases GI motility
   b. Eat slowly in order to decrease GI motility and hyperosmolarity

Small Intestine

Functions

- Acidic chyme entering the duodenum stimulates release of hormones and enzymes from the gallbladder, pancreas, and intestinal glands
- The small intestine acts to hydrolyze nutrients into their smallest fragments
  1. Carbohydrates are absorbed through the portal bloodstream in the form of glucose, galactose, and fructose

2. Proteins are absorbed into the portal bloodstream as amino acids and ammonia

3. Fats are absorbed into the lacteals (lymphatic vessels) as fatty acids and glycerol

4. Water-soluble vitamins and minerals are absorbed into the portal bloodstream

5. Fat-soluble vitamins (A, D, E, and K) are absorbed into the lacteals

Common Dysfunctions

Lactose Intolerance

- Description. A condition induced by an individual's inability to hydrolyze lactose (a sugar found in milk; 1 cup = 12 g of lactose) into glucose and galactose
- Etiology. A hereditary autosomal recessive trait with a delayed clinical expression
- Characteristics. If the quantity of ingested lactose exceeds the individual's available lactase (a disaccharide enzyme found in the brush-border lining of the small intestine), the unhydrolyzed lactose moves down the intestine, carrying with it water and some electrolytes drawn by osmotic action, into the large bowel. This net fluid accumulation, or volume overload, plus fermentation of the sugar by colonic bacteria, causes distention of the bowel, rapid transit time, and other symptoms.
- Classifications
    1. Congenital Lactase Deficiency (rare)
    2. Secondary Lactase Deficiency. Inactivity of the enzyme caused by other conditions that impair the bowel mucosa, including celiac sprue, protein–calorie malnutrition, Crohn's disease, excessive use of antibiotics
    3. Developmental Lactase Deficiency. Enzyme levels normal throughout infancy but decrease with age; populations most affected by this decline are blacks, Orientals, American Indians, and those of Central European and Mediterranean ancestry
- Symptoms. Abdominal distention (bloated feeling) and cramps, belching, flatulence, and watery osmotic diarrhea; failure of children to thrive
- Drug Therapy. Drugs that relieve symptoms, such as antidiarrheals (see Table 7-1)
- Diet Therapy
    1. Nutritional Care Plan. Lactose-restricted diet (8 g or less/day)
        a. Methodology. Oral feedings
        b. Nutrients Increased. Protein, calcium, vitamin B_{12}, vitamin D and vitamin B_2

c. Nutrients Decreased. Carbohydrates that contain lactose

d. Dietary Adaptations. Individuals vary in their ability to utilize lactose; therefore they must be individually tested for tolerance

    (1) Dairy products usually tolerated by individuals with some lactase activity are buttermilk; yogurt; cheese, including some cottage cheese; milk and milk solids in breads, cakes, and sherbet; margarine; butter; and acidophilus milk (a milk treated with commercial enzymatic products that hydrolyze the lactose)

    (2) Products usually omitted, even with some lactase activity, are milk, whole and skim (the latter has fat removed, not lactose); milk drinks such as malted milk, milkshakes, and chocolate milk (the last is tolerated by some individuals); creamed soups and sauces; ice cream; and puddings*

    (3) Lact-Aid (a lactase enzyme powder) can be added to milk before ingestion; this commercial lactase preparation, derived from yeast, will hydrolyze lactose, and malabsorption symptoms will be eliminated

    (4) The calcium content of the diet is increased by greater consumption of foods such as soy milk, sardines, herring, and some leafy vegetables; calcium supplements (400–1000 mg/day) may also be used

e. Meal Plan Modifications

    (1) Do not consume milk by itself as a snack, even if some milk is tolerated

    (2) Drink only small amounts of milk with meals or mix with other foods such as mashed potatoes, scrambled eggs, and meat loaf (the meal delays gastric emptying and dilutes the lactase load in some individuals, but not all)

2. Behavioral Modifications.

a. Read food product labels; products containing milk, milk solid, curds, or whey must be avoided

b. Products containing lactalbumin, lactic acid, and calcium lactate are allowed, because these substances are chemically different from lactose

Other Carbohydrate Intolerances

• Description. Some individuals cannot absorb isomaltose, sucrose, glucose, or fructose; these conditions have symptoms similar to

---

* Individuals with no lactase activity will have to omit all products listed in (1) and (2).

those found with lactose intolerance; however, these disorders are rare

Celiac Sprue (Nontropical Sprue, Celiac Disease, Gluten-Sensitive Enteropathy)

- Description. A primary malabsorptive disorder
- Etiology. Hypothesized to be due to an abnormal (either defective or deficient) enzyme in the mucosal cell, a defect in immunity, or a defect in the mucosal cell membrane
- Characteristics. A toxic substance called gliadin causes atrophy of the mucosal villi, hyperplasia of the cells of the mucosal glands, and lymphocytic infiltration in the lamina propria in sensitive individuals. These mucosal changes lead to malabsorption of many nutrients. (Gliadin is a component of the protein gluten found in wheat, barley, rye, oats, and malt)
- Symptoms. Steatorrhea, diarrhea (light-colored, malodorous, bulky, greasy stools), and abdominal pain and distention; secondary symptoms, related to malabsorption, are often evident, such as weight loss, malnutrition, clotting abnormalities (due to vitamin K malabsorption), edema (due to protein–calorie malnutrition), anemia (due to vitamin B_{12}, folic acid, or iron malabsorption), osteoporosis (due to calcium, phosphorus, vitamin D, and protein malabsorption), hypokalcemia (due to potassium malabsorption), and secondary disaccharidase deficiency symptoms (*e.g.*, lactose intolerance); in children, linear growth and weight is retarded*
- Drug Therapy. Corticosteroids and antidiarrheal agents (see Table 7-1)
- Diet Therapy
  1. Nutritional Care Plan. Gluten-free diet
     a. Methodology. Parenteral, enteral, or oral feedings, depending on severity of disease
     b. Nutrients Increased. Vitamins and minerals (by supplements), especially iron, folate, and vitamin B_{12} (parenterally) until the condition is under control; calories and protein, other than gluten, are also increased to prevent malnutrition with subsequent increased intestinal mucosal damage
     c. Nutrients Decreased. Gluten, protein, and fat, until the condition improves (because fat enhances steatorrhea); refined carbohydrates (because disaccharide enzymes are usually inac-

---

* These symptoms can be totally reversed, over time, by removing gluten from the diet.

tive); complex carbohydrates that contain excess fiber or gluten (because they enhance diarrhea)

d. Dietary Adaptations

(1) Eliminate all cereal and bakery products that contain wheat, barley, rye, oats, and malt

(2) Eliminate all products that contain hidden sources of these foodstuffs, such as instant coffee, mustard, candy bars, ice cream, salad dressings other than oil- and vinegar-based ones, cream soups, cold cuts, gravies, biscuits, puddings, beer, and ale

(3) Lactose intolerance often develops in clients with celiac sprue because lactase is the first enzyme impaired and the last to be replenished (see Lactose Intolerance for dietary adaptations needed)

(4) Portagen, a commercial product that contains sodium caseinate, corn oil, corn syrup solids, sugar, vitamins, and minerals, less than 0.15% lactose, and MCT (medium-chain triglycerides), can be added to the diet to increase calories because the fatty acids found in MCT can be absorbed directly into the portal bloodstream rather than the lacteals (like long-chain triglycerides [LCT]); therefore, they become a source of calories for individuals with biliary, pancreatic, or small intestinal dysfunctions (see Table 8-2); foods that contain LCTs, which are absorbed through the lacteals, include margarines, corn oil, meat fat, and whole milk fat

(5) Products that can be substituted for the foodstuffs omitted are corn meal flour and corn, potato, rice, soybean, and wheat-starch flours that have had the gliadin removed commercially*

e. Meal Plan Modifications.

(1) Eat small meals frequently to enhance absorption and caloric intake

(2) When diet restrictions are liberalized, add new foods to the diet one at a time

2. Behavioral Modifications. *Always read food product labels*

---

* These flours have some texture and leavening abnormalities. Preparation suggestions that may alleviate these are to use only ⅝ cup of potato flour, ⅞ cup of rice flour, and ¾ cup of coarse corn meal for 1 cup wheat flour (other substitutes can be used in the same proportions as for wheat flour). Also, soy flour must always be combined with another flour in recipes. Portions of all baked products should be smaller and baked at a lower temperature for a longer period of time. Leavening agent (*e.g.*, baking powder) proportions should be increased. Frostings should be added to baked products, whenever possible; they increase moisture, add calories, and enhance palatability.

Small Intestinal Resections

Treatment, including nutritional care plans, needed for individuals after surgical resection of the intestines is set forth in the section on the large intestine.

Large Intestine

Functions

- Acts as a recycling plant that enables the body to regain, from waste fluids, metabolites that would otherwise be lost; recycles half the body's extracellular fluids and two thirds of its total salts
- Produces bacteria that ferment carbohydrates into organic acids and gases and enhance the production of vitamin K and some B-complex vitamins
- Acts as a reservoir for the waste products of digestion, which the host can eliminate at will

Terminology Related to Intestinal Digestion

- Crude Fiber. Residue of plant food after extraction by dilute acid and then dilute alkali in the laboratory
- Dietary Fiber. All the dietary constituents derived from plant cell walls, including cell wall protein, that are not digested by human digestive secretions; these constituents, however, may be somewhat digested by microorganisms; they are cellulose, hemicellulose, lignin, and pectin, also called plantix or plant fiber
- Dietary Residue. Residue refers to the volume (bulk) of material (dietary fibers, cells sloughed from the intestinal mucosa, intestinal bacteria, and their residues) present in the colon after digestion; in general, in order of increasing fecal output from lowest to highest: protein, fat, milk,* digestible carbohydrate, and carbohydrate with nondigestible fiber.
- Bran. Outer layer of the grain kernel, which is largely removed during the refining process but retained in whole-grain products. Rapidly increasing amounts of bran in the diet may irritate a sensitive GI tract or cause flatulence, loose stools, or intestinal blockage; increasing intake slowly may prevent these adverse effects; excessive intake may cause malabsorption of some nutrients such as protein, calcium, iron, and zinc

---

* Milk does not contain fiber, but it does increase stool weight by expanding fluid content; therefore, it is restricted on low-residue nutritional care plans.

Common Dysfunctions

Diarrhea

- Description. An increase in volume, fluidity, and frequency of bowel movements over the usual pattern of the individual
- Etiology. See Table 7-4
- Characteristics. Passage of food through the intestine is abnormally rapid; therefore, the complete digestion and absorption of nutrients are impaired (see Table 7-4 on other characteristics)
- Classifications. See Table 7-4
- Symptoms. Diarrhea itself is a symptom, not a disease, which is instituted by the body to rid the system of toxic agents; weight loss and general malnutrition may occur if diarrhea is chronic
- Drug Therapy. Antidiarrheals (see Table 7-1)
- Diet Therapy
  1. Acute Phase
     a. Nutritional Care Plan
        (1) Methodology
            (a) Nothing by mouth for 24 to 48 hours to "rest" the intestine
            (b) Intravenous feedings that include fluids, electrolytes, glucose, vitamin C, and vitamin B complex may be given during this time to replace fluids and electrolytes and prevent further lean tissue catabolism
            (c) After 48 hours, foods high in sodium and potassium (fruit juices, tea, and broth) are given as tolerated
            (d) As tolerance improves, foods low in residue are added to the diet (Table 7-5)
  2. Chronic Phase
     a. Nutritional Care Plan
        (1) Methodology. Oral feedings, plus enteral supplements (low in residue) if nutritional status severely impaired
        (2) Nutrients Increased. Protein (150 g), potassium, sodium, iron, calcium, vitamin B_{12}, folic acid, vitamin C, and fat-soluble vitamins, if steatorrhea is evident; caloric intake increased to 3000 to 4000 kcal/day.
        (3) Nutrients Decreased. Complex, natural, and refined carbohydrates; fat, if steatorrhea is evident
        (4) Dietary Adaptations
            (a) Foods low in residue allowed (Tables 7-5 to 7-7)
            (b) Foods high in fiber avoided (see Tables 7-6 and 7-7)
            (c) To achieve the high protein and calorie levels rec-

ommended, increase intake of foods that have concentrated sources of protein and calories, such as skim milk powder, creamed dishes, and puddings as tolerated

(d) Increase intake of foods that contain high levels of vitamin C, such as fruit and vegetable juices, as tolerated

(e) MCTs given instead of fats that contain LCTs (margarine, oils, and others), if steatorrhea is evident (see Table 8-2 and dietary adaptations for pancreatitis in Chap. 8)

(4) Lact-Aid may be necessary

(5) Meal plan modifications: 6 small, rather than 3 large, meals

b. Behavioral Modifications

(1) Eat slowly

(2) Eat at regular times

(3) Obtain adequate rest

(4) Establish regular evacuation times

Constipation

- Description. Retention of small, dry, hard stools in the colon beyond the individual's normal emptying time
- Etiologic Risk Factors
  1. Environmental. Excessive intake of refined carbohydrates and reduced intake of complex carbohydrates and fluids; sedentary living; ignoring call to defecate; poor eating habits (*e.g.,* skipping breakfast, eating on the run); excessive intake of medications such as laxatives, iron tablets, and calcium compounds
  2. Physiological. Irritable colon (alternating with diarrhea), diverticulosis, pregnancy, advanced age, obesity, polio, and obstructive bowel lesions
- Characteristics. Stools become hard and static when nonpropulsive segmental contractions increase pressure and drying of stool without moving colon contents into the rectum where normal defecation occurs; urge to move stools depressed
- Symptoms. Malaise, headache, foul breath, abdominal distention, anorexia, flatulence
- Drug Therapy. Bulk laxatives, which should be used only on the advice of the physician because they are habit forming and may do more harm than good (see Table 7-1)
- Diet Therapy
  1. Nutritional Care Plan. High fiber diet with increased fluids
     a. Methodology. Oral feedings

   b. Nutrients Increased. Complex carbohydrates that contain fiber (25 g/day); fluids increased from 4 to 6 glasses/day to 8 to 10 glasses/day, because fiber and fluid add volume and bulk to stools, which stimulate normal propulsive contractions of the colon; these, in turn, decrease intestinal transit time, decrease intraluminal pressure, and change intestinal flora

   c. Nutrients Decreased. Refined carbohydrates; "What goes in soft comes out hard"

   d. Dietary Adaptations

     (1) Increase intake of foods high in fiber (see Tables 7-6 and 7-7)

     (2) Decrease intake of foods low in residue (see Tables 7-5 and 7-7)

     (3) Decrease intake of refined sugars, such as desserts, candies, and table sugar

     (4) Increase fluid intake by drinking more fluids, adding fluids to sauces, eating fruits and vegetables high in fluid content such as watermelon, lettuce, and spinach

     (5) Add bran (2 tsp = 2–3 g of fiber) to meat loaves, stew, baked goods, and cereals

     (6) Drink prune juice or eat prunes in the morning; they contain a natural laxative, dihydroxyphenyl isatin

     (7) Add figs or raisins to food to increase bulk

   e. Meal Plan Modifications. Eat a large breakfast with some type of hot beverage (tea, hot water, or coffee) and allow time to defecate

2. Behavioral Modifications

   a. Eat in a relaxed atmosphere

   b. Eat at regular times

   c. Obtain adequate exercise

   d. Obtain adequate rest

   e. Establish regular elimination times

   f. Read food labels (*e.g.*, first ingredients on foodstuffs should include the words whole-wheat flour or grain and bran)

Diverticulosis and Diverticulitis

- Description. Diverticulosis is the herniation of the mucosa through the muscular layers of the colon. Diverticulitis is the inflammation of a diverticulum, usually resulting from the collection of bacteria or other irritating agents trapped in the diverticula.

- Etiologic Hypothesis. Conditions that enhance intraluminal pressure and colonic wall weakness such as the irritable bowel syndrome, spastic colon, and increased age

- Characteristics
    1. Diverticulosis. Diverticula (small sacs or pouches of mucous membrane) are protruded through weak spots in the muscular layers of the colon (usually sigmoid) by high intraluminal pressure, which leads to eventual narrowing of short segments of the colon.
    2. Diverticulitis. Diverticula may become inflamed by the entrance and stasis of food residues and bacteria (fecal material) causing perforation of the diverticula.
- Symptoms
    1. Diverticulosis. Individual may be asymptomatic or have mild symptoms such as constipation, abdominal discomfort, or distention.
    2. Diverticulitis. Left lower quadrant pain, fever, leukocytosis, and occasionally bloody stools
- Drug Therapy
    1. Acute Phase. Antibiotics. See Table 7-1
    2. Chronic Phase. Bulk laxatives, when prescribed by a physician; avoid harsh laxatives and enemas. See Table 7-1
- Diet Therapy
    1. Acute Phase
        a. Nutritional Care Plan. Table 7-8
        b. Behavioral Modifications. Table 7-8
    2. Chronic Phase
        a. Nutritional Care Plan. Table 7-9
        b. Behavioral Modifications. Table 7-9

Ulcerative Colitis

- Description. A chronic nonspecific inflammation and ulceration of the colonic mucosa
- Etiologic Hypotheses. Nervous tension, autoimmune disorder, allergic condition, infection; incidence higher in women aged 20 to 25 years; incidence higher in Jews
- Characteristics. Chronic with repeated exacerbations and remissions; the colon, especially the descending colon, as seen by sigmoidoscopy, reveals a spongy mucosal surface dotted with many tiny blood- and pus-oozing ulcerations; ulcerative colitis is related to an increased incidence of colon cancer
- Symptoms. Frequent movement of watery stools that contain blood, pus, and mucus but no fat; abdominal cramps; anemia; hypoalbuminemia; fever; hemorrhage; malnutrition; weight loss

- Drug Therapy. Anti-inflammatory agents such as azulfidine and prednisone (see Table 7-1)
- Diet Therapy
  1. Acute Phase
     a. Nutritional Care Plan. See Table 7-8
     b. Behavioral Modifications. See Table 7-8
  2. Chronic Phase
     a. Nutritional Care Plan. Table 7-9
     b. Behavioral Modifications. Table 7-9

Crohn's Disease (Regional Enteritis)

- Description. A nonspecific chronic granulomatous inflammatory disease
- Etiologic Hypotheses. Genetic disorder, autoimmune disorder, infection; incidence higher in women aged 15 to 35 years; incidence higher in Jews
- Characteristics. Bowel, especially the proximal portion of the colon and the ileum, as seen by barium enema and other procedures, reveals patchy ulcerations on mucosa that resemble "cobblestones"; these ulcerations may be continuous, but they are usually only seen in segments of the colon, thus the name "regional enteritis." Complications of the disorder include fistulas, abscesses, or obstruction.
- Symptoms. Three to four semisoft fatty stools per day (no blood usually), colicky abdominal pain after a meal, anorexia, fever in the acute phase, fatigue, weight loss, rough skin (due to impaired fat-soluble vitamin absorption), and malnutrition
- Drug therapy. Anticholinergic drugs, narcotic analgesics (tincture of opium or codeine), anti-inflammatory drugs (see Table 7-1)
- Diet Therapy
  1. Acute Phase
     a. Nutritional Care Plan. See Table 7-8
     b. Behavioral Modifications. See Table 7-8
  2. Chronic Phase
     a. Nutritional Care Plan. See Table 7-9
     b. Behavioral Modifications. See Table 7-9

Carcinoma of the Colon

See Tables 7-8 and 7-9 and Chapter 4 for details on diet therapy in the treatment of cancer.

Colostomy and Ileostomy

- Description. Surgical procedures in which a segment of the large bowel or the entire bowel is removed and an artificial opening to the outside of the body is created for the elimination of fecal waste products. In an ileostomy, the entire colon, rectum, and anus are resected. In a colostomy, the rectum and anus are resected.
- Indications. Intractable cancer, ulcerative colitis, Crohn's disease
- Adverse Nutritional Effects. Impairment of electrolyte and fluid recycling, curtailment of production of vitamin K and B-complex vitamins by bacteria. With an ileostomy, oral intake of vitamin B_{12} can no longer be absorbed through the ileum. Watery or heavy discharge, odor, gas, belching, and diarrhea or constipation may occur. Nutrient absorption and utilization may be impaired by diarrhea or constipation.
- Drug Therapy. Laxatives (*e.g.*, Metamucil) or antidiarrheal agents (*e.g.*, Lomotil), depending on symptoms (see Table 7-1)
- Diet Therapy
  1. Nutritional Care Plan
     a. Methodology. Total parenteral nutrition, followed by enteral feedings, then oral feedings, depending on client's recovery rate
     b. Nutrients Increased. All nutrients are increased, as tolerated after surgery, to improve nutritional status, enhance weight gain, and promote healing. Special emphasis on increasing protein, water, vitamin C, B-complex vitamins, vitamin K, potassium, and iron.*
     c. Nutrients Decreased. Carbohydrates—complex, refined, and those containing lactose if they cause distress (see Table 7-10); if steatorrhea is evident, fat (LCTs) is decreased; MCTs may be substituted
     d. Dietary Adaptations.† See Table 7-10
     e. Meal Plan Modifications
        (1) Small portions eaten slowly may eliminate distention and gas
        (2) Meals should be adapted to convenient defecation times
  2. Behavioral Modifications
     a. Eat in a relaxed atmosphere

---

* Vitamin B_{12} and sometimes vitamin K will need to be given parenterally in clients with an ileostomy.

† Individuals with flatulence may also be advised to follow some of the dietary adaptations, meal plan modifications, and behavioral modifications suggested in this section.

   b. Chew foods thoroughly

   c. Try not to swallow air when swallowing foods (often a nervous habit)

   d. Avoid reclining after meals

Nurses' Responsibilities in the Nutritional Care of Clients With Gastrointestinal Dysfunctions

Oral Nutritional Care Plan

- Initiate Good Care
    1. Procure instructions from trained professionals, including rationale for treatment by diet (*e.g.,* relief of pain and symptoms) and dietary adaptation suggestions immediately following diagnosis
    2. Procure advice from nonprofessional individuals who have learned to cope with similar conditions (*e.g.,* colostomy), when client is receptive
    3. Client compliance is often enhanced by knowing why the diet has been prescribed, and/or how long dietary restrictions will be stringent (acute phase); assure him that most regimens will be liberalized upon discharge (*e.g.,* low-residue regimens [diverticulitis] change to high-fiber regimens [diverticulosis] on discharge)
- Participate in Care
    1. Weigh client upon admittance, in the clinic or outclient clinic; weigh frequently after dietary regimen is instituted to evaluate progress and efficacy of treatment. Remember that edema may mask weight loss.
    2. Motivate and encourage client to eat all the foods on his tray; clients with GI or accessory organ dysfunctions often associate pain and unpleasant symptoms with food consumption; still these fears by assurances that the prescribed nutritional care plan is designed to relieve these adverse side-effects and promote healing. If food induces diarrhea, however, remove tray until client is ready to resume eating.
    3. Observe
        a. Client's food consumption: What foods is client still avoiding even though he has been assured they will probably not cause distress (*e.g.,* traditional vs. liberal ulcer dietary adaptations)?
        b. Behavior while eating (*e.g.,* how quickly does he eat?)
        c. Mental status before and after meals: Is he depressed or angry because he can no longer consume his traditional foods

    or anxious that food will still precipitate pain? (Additionally, if alternative methods of feeding are being instituted [*e.g.*, TPN], what are his reactions?)

    d. Physiological status after meals: Does the client have adverse effects such as pain, rapid pulse, diarrhea, colicky abdominal pain, or nausea after eating? If so, record what foods he ate so that the food causing distress may be determined and eliminated.

    e. Reactions to medications: Are they creating symptoms such as diarrhea that may have adverse effects on nutritional status?

    f. Compliance: Is client "cheating"? For example, food as a means of treatment in liver and other GI dysfunctions will be of no account if alcohol consumption continues. Cheating is also a problem when a client has severe renal dysfunction, for he feels the condition cannot be reversed by dietary treatment so why not eat what he desires?

4. Enhance compliance with the new nutritional care plan by making sure foods are palatable; serve hot foods hot, cold foods cold, and so on

5. Collect urine or stool specimens

6. Record fluid intake and output

- Coordinate Care

The overall responsibility of the nurse to clients with GI or accessory organ dysfunctions is to help relieve adverse symptoms and promote healing. She can accomplish this by organizing health-team conferences and by observing and reporting subjective as well as objective information.

1. Subjective information to be reported. Any information the client reveals about appetite and usual eating and drinking habits (especially important in these conditions), place of eating, and other observations that will influence nutritional status

2. Objective information to be reported. Present weight (does this constitute a weight gain or loss?), fluid intake and output recordings, and new laboratory findings that may affect nutritional status or indicate that a new nutritional care plan should be instituted (see General Factors in Developing a Nutritional Care Plan at the beginning of this chapter for information that should be reported)

3. Clinical signs to be reported. Weight gain or loss; general malnutrition; decubitus ulcer, rough skin, mouth disorders; these adverse signs may indicate that nutritional treatment should be adjusted or enhanced

- Reinforce and Follow Up Care

1. Empathize with the client because many of the dietary adjustments designed to relieve symptoms will have to be followed for

a lifetime. Help make these dietary adaptations as palatable as possible by assisting in food selections. Assure him he is not alone. Seek advice from others with the same condition whenever possible.

2. Compliment clients who try new foods although they may associate them with adverse effects. Also compliment clients who consume foods they find unpalatable in order to enhance recovery.

3. Obtain a working knowledge of the rationales behind dietary treatment in GI and accessory organ dysfunctions. Compliance is enhanced when client knows why a certain treatment is being instituted. Rationales can be obtained from information in this book, from advanced nutritional care books, and from most hospital diet manuals. Also included in this responsibility is being medically up to date. The nurse should know what nutritional care plans are obsolete, what care plans have been substituted, and why the substitutions have been made.

Enteral and Parenteral Care Plans

The nurse's responsibilities to clients with GI or accessory organ dysfunctions, on specialized care plans, are the same as those to any individual receiving these care plans. Consult Chapter 2 for details on responsibilities.

Table 7-1
Interactions Among Medications Used in
Gastrointestinal Disorders, Nutrients, and Nutritional Status

Medication Category	Mechanism of Action	Adverse Side-Effects With Nutritional Implications	Dietary Suggestions
Antacids			
Aluminum hydroxide (Amphojel), magnesium hydroxide (Phillips' Milk of Magnesia), combinations of aluminum hydroxide, magnesium hydroxide, and simethicone (Gelusil II, Maalox Plus), sodium bicarbonate (baking soda)	By elevating stomach *p*H to a level that decreases pepsin activity, they reduce acidity and provide relief from peptic ulcer symptoms; may also relieve flatulence	Common Side-Effects Edema (most antacids contain sodium; magaldrate [Riopan] is an exception) Thiamine deficiencies (most antacids inactivate thiamine) Generalized nutrient imbalances due to decreased absorption, especially of vitamin A, and iron malabsorption Hypercalcemia, especially when taken with milk (called the "milk–alkali" syndrome), manifested by vomiting, nausea, anorexia, and metabolic alkalosis	Sodium intake may have to be limited if antacids are taken over long periods of time. Foods with high thiamine content should be taken frequently (*e.g.*, wholewheat and enriched grain products). Supplements may also be needed. A well-balanced diet with added vitamin and mineral supplements is indicated. Milk and milk products (*e.g.*, cheese) may be limited.

(continued)

Table 7-1 275

Table 7-1
Interactions Among Medications Used in
Gastrointestinal Disorders, Nutrients, and Nutritional Status (continued)

Medication Category	Mechanism of Action	Adverse Side-Effects With Nutritional Implications	Dietary Suggestions
Antacids *(continued)*		Specific Side-Effects	Foods with high phosphorus content may be indicated (*e.g.*, meat). Fluids and fibrous foods (*e.g.*, raw vegetables) are indicated.
		Aluminum hydroxide decreases phosphorus absorption, with resultant osteomalacia; constipation.	Foods high in fiber and fat are limited.
		Magnesium hydroxide induces diarrhea and steatorrhea.	Foods high in sodium are limited. Foods with a high calcium content are limited.
		Sodium bicarbonate is not recommended since it induces sodium retention and metabolic acidosis.	Give all antacids 1–3 hr after meals and at bedtime. Administer tablets with a full glass of water or milk, or suggest chewing tablets well before swallowing. Small frequent meals will augment medications.
Antiulcers Sucralfate (Carafate)	A sulfonated disaccharide that complexes with proteins, it combines with proteins at the base of a peptic ulcer,	Constipation	Increase the fiber content of the diet (*e.g.*, whole grains and raw fruits and vegetables with skins and seeds); increase fluid intake.

(continued)

Table 7–1
Interactions Among Medications Used in Gastrointestinal Disorders, Nutrients, and Nutritional Status (continued)

Medication Category	Mechanism of Action	Adverse Side-Effects With Nutritional Implications	Dietary Suggestions
Antiulcers (continued)	forming a protective coat that prevents further digestive action of both acid and pepsin and promotes healing, especially of duodenal ulcers.	Xerostomia (dry mouth)	Suggest sucking on ice cubes or hard candy if calories are not limited. These may be given 1 hr before meals and ½ hour before antacids at bedtime as needed for pain.
Histamine Blockers Cimetidine (Tagamet)	Antagonist of histamine at the histamine (H_2) receptors on the parietal cells. Decrease HCl acid production, inhibit gastric acid secretion, reduce pain and promote healing.	Hydrochloric acid production is decreased; consequently, protein, calcium, iron, and vitamin B_{12} absorption may be impaired. Diarrhea or constipation is induced in some clients; therefore, absorption of nutrients may be impaired even more.	Increase intake of these nutrients to offset malabsorption; supplements may be needed. Limit or increase fluids and fiber, depending on client's symptoms; give medication before meals and at bedtime, but not with antacids.
Cholinergics Metoclopramide (Reglan)	Increase tone and amplitude of gastric (especially antral) contractions, relax pyloric sphincter, and increase persistalsis with resultant	Diarrhea is often induced, which can enhance malabsorption of some nutrients.	A well-balanced diet, somewhat limited in fiber, may be indicated. Administer ½ hr before meals and at bedtime.

(continued)

Table 7–1 277

Table 7–1
Interactions Among Medications Used in Gastrointestinal Disorders, Nutrients, and Nutritional Status (continued)

Medication Category	Mechanism of Action	Adverse Side-Effects With Nutritional Implications	Dietary Suggestions
Cholinergics *(continued)*	accelerated gastric emptying and intestinal transit.		
Anticholinergics			
Atropine sulfate (Antrocol [also contains phenobarbital], Donnatal [also contains phenobarbital, hyoscyamine sulfate, and scopolamine hydrobromide]); propantheline bromide (Pro-Banthine)	Depress postganglionic fibers of smooth muscle and secretory gland activity.	Xerostomia (dry mouth) Nausea, vomiting, or constipation with some	Give client ice or hard candies to suck or sugar-free gum to chew; moisten foods. Small frequent meals that have adequate fiber are indicated. Fluids should be taken with and between meals. Exercise should be increased. Antacids given concomitantly should contain magnesium. Give ½ hr before meals and at bedtime.
Antidiarrheals			
Diphenoxylate with atropine sulfate (Lomotil); loperamide (Imodium)	Slow intestinal motility.	Abdominal discomfort, swelling of gums, dry mouth, and nausea; excessive	Diet should be limited in fiber (*e.g.*, whole grains) and lactose (*e.g.*, milk) to augment *(continued)*

Table 7-1
Interactions Among Medications Used in
Gastrointestinal Disorders, Nutrients, and Nutritional Status (continued)

Medication Category	Mechanism of Action	Adverse Side-Effects With Nutritional Implications	Dietary Suggestions
Antidiarrheals (continued)		amounts may induce constipation.	medication. However, fluid intake must be adequate to prevent dehydration. Dry mouth can be relieved by sucking ice or hard candy. Small frequent meals are better tolerated.
Laxatives	Promote fecal evacuation from the bowel.	Dehydration is possible when laxatives are used too frequently. Electrolyte imbalances may be induced. Malabsorption syndromes are possible.	Fluid intake may need to be increased to prevent obstruction. Clients should be monitored for signs of electrolyte imbalances and malabsorption syndromes. If symptoms are evident, give increased amounts of essential nutrients in foods or supplements.

(continued)

Table 7-1 279

Table 7-1
**Interactions Among Medications Used in
Gastrointestinal Disorders, Nutrients, and Nutritional Status** (continued)

Medication Category	Mechanism of Action	Adverse Side-Effects With Nutritional Implications	Dietary Suggestions
Saline Laxatives			
Magnesium hydroxide (Phillips' Milk of Magnesia); sodium phosphate with sodium biphosphate (Phospho-Soda)	Hypersmolar compounds, they retain water in intestinal lumen.	Electrolyte imbalances; high in sodium. Dehydration is possible with excessive intake	Clients on low-sodium diets should not use these laxatives. Give fluids with and between meals.
Irritant or Stimulant Laxatives			
Castor oil (Neoloid); phenolphthalein (Feen-A-Mint, Prulet); bisacodyl (Dulcolax)	Increase intestinal motility by direct action on the smooth mucosa, with loss of structural integrity.	Loss of mucosal structural integrity may cause malabsorption of many nutrients, especially calcium.	A well-balanced diet high in fluids and fiber is indicated. If malabsorption or nutrient deficiency symptoms occur, replace nutrients by food or supplements. Recommend increased exercise to augment medication.

(continued)

Table 7-1
Interactions Among Medications Used in Gastrointestinal Disorders, Nutrients, and Nutritional Status (continued)

Medication Category	Mechanism of Action	Adverse Side-Effects With Nutritional Implications	Dietary Suggestions
Bulk-Producing Laxatives			
Methylcellulose (Cologel); psyllium hydrophilic mucilloid (Konsyl, Metamucil)	Soften stool by holding water; slowly increase frequency of bowel movements.	Intestinal or esophageal obstruction possible; also flatulence.	*Give with a full glass of water.* Give a high-fiber diet to augment medication. Recommend moderate exercise. Limit foods that may induce flatulence (see Table 7–10).
Lubricant Laxatives			
Mineral oil (Agoral Plain)	Lubricate intestinal mucosa and soften stool; nutrients dissolve in oil.	Malabsorption of vitamins A, D, E, and K	Mineral oil is not recommended. However, it may be used by older adult clients who refuse other medications. Encourage moderate exercise. Encourage client to take hot water before breakfast; this may have the same laxative effect. Give a high-fiber diet when tolerated. Give mineral oil between meals, never with meals.

(continued)

Table 7–1

Interactions Among Medications Used in
Gastrointestinal Disorders, Nutrients, and Nutritional Status (continued)

Medication Category	Mechanism of Action	Adverse Side-Effects With Nutritional Implications	Dietary Suggestions
Fecal Softeners			
Dioctyl sodium sulfosuccinate (Colace)	Surfactants Promotes water retention in fecal mass to soften it for easier passage.	Bitter taste, throat irritation, and nausea; consequently, nutrient ingestion may be impaired.	Take a diet history to discover which foods cause adverse symptoms. Individualize diet to client's likes and dislikes but emphasize the importance of fibrous and fluid-containing foods.
Antimicrobials			
Neomycin sulfate tablets, tetracycline (Panmycin)	Alter intestinal flora by inhibiting or killing microorganisms.	Inhibit pancreatic lipase; thus maldigestion and malabsorption syndromes, including steatorrhea and malnutrition, develop. Impair absorption of fat, carotene, xylose, sodium, potassium, magnesium, calcium, iron, zinc, and vitamin B_{12} Impair absorption of nitrogen, which may be beneficial in hepatic disorders	Parenteral or oral supplements of affected nutrients may be necessary. Enteral feedings high in these nutrients that do not induce increased diarrhea may be necessary. (See Chap. 2 for the composition of enteral feedings.)

(continued)

Table 7–1
**Interactions Among Medications Used in
Gastrointestinal Disorders, Nutrients, and Nutritional Status** (continued)

Medication Category	Mechanism of Action	Adverse Side-Effects With Nutritional Implications	Dietary Suggestions
Antimicrobials (continued)			The calcium in dairy products may impair tetracycline absorption. Dairy products are not limited, however; merely advise client to take medication with water 1 hr before or 2 hr after meals. Enteral supplements such as MCT oil may be necessary.
Anti-inflammatory Agents *Nonsterod anti-inflammatory agents* Sulfasalazine (Azulfidine)	Reduce inflammation along intestinal tract.	Impaired folate absorption. Over a period of time, megaloblastic anemia may develop. Nausea and vomiting are possible.	Give foods high in folate (*e.g.,* fruits and vegetables) or supplements. Small frequent meals may be better tolerated.

(continued)

Table 7-1 283

Table 7-1
**Interactions Among Medications Used in
Gastrointestinal Disorders, Nutrients, and Nutritional Status** (continued)

Medication Category	Mechanism of Action	Adverse Side-Effects With Nutritional Implications	Dietary Suggestions
Anti-inflammatory Agents (continued)			
Aspirin (*see Table 9-1*)			
		Profound Metabolic Effects	
Steroid anti-inflammatory agents Cortisone, hydrocortisone, prednisone, prednisolone, betamethasone	Anti-inflammatory action may be due to lysosomal stabilization, inhibition of leukocyte response, biosynthesis, and alteration of immune response.	Gluconeogenesis at the expense of lean tissue, with resultant hyperglycemia	High-protein diabetic diet is advised (see Chap. 5).
		Lipolysis of adipose tissue with resultant hypertriglyceridemia	Type IV hyperlipoproteinemia diet is advised (*e.g.*, limit refined sugars, such as cane; see Chap. 3).
		Changes in cholesterol metabolism with resultant hypercholesterolemia	Foods high in cholesterol (*e.g.*, beef and eggs) are limited (see Chap. 3).
		Retention of sodium with resultant edema and hypokalemia	Low-sodium diet is recommended. Increase intake of potassium-containing foods (*e.g.*, fruits and vegetables) or give potassium chloride (see Chap. 3).

(continued)

Table 7-1
Interactions Among Medications Used in
Gastrointestinal Disorders, Nutrients, and Nutritional Status (continued)

Medication Category	Mechanism of Action	Adverse Side-Effects With Nutritional Implications	Dietary Suggestions
Anti-inflammatory Agents (continued)			
		Impaired absorption of calcium, with resultant osteoporosis	Calcium and vitamin D supplements may be necessary because milk products often enhance lactose disorders (see Chap. 8).
		Increased excretion of vitamin C, potassium, and zinc	Give foods high in vitamin C (*e.g.*, citrus fruits); give foods high in potassium (*e.g.*, fruits and vegetables); give foods high in zinc (*e.g.*, wheat germ and meats low in cholesterol).
		Peptic ulcer	Supplements may be needed. Liberal bland diet unless actively bleeding.

* Corticosteroids are used in gastrointestinal disorders only in severe cases (*e.g.*, severe flare-up of ulcerative colitis)

Table 7-2 285

Table 7-2
Characteristics and Symptoms of Duodenal and Gastric Ulcer

Characteristics and Symptoms	Chronic Duodenal Ulcer	Chronic Gastric Ulcer
Prevalence	More common	Less common
Age	5th–6th decades	6th–7th decades
M:F ratio	3:1	3:4
Seasonal trend	Spring and fall	No seasonal trend
Blood group	Most frequently 0	No differentiation
General nourishment	Usually well nourished	Often malnourished, underweight
Location	Mostly within 3 cm of pylorus	Most occur in antrum of stomach
Gastric acid production	Hypersecretion	Normal to hyposecretion but backward diffusion of H_2 ions causes mucosal damage
Etiology	Rapid entry of acidified chyme into the duodenum that cannot be neutralized rapidly enough	Backward reflux of bile acids from the duodenum into the stomach can cause mucosal damage that is irritated by even small amounts of acid
Pain	2–3 hr after meals and during night; ingestion of food relieves pain	½–1 hr after meals, seldom during night; vomiting relieves pain but ingestion of food does not
Vomiting	Uncommon	Common
Hemorrhage	Melena (passage of tarry stools) more common than hematemesis (vomiting of blood)	Hematemesis more common than melena
Anemia	Common	Common

Table 7-3
Traditional and Liberal Chronic Ulcer Nutritional Care Plans

	Traditional Care Plan	Liberal Care Plan	Rationale for Modifications
Nutrients Increased			
Protein	Especially milk protein, because protein neutralizes gastric juice	Moderate amounts of protein still emphasized for wound healing but egg, meat, and cheese protein considered as effective as milk protein; meat also contains heme iron.	Protein neutralizes gastric acid for approximately 20 min but stimulates its secretion for 3 hr. Excessive milk intake may cause lactose intolerance. The calcium in milk stimulates gastrin secretion. Additionally, in conjunction with antacids, it causes the Burnett milk–alkali syndrome (hypercalcemia, hypophosphatemia, renal stones, and other complications).
Fat	Especially in the form of cream, because fat decreases hunger, which inhibits the vagus nerves and retards gastric acid secretion and gastric motility	Total fat intake is limited to 30%–35% of total calories; fats in other foods, such as eggs, oil, meat, and margarines, retard gastric acid secretion, as does cream.	Fat retards gastric acid secretion, but it also increases distention, which stimulates gastrin secretion. Excess fat raises blood lipid levels and enhances obesity, which may induce hypertension, atherosclerosis, and coronary heart disease.
Iron	Supplements often given to counteract anemia, because dairy products are a poor source of iron; antacids decrease HCl, which enhances iron absorption	Same as for traditional; however, meat, fruits, and vegetables that also supply iron are allowed; meat is the best source of heme iron.	Ulcer clients develop not only nutritional anemia (iron deficiency) but also macrocytic anemias (inadequate vitamin B_{12} and folate) after some surgical procedures.

(continued)

Table 7–3 287

Table 7–3
Traditional and Liberal Chronic Ulcer Nutritional Care Plans (continued)

Traditional Care Plan	Liberal Care Plan	Rationale for Modifications
Nutrients Decreased		
Complex carbohydrates Considered mechanically irritating to the damaged mucosa, whole grains, raw fruits and vegetables, seeds, nuts, and "gassy" vegetables such as beans and cabbage are avoided	Not limited but, rather, emphasized, for these foods provide the nutrients necessary for healing. Client is advised to chew these foods well and avoid only foods known to cause distress; pureed foods only recommended when client cannot chew properly.	No food has scientifically been proven to scrape the mucosa as long as mucin is being produced and the food has been chewed well and mixed with saliva before swallowing. Eliminating complex carbohydrate from the diet, however, may induce constipation and vitamin and mineral deficiencies.
Other Dietary Adaptations		
Chemically irritating foods Avoided because they stimulate the production of gastrin and gastric juice and irritate mucosal lining. Also, some cause a backward diffusion of H_2 ions, which irritates the mucosal lining (*e.g.,* alcohol, wine, and beer, to a lesser extent). All spices and condiments (except salt), caffeine drinks, and alcohol avoided	Some foods in this category have proved to be chemically irritating; they are avoided on the liberal bland diet as well as on the traditional. Foods avoided are pepper, chili powder (other spices may be used with food sparingly), and caffeinated drinks as well as decaffeinated coffee, bouillon, and alcohol.	The only spices proved to irritate the mucosa, when applied directly, are chili powder and pepper. At present no scientific evidence shows that a bland diet is more effective than a regular diet in healing ulcers.
Thermally irritating food Avoided because they stimulate gastric secretion and increased tone and motility. Hot and cold drinks and frozen food avoided.	Hot and cold drinks may be consumed as long as they do not cause distress	No scientific evidence shows that hot or cold foods stimulate or increase stomach activity.

(continued)

Table 7–3
Traditional and Liberal Chronic Ulcer Nutritional Care Plans (continued)

Traditional Care Plan	Liberal Care Plan	Rationale for Modifications
Meal Plan Modifications		
Frequency of meals is increased from 3 to 6 because some foods neutralize acids and food eliminates hunger, which stimulates the vagus nerve ("stress ulcers" are thought to be the result of persistent stimulation of the vagus nerve). Meal size is reduced because small meals avoid distention of antrum and consequent secretion of gastrin	Same meal plan modifications; however, bedtime snacks may be discouraged.	Food in the stomach seems to enhance the well-being of most ulcer clients, with the exception of some clients with gastric ulcers. Bedtime snacks may be discouraged, for they delay the natural basal secretory state, thus producing higher nocturnal acidity. Small meals seem to alleviate distress.
Behavioral Modifications		
Eat regularly, do not skip meals, eat slowly in a relaxed atmosphere. Rest frequently; cease smoking; avoid alcohol or, if a cocktail is consumed, drink it with food, never on an empty stomach; and ask your physician which drugs can be used that do not irritate or stimulate stomach activities.	Same behavioral modifications	Drugs that are presently known to damage the gastric mucosa are salicylates (aspirin), corticosteroids, phenylbutazone, and reserpine.

Table 7-4

Classification, Characteristics, Etiology, and Adverse Nutritional Effects of Diarrhea

Table 7-4 289

Classification	Characteristics	Etiology	Adverse Nutritional Effects
Watery Diarrhea Excessive volumes of water and electrolytes are delivered to colon. Transit time of foodstuffs is increased.	Stool volume usually more than 1 liter, does not decrease with fasting; sodium, potassium, and bicarbonate found in excess; *p*H of stool neutral	Dietary indiscretions, food poisoning (*e.g.*, *E. coli*, salmonellosis), cholera, laxative abuse, anxiety, regional ileitis, ulcerative colitis, protein-calorie malnutrition (PCM), irritable colon	Water, sodium, and potassium lost in excess; also water-soluble vitamins (*e.g.*, vitamin C, vitamin B$_{12}$, and folate). Lean tissue catabolism enhances protein and potassium excretion. Glucose needed to prevent further malnourishment, especially when PCM is the cause. Excessive weight loss and anemia over time.
Osmotic Diarrhea A watery diarrhea secondary to the osmotic effect created by unabsorbable ingested solutes. Fermentation of these solutes enhances diarrhea.	Stool volume usually less than 1 liter, decreases with fasting; potassium found in excess; stool is acidic owing to fermentation of nutrients	Fermentation caused by incomplete digestion of foodstuffs (*e.g.*, lactase deficiency), excessive antacid ingestion, GI resections, hyperosmolar tube feedings.	Water and potassium lost in excess, also water-soluble vitamins. Weight loss and anemia, if nutrients causing distress are not eliminated.

(continued)

Table 7–4
**Classification, Characteristics, Etiology, and
Adverse Nutritional Effects of Diarrhea** (continued)

Classification	Characteristics	Etiology	Adverse Nutritional Effects
Steatorrhea			
Passage of large amounts (60 g *vs* 2–5 g normal) of fat in the stool daily	Stool is frothy, greasy, bulky, and voluminous. Increased numbers of muscle fibers indicate impaired intraluminal digestion.	Pancreatic insufficiency, gastric resection, biliary disorders, cirrhosis, blind loop syndrome, celiac sprue, cystic fibrosis	Multiple vitamin losses, especially fat-soluble vitamins (*e.g.*, A,D,E, and K), vitamin B_{12}, and folate. Multiple mineral losses, especially calcium, zinc, magnesium, iron, and potassium. Severe weight loss, over time, if condition not corrected.
Small-Volume Diarrhea			
Passage of small, poorly formed stools	Three to four poorly formed stools passed daily; episodes of constipation and mucus-containing watery diarrhea may also occur. Possible fever.	Ulcerative colitis, Crohn's disease, diverticular disease, carcinoma of the colon	All nutrients lost in excess unless constipation is frequent (*e.g.*, in diverticulosis). Weight loss excessive, except in diverticulosis; clinical signs of PCM evident if condition not corrected.

Table 7–5 291

Table 7-5
Restricted-Residue Diet*

Food Group	Foods Allowed	Foods Limited or Avoided
Milk	Milk and cottage, cream, and mild cheddar cheese	All foods in the milk group in excess of 2 servings/day
Fruits	Fruit juices (preferably citrus), cooked and canned fruits (without skin, seeds, or fiber), ripe banana	Raw fruits (except ripe bananas) with and without skins
Vegetables	Cooked vegetables (e.g., asparagus tips, string beans, carrots, winter squash, potatoes, and beets)	Raw or fried vegetables and those with extensive fiber (e.g., celery)
Breads and cereals	Refined, enriched rice, bread, cereals, pasta, and crackers	Whole-grain or bran flour, rice, bread, cereals, pasta, and crackers
Meat	Tender chicken, fish, ground beef, and lamb; eggs (other than fried), and smooth peanut butter	Tough stew meats, seasoned meats, fried meats, fried eggs, all nuts, dry beans, and peas
Miscellaneous	Fat (margarines, butter), mild sauces, broth, gelatin, salt, sugar, pepper (in moderation), tea, and coffee	Fats in excess if steatorrhea is evident, highly seasoned foods, pickles, garlic, and jams with seeds

* This regimen can be made lower in residue by (1) limiting the milk group servings to 1 per day, (2) avoiding all fruits except fruit juices (may be better tolerated with a meal), (3) avoiding all vegetables except unseasoned vegetable juices, (4) grinding all meats and fish, (5) avoiding all spices and condiments except salt, (6) avoiding all foods that cause individual distress. A low- or minimal-residue diet is not nutritionally balanced; therefore, it should not be used for extended periods of time. If long-term use of a low-residue regimen is indicated, elemental or chemically defined enteral formulas or parenteral solutions should be considered. (After Anderson L, Dibble MV, Turkki PR et al: Nutrition in Health and Disease, 17th ed, p 448. Philadelphia, JB Lippincott, 1982)

Table 7-6
Dietary Fiber Content of Common Foods*

Food	Household Measure	Grams	Fiber Content (g)
Fruits			
Apple, peel only	1 small	100	3.71
Apple, flesh only	1 small	100	1.42
Grapefruit	½ medium	100	0.44
Plums	2 medium	100	1.52
Pear, peel only	½	100	8.59
Pear, flesh only	½	100	2.44
Strawberries, whole	10 large	100	2.12
Banana	1 small	100	1.75
Vegetables			
Lettuce, romaine	2 leaves	50	0.76
Brussels sprouts	6–7 cooked	100	2.86
Cabbage	1 cup shredded	100	2.83
Celery	½ cup diced	50	0.36
Carrots	1 large	100	3.70
Potato, peeled	1 small	100	3.51
Tomato, raw	1 small	100	1.40
Onion, 2¼ inch diameter	1 small	100	2.10
Cereals			
All Bran, Kellogg's	1 cup	56	13.30
Puffed wheat	1 cup	14	1.51
Shredded wheat	1 biscuit	25	3.06
Bran	7 tablespoons	100	44.00

(continued)

Table 7-6

Dietary Fiber Content of Common Foods* (continued)

Food	Household Measure	Grams	Fiber Content (g)
Breads			
White, enriched	1 slice	23	0.68
Whole wheat	1 slice	23	2.10
Meat Group			
Peas, split, dried, raw	½ cup	100	11.9
Brazil nuts	⅓ cup, 25 nuts	100	7.73
Peanut butter	3 tablespoons	45	3.77
Meats and fish	3½ oz serving	100	trace
Milk Group			
Milk	1 cup	244	residue

* The recommended dietary fiber intake for an individual on a high-fiber diet is 25–30 g/day. Dietary suggestions that will help an individual obtain this amount of fiber daily are (1) change from refined breads and cereal products to whole wheat; (2) eat at least 4 servings of fruits and vegetables daily, preferably raw; (3) eat beans and lentils more frequently than meats; (4) add bran to foods gradually. Upper limit suggested is ¼ to ½ cup of bran daily. (Adapted from Shipley EA: Dietary fiber content of foods, pp 203–212. In Spiller GA, Amen RJ [eds]: Dietary Fiber Research. New York, Plenum Press, 1978; and Pennington JAT, Church HN: Food Values of Portions Commonly Used, 13th ed. Philadelphia, JB Lippincott, 1980)

Table 7-6 293

Table 7-7
Comparison of Daily Menus for High-Fiber and Restricted-Residue Diets

High-Fiber Menu	Restricted-Residue Menu
Breakfast	
Grapefruit, ½ whole	Grapefruit juice (canned), ½ cup
Shredded wheat, 1 biscuit	Cream of wheat (cooked), ½ cup
Bran, 2 teaspoons	Sugar (no bran), 1 teaspoon
Skim milk, 1 cup	Skim milk, ½ cup
Coffee or tea	Coffee or tea
Lunch	
Tuna salad sandwich on whole-wheat toast (tunafish, diced celery, mayonnaise, 2 lettuce leaves)	Mild cheddar cheese sandwich on enriched white bread
Apple with skin, 1 small	Applesauce
Coffee or tea	Coffee or tea
Dinner	
Roast turkey with skin and turkey stuffing (whole-wheat bread crumbs, diced celery, 2 teaspoons of bran, and nuts)	Roast turkey (white meat, no skin)
	Enriched white bread, 1 slice
Baked potato with skin	Baked potato without skin
Carrot and raisin salad	Sliced carrots (cooked) with butter
Whole berry cranberry sauce	Jellied cranberry sauce
Fresh strawberries	Sliced banana
Skim milk, 1 cup	Skim milk, ½ cup
Coffee or tea	Coffee or tea

Table 7–8 295

Table 7–8
Nutritional Care Plans for Acute Ulcerative Colitis, Crohn's Disease, and Diverticulitis

Nutritional Care Plan	Rationale
Methodology	
Severe	
NPO with parenteral solutions or TPN for brief periods; elemental enteral feedings (Vivonex or Vipep) instead of parenteral solutions if tolerated.	Rests the bowel Provides all nutrients in the quantities and balance needed to restore nutritional status and promote healing Relieves symptoms and pain (any bowel movement induces pain) Prevents complications such as fistulas and obstructions
Acute but less severe	
Oral feedings, clear liquid diet, or soft low-residue diet (see Table 7–5)*	Same as above, except that these diets seldom supply the nutrients needed for nutritional status restoration or healing
Nutrients Increased	
All, including carbohydrates, if they do not need digestion (see Methodology); caloric content is also increased.	Increased amounts of nutrients, even above normal requirements, in some instances, will restore nutritional status and promote healing. Fluids and electrolytes will replace those excreted and prevent dehydration.
Nutrients Decreased	
Complex carbohydrates with fiber, natural carbohydrates with lactose (e.g., milk) Refined carbohydrates (sugar)	Eliminating complex carbohydrates reduces fecal material and bowel movements; limiting lactose may reduce symptoms such as diarrhea; eliminating sugar curtails fermentation and diarrhea.
	(continued)

Table 7-8
Nutritional Care Plans for Acute Ulcerative Colitis, Crohn's Disease, and Diverticulitis (continued)

Nutritional Care Plan	Rationale
Dietary Adaptations Consult Chapter 2 for details of dietary adaptations in TPN, elemental diets, and clear liquid diets. Consult this chapter for dietary adaptations suggested in lactose intolerance, celiac sprue, diarrhea, and constipation.	Proper administration of TPN and enteral feedings will prevent symptoms such as cramping, diarrhea, and distention; small oral feedings will also prevent distention.
Meal Plan Modifications See TPN and enteral feedings (Chap. 2) for proper administration (flow rate and so on) of these feedings; advise eating 6 small, rather than 3 large, meals a day; see meal plan modifications for related disorders (*e.g.*, diarrhea and constipation)	
Behavioral Modifications Psychological adjustments to alternative feeding methods necessary in some of these disorders; see behavioral modifications for related disorders (*e.g.*, diarrhea and constipation).	Consult Chapter 2 for details on how to help individuals cope when alterations in feeding methods are necessary.

* This is the care plan usually used for clients with diverticulitis.

Table 7-9 297

Table 7-9
Nutritional Care Plans for Chronic Ulcerative Colitis, Crohn's Disease, and Diverticulosis

Nutritional Care Plan	Rationale
Methodology Oral feedings → low in residue → liberalized in residue → high in fiber (diverticulosis)	Low-residue diets are believed to prevent irritation of the colon; residue can be increased when inflammation decreases, but only according to individual tolerance. High-fiber diets, in contrast, are thought to prevent high intraluminal pressure and prevent retention of feces and perforation.
Nutrients Increased Protein (1.5 g/kg/body weight), vitamins and minerals, especially vitamin C, folic acid, vitamin B_{12}, fat-soluble vitamins (A, D, E, and K), calcium, iron, and zinc (supplements may be needed) Caloric intake increased to 2500 or 3000 calories Fluids increased to the equivalent of 8 to 10 glasses/day	Increased protein provides the nitrogen necessary for new tissue synthesis and healing; vitamins and minerals enhance tissue synthesis and healing and aid medical treatment of many deficiency diseases such as anemia. Calories from other sources (carbohydrate and fat) spare protein for tissue synthesis and enhance weight gain. Fluids restore fluids lost during periods of hemorrhage or diarrhea.
Nutrients Decreased Complex carbohydrates with fiber in colitis and Crohn's disease.* Natural sugars with lactose (milk) if lactose intolerance is evident LCTs. Fat of this type is limited to 10%–25% (50 g) of total calories, if steatorrhea evident.	Complex carbohydrates are believed to be colon irritants but there is no need to limit them if obstruction or fistulas are not imminent. Lactase is the first enzyme to be impaired in intestinal disorders and the last to be restored; consequently, lactose intolerance may develop in intestinal disorders. LTCs need bile salts and enzymatic action to be absorbed; these may be lacking or inactive in intestinal disorders.

(continued)

Table 7–9
Nutritional Care Plans for Chronic Ulcerative Colitis, Crohn's Disease, and Diverticulosis (continued)

Nutritional Care Plan	Rationale
Dietary Adaptations	See rationales for dietary adaptations in related conditions. Cold or spicy foods may irritate or stimulate colon motility; fibrous foods may cause obstructions in sensitive intestinal conditions; LCTs may cause steatorrhea.
See dietary adaptations for related disorders: lactose intolerance, celiac sprue, diarrhea, and constipation	
Limit intake of cold foods, spicy foods, and foods high in fiber, in individuals who find them distressing. Limit LCT intakes, substitute MCTs.	
Meal Plan Modifications	
See meal plan modifications in related disorders	
Behavioral Modifications	
See behavioral modifications in related disorders	

* Complex carbohydrates with fiber are not limited in diverticulosis; instead, they are increased.

Table 7–10 299

Table 7-10
Dietary Adaptations for Clients With a Colostomy or an Ileostomy

Symptom	Dietary Adaptations*	Rationale
Blockage	**Foods Limited or Avoided** Nuts, corn, seeds, dried beans, and foods high in fiber (celery) or with heavy skins	Blockage of the artificial opening can cause multiple complications.
Heavy discharge	**Foods Limited or Avoided** Beans, broccoli, spinach, raw fruits, and heavily spiced foods	May prevent a watery or inconvenient discharge, especially if client has an ileostomy
Gas and odor	**Foods Limited or Avoided** Broccoli, cauliflower, milk, onions, Brussels sprouts, highly spiced foods, cabbage, beer, carbonated beverages, fish, legumes, asparagus, melons, and eggs. Fat limited if steatorrhea evident The physician may also advise limiting antibiotics and some vitamin and mineral supplements or giving medications that limit odor (*e.g.*, chlorophyll). Spinach and parsley may help minimize odor; however, spinach may induce a heavy discharge or diarrhea.	Excess gas is caused by aerophagia (swallowing of air while eating or drinking), increased intestinal motility (rapid transit time), or excessive bacterial fermentation of bowel contents; the gases produced are N_2, O_2, CO_2, H_2, and CH_4 (methane). Limiting the foods listed may prevent rapid transit time and fermentation. Odor is caused by steatorrhea or by bacterial action on a particular foodstuff.
Diarrhea	**Foods Limited or Avoided** Raw fruits, broccoli, highly spiced foods, beans, and spinach	Limiting these foods may decrease GI motility and increase transit time.

(continued)

Table 7–10
Dietary Adaptations for Clients With a Colostomy or an Ileostomy (continued)

Symptom	Dietary Adaptations*	Rationale
Constipation	*Foods Limited or Avoided* Refined foods such as refined cereal, white breads, refined pastas, sugar, and rich desserts	If adequate fluids are consumed, constipation may be less severe.

* After these surgical procedures are performed, the client should be encouraged to eat a well-balanced diet in small portions at intervals that suit his lifestyle. These suggestions should be made only if a client expresses discomfort or is in obvious distress after eating one or several of these foods. The nurse should avoid mentioning these symptoms in advance, because the client is apt to imagine symptoms if he has been told they might occur.

Bibliography

American Dietetic Association: Position paper on bland diet in the treatment of chronic duodenal ulcer disease. J Am Diet Assoc 59:244, 1971

Anderson L, Dipple MV, Turkki PR et al: Nutrition in Health and Disease, 17th ed. Philadelphia, JB Lippincott, 1982

Brunner LS: What to do (and what to teach your patient) about peptic ulcer. Nursing 6:27, 1976

Castell DO, Frank BB: How to treat heartburn with diet therapy. Nutrition Today 14:12, 1979

Chernoff R, Dean JA: Medical and nutritional aspects of intractable diarrhea. J Am Diet Assoc 76:161, 1980

Coale MS, Robson JRK: Dietary management of intractable diarrhea in malnourished patients. J Am Diet Assoc 76:444, 1980

Dolin BJ, Boyce HW: Dietary management of gastrointestinal disorders. J Fla Med Assoc 66:305, 1979

Gannon RB, Pickett K: Jaundice. Am J Nurs 83:404, 1983

Greenberger NJ: Gastrointestinal Disorders: A Pathophysiologic Approach, 2nd ed. Chicago, Year Book Medical Publishers, 1981

Hunt SM, Groff JL, Holbrook JM: Nutrition: Principles and Clinical Practice. New York, John Wiley & Sons, 1980

Ippoliti AF, Maxwell V, Isenberg JI: The effect of various forms of milk on gastric-acid secretion. Ann Intern Med 84:286, 1976

Krause MV, Mahan LK: Food, Nutrition and Diet Therapy. Philadelphia, WB Saunders, 1979

Levitt MD: Foods that produce gas. Nutrition and the M.D. 8:1, 1982

Levitt MD, Bond JH: Flatulence. Annu Rev Med 31:127, 1980

Morain CO, Segal AW, Levi AJ: Elemental diets in treatment of acute Crohn's disease. Br Med J 281:1173, 1980

Mullen BD, McGinn KA: The Ostomy Book: Living Comfortably with Colostomies, Ileostomies, and Urostomies. Palo Alto, CA, Bull Publishing, 1980

Pennington JAT, Church HN: Food Values of Portions Commonly Used, 13th ed. Philadelphia, JB Lippincott, 1980

Phillips SF, Stephen AM: The structure and function of the large intestine. Nutrition Today 16:4, 1981

Roe DA: Drug-nutrient interactions. Med Times 109:66, 1981

Smith CH, Bidlack WR: Food and drug interactions. Food Technology 36:99, 1982

Southgate DAT, Van Soest PJ: Fiber analysis tables. Am J Clin Nutr 31 (Suppl):281, 1978

Spiller GA, Amen RJ (eds): Dietary Fiber Research. New York, Plenum Press, 1978

Spiller GA, Freeman HJ: Recent advances in dietary fiber and colorectal diseases. Am J Clin Nutr 34:1145, 1981

Wiener MB, Pepper GA, Kuhn–Weisman G et al: Clinical Pharmacology and Therapeutics in Nursing. New York, McGraw–Hill, 1979

Willoughby JMT: The management of Crohn's disease. Practitioner 225:345, 1981

Winick M (ed): Nutritional Management of Genetic Disorders. New York, John Wiley & Sons, 1979

chapter 8

Gastrointestinal Accessory Organs and Kidneys

Gastrointestinal accessory organs are located within close proximity of the gastrointestinal tract (GI), and contribute to the tract's performance. The organs discussed here are the pancreas, gallbladder, liver, and kidneys. The kidneys, although not distinctly GI accessory organs, are included in this chapter for the sake of completeness.

Functions

In general, the GI-related functions of these organs are as follows:

- The pancreas provides the chemical secretions, enzymes, and hormones necessary for chemical digestion of food molecules into their smaller counterparts in order that they may be absorbed. In addition, it secretes hormones (insulin and glucagon) that assist in the utilization of absorbed nutrients.
- The gallbladder stores the bile produced by the liver and releases it into the duodenum, where it enhances the digestion and absorption of fats.
- The liver, besides producing bile, receives the absorbed nutrients through the portal blood, which it stores, activates, reconstructs, and releases into the bloodstream. The bloodstream then transports the nutrients to the body sites where they are used for energy or tissue synthesis.
- The kidneys' relation to the GI tract is to excrete toxins produced by nutrient breakdown (*i.e.,* urea and ammonia) and toxins ingested with foods. The kidneys also reabsorb certain nutrients and elements to maintain homeostasis.

General Etiologies

Etiologies of organ dysfunctions are listed in the section on each organ.

Drug Therapy

See discussions of specific dysfunctions and Table 7-1.

Principles of Diet Therapy

Goals

See the discussion of goals of diet therapy in gastrointestinal dysfunctions in Chapter 7 and specific dysfunctions in this chapter.

Nutritional Care Plan

Factors in General GI Accessory Organ Dysfunctions

Interview Chart

See components with special significance in GI dysfunctions, Chapter 7.

Nutritional Assessment Data

See data requiring specific emphasis in GI dysfunctions, Chapter 7.

Factors in Specific GI Accessory Organ Dysfunctions

All the general factors in developing any gastrointestinal care plan are included, as well as

- Location of the dysfunction
- Normal functions of the organ involved
- Etiology and risk factors
- Characteristics, symptoms, and clinical signs of the disorder
- Treatment of the disorder (*e.g.,* drug therapy, drug–diet interactions)

Pancreas

Functions

- Produces a digestive juice (pancreatic juice), which it secretes into the small intestines when stimulated by a hormone (secretin); this secretion, which contains bicarbonate (HCO_3), functions to neutralize the acidic chyme released from the stomach into the duodenum
- Secretes insulin and glucagon directly into the bloodstream (see Chaps. 1 and 5)
- Secretes digestive enzymes into a collecting duct, which empties into the small intestine. The release of these enzymes is stimulated by a hormone (cholecystokinin–pancreozymin [CCK–PZ]), which is produced by the duodenum. Liberation of this hormone into the bloodstream is stimulated by the presence of amino acids and fatty acids in the duodenum. The enzymes secreted include trypsin, which converts protein into polypeptides and amino acids; amylase, which breaks down polysaccharides (complex sugars) into disaccharides (less complex sugars); and lipase, which, along with bile, changes neutral fats (long-chain triglycerides) into free fatty acids and glycerol. Information about other enzymes released by the pancreas can be obtained in advanced nutrition texts.

Common Dysfunctions

Pancreatitis

Description

An inflammatory disease of the pancreas, which may be acute or chronic

Etiological Hypotheses

1. Primary organ dysfunctions, such as a reflux of duodenal contents into the pancreatic duct, regurgitation of bile from the common duct up the pancreatic duct, or obstruction of the pancreatic duct
2. Secondary to other disorders, such as alcoholism, biliary tract disease, penetration duodenal ulcer, metabolic disorders (*e.g.,* hyperlipoproteinemia), infections (*e.g.,* mumps and viral hepatitis), cystic fibrosis, postoperative trauma, and excessive use of certain drugs (*e.g.,* corticosteroids and thiazide diuretics)

Characteristics

Progressive inflammatory destruction, edema, fibrosis, and calcification. (May be asymptomatic even with 90% reduction in the secretion of lipase and trypsin). Results in pancreatic insufficiency with reduced production and release of enzymes and hormones, leading to impaired degradation of foodstuffs. Additionally, when extensive damage occurs in the pancreas or the ducts become blocked, large quantities of pancreatic secretions are held within the pancreas. Consequently, the proteolytic enzymes (normally as bland as pablum within the pancreas) penetrate their lipoprotein membranes, become activated, and begin autodigestion of the cellular tissues.

Symptoms

Vomiting, nausea, epigastric pain, anorexia, weight loss, steatorrhea (see Table 7-4), azotorrhea (nitrogen in the urine or feces), hypotension, hypocalcemia, hypoalbuminemia, possible hypoglycemia, fever, ileus, and shock

Drug Therapy

- Acute Pancreatitis. Analgesics and narcotics (*e.g.*, meperidine hydrochloride) for pain; insulin if necessary
- Chronic Pancreatitis. Antacids; anticholinergics; cimetidine with antacids (see Table 7-1); supplements such as pancreatin capsules; multiple vitamin supplements including water-soluble forms of vitamins A, E, D, and B_{12} (parenterally if necessary); and mineral supplements, especially iron (pancreatic supplements decrease its absorption) and zinc

Diet Therapy

- Acute Phase
  1. Nutritional Care Plan. Methodology is to give nothing by mouth (NPO) until symptoms subside. Homeostasis is maintained by intravenous (IV) solutions of fluids, dextrose, and electrolytes. As symptoms subside, progress to carbohydrate liquid feedings such as fruit juice and gelatin.

     Clients who have severe symptoms (*e.g.*, shock) or are recovering slowly, however, may need to be maintained on central vein total nutritional support solutions or chemically defined elemental diets (consult Chap. 2 for details on the nutrient content and administration of these nutritional support systems).
- Chronic Phase
  1. Nutritional Care Plan. High-calorie, high-protein, high-carbohydrate, low-fat (25 g–30 g), bland diet, as tolerated; designed to prevent malnutrition and overstimulation of the pancreas
     a. Methodology. Oral feedings
     b. Nutrients Increased. Protein; all vitamins and minerals, especially fat-soluble vitamins (A, D, E, and K), vitamin B_{12} and

iron; electrolytes (especially potassium) and fluids increased to replace losses; carbohydrates increased to enhance weight gain and allow protein to be used for tissue synthesis instead of for energy

c. Nutrients Decreased

(1) Fats containing long-chain triglycerides (LCTs) because LCTs require pancreatic lipase plus bile for digestion

(2) Complex carbohydrates because complex carbohydrates require amylase for digestion

(3) Refined carbohydrates, if insulin is insufficient

d. Dietary Adaptations

(1) Avoid gastric stimulants such as beverages containing caffeine, meat extracts, spices limited on the liberal ulcer regimen (see Table 7-3), and alcohol, which is believed to stimulate pancreatic secretions, irritate the intestinal mucosa, and encourage exacerbations

(2) Limit foods containing starch such as pastas, breads, and cereals unless pancreatin is administered

(3) If insulin is insufficient, limit foods containing refined sugars such as candies, sugar, and sodas; otherwise increase these foods in order to increase calories

(4) Limit foods containing LCTs (Table 8-1),* unless pancreatin is administered

(5) When food variety is limited, owing to intolerance, administer oral solutions of water-soluble vitamins and fat-soluble vitamins A, D, E, and K

(6) Administer capsules or tablets† containing pancreatin (Cotazym), pancreatic enzymes extracted from porcine pancreas, with meals and snacks; these enzymes will enhance nutrient absorption but they will not completely eliminate maldigestion because some of the pancreatin is destroyed by gastric pepsin; client must be closely monitored

(7) Substitute medium-chain triglyceride (MCT) oils, MCT margarines, or other preparations that combine sugar, vitamins, essential fatty acids, and minerals with MCT oils (*e.g.,* Portagen or Pregestimil; see Tables 8-1 and 8-2); approximately 3 tablespoons of MCT oil can be added, each day, to foods such as skim milk, homemade salad dressing, and milkshakes made of whole milk, sugar, and vanilla; the oil can also be used for frying if the heat is low and slow;

---

* See tables at the end of this chapter.

† Tablets must not contact lips or skin, because they will digest the protein in those tissues.

        solids can be used in food preparation or at the table if tolerated

   (8) If hyperglycemia is evident, use dietary adaptations recommended for diabetes mellitus (see Chap. 5); if flatulence evident, limit foods that may produce excessive gas (see Table 7-10)

  e. Meal Plan Modifications

    (1) Advise 6 small meals a day rather than 3 large ones

    (2) Introduce foods that may cause discomfort one at a time, so that individual intolerances can be detected rapidly

2. Behavioral Modifications

  a. Obtain adequate rest

  b. Avoid alcohol

Cystic Fibrosis—Mucoviscidosis

Description

Systemic disorder caused by dysfunction of mucus-producing exocrine glands

Etiologic Hypothesis

Mendelian recessive trait by which low plasma levels of essential fatty acids impair synthesis of prostaglandins

Characteristics

Mucin-producing exocrine gland dysfunction is believed to cause a buildup of abnormally thick viscous mucus in the bronchi, pancreas, liver, and intestines, which ultimately blocks passage of exocrine gland secretions. Blockage in the pancreatic duct causes dilatation of the secretory acini, degeneration and infiltration of exocrine parenchyma by adipose tissue, pancreatic insufficiency, and malabsorption

Symptoms

Chronic pulmonary disease; abnormal concentration of electrolytes in sweat, salivary, and lacrimal secretions; pancreatic insufficiency with maldigestion and steatorrhea; voracious appetite until treated, after which the child becomes a picky eater, leading to weight loss and malnutrition; dry hacking cough; secondary symptoms created by secondary dysfunctions such as liver disease, heart disease, respiratory disease, and disorders of the small intestine

Drug Therapy

Potassium iodide (liquefies mucus and minimizes its formation); antibiotics; multiple vitamin and iron supplements; pancreatin tablets, capsules, or powder (Pancrease, Cotazym, Viokase); and, in hot climates or when exercise is excessive, salt tablets

Diet Therapy

- Acute Phase. Nutritional care plan is same as for pancreatitis
- Chronic Phase
  1. Nutritional Care Plan. High-calorie, high-protein, high-carbohydrate, low-or moderate-fat, increased-fluid, bland diet, as tolerated; designed to prevent overstimulation of the pancreas, malnutrition, and growth retardation
     a. Methodology. Oral feedings
     b. Nutrients Increased. Protein (6–8 g/kg IBW/day or $2\frac{1}{2}$ times the normal requirement); carbohydrates (grams given determined by caloric requirements); all vitamins (especially A, D, E, and K); all minerals (especially iron [pancreatic enzymes decrease absorption]); all electrolytes (especially sodium); fluids also increased to replace losses and thin mucus; caloric intake increased to 150 kcal/kg IBW/day or approximately 50% to 100% above normal requirements to offset malabsorption, increased basal metabolic rates (increased respiratory and heart rates and infection), malnutrition, and undesirable growth rates
     c. Nutrients Decreased. Fat, moderate reduction (70 g/day) to enhance caloric intake, but a more strict plan (25 g–30 g of fat) may be necessary if steatorrhea and abdominal pain are severe; complex carbohydrates (*e.g.,* starches) because complex carbohydrates need amylase for digestion; refined carbohydrates when hyperglycemia is apparent
     d. Dietary Adaptations. Same as the adaptations used for pancreatitis with the following modifications
        (1) Pancreatic powder (Viokase) may be used, in carbohydrate foods, instead of tablets; powder can be added to cereals or applesauce (*e.g.,* $\frac{1}{3}$–1 teaspoon Viokase per serving)
        (2) Infant formulas that are high in protein and carbohydrate but low in fat may be used rather than other infant formulas; commercial formulas with this composition are Probana, which contains LCTs, Pregestimil and Portagen, which contains a high percentage of MCTs and some LCTs (*e.g.,* corn oil). The latter provides linoleic acid.
        (3) Extra salt may be added to foods to make up for losses
        (4) Liquid supplements that are low in fat such as sweetened fruit juices or milkshakes made with skim milk and sherbet may be necessary to meet caloric needs in older children (supplements high in protein must have enzymes added; when foods have enzymes added they must not contact

lips [use straws] or skin because the enzymes will digest the protein in these tissues)

(5) Administer iodine medications with grape juice to enhance palatability

(6) Increase fluid intake to liquefy secretions

e. Meal Plan Modifications. Same as for pancreatitis

2. Behavioral Modifications

a. Obtain adequate rest

b. Take salt tablets (on the advice of a physician) before extensive exercise

c. Eat in an upright position to enhance pulmonary function

d. Practice good dental hygiene. Malnutrition and altered saliva contents enhance dental caries

Zollinger–Ellison Syndrome

Description

Disorder of the pancreas that causes extensive secretion of gastrin

Etiology

A tumor in the non-beta islet cells of the pancreas

Characteristics

High levels of gastrin cause hypersecretion of gastric acid with the resultant development of duodenal ulcers. The lower pH in the intestines also stimulates intestinal motility, which causes diarrhea and steatorrhea

Symptoms, Drug Therapy, and Diet Therapy

Same as for duodenal ulcers, diarrhea, and steatorrhea (consult Chap. 7 for details on the treatment of these disorders)

Carcinoma of the Pancreas

Consult Chapter 4 for details on the nutritional management of clients with cancer

Gallbladder

Functions

• Stores a limited amount of bile, which is produced by the liver

• Concentrates bile by removing water and inorganic electrolytes; bile composed of bile salts, bilirubin, organic anions, cholesterol, lecithin, water, cations, and anions

- Delivers bile to the small intestines when stimulated by cholecystokinin-pancreozymin (CCK-PZ), a hormone produced in the small intestines. The hormone travels by way of the bloodstream to the gallbladder where it simultaneously stimulates gallbladder musculature contraction and sphincter of Oddi relaxation. Foods that stimulate the hormone's release contain high concentrations of LCTs. In the small intestines, bile acts to emulsify fats so that they can be broken down by the enzyme lipase and absorbed through the lymph system.

Common Dysfunctions

Cholelithiasis and Cholecystitis

Description

In cholelithiasis, bile is crystallized and gallstones are formed. These stones usually have a high cholesterol content. Cholecystitis (inflammation of the gallbladder) occurs when a gallstone becomes impacted in the cystic duct. Impaction may be precipitated by obesity, dietary indiscretions, pregnancy, and constricting clothing. Trauma and surgery in other areas of the body may also cause cholecystitis.

Etiologic Hypotheses

Advanced age; sex (higher in females); obesity (fat intake may be increased); hormonal imbalance (estrogen, progestin, and insulin); excessive use of certain drugs (*e.g.,* clofibrate, cholestyramine, oral contraceptives); a dual defect involving the enzyme 3-hydroxy-3-methylgluryl C_o A (HMG C_oA), an enzyme concerned with cholesterol synthesis, and cholesterol 7-a-hydroxylase, an enzyme concerned with bile salt synthesis

Characteristics

Gallstones are believed to develop when bile salts are insufficient and the cholesterol content of bile is too high. Consequently, the cholesterol crystallizes and gallstones are formed. When these stones slip into the common bile duct, they prevent the passage of sufficient bile into the duodenum. The end result is that absorption of fats and fat-soluble vitamins (A, D, E, and K) is impaired. When a gallstone becomes impacted in the cystic duct, the bile becomes imprisoned, the gallbladder becomes distended, bacteria proliferate, and inflammation occurs.

Symptoms

Gallstones may be asymptomatic, or there may be intermittent epigastric pain, indigestion, intolerance to fatty and spicy foods, nausea, vomiting, flatulence, belching, and heartburn. Stools may be light-colored (because of a lack of bile pigments). When the common duct becomes obstructed, jaundice and steatorrhea usually become apparent.

Drug Therapy

Antispasmodics, analgesics, antacids, and chemodeoxycholic acid (CDCA), which is administered to dissolve gallstones that are predominately cholesterol

Diet Therapy

- Acute Phase
  1. Severe Inflammation. Methodology of the nutritional care plan is NPO for 12 to 24 hours. Homeostasis maintained by IV solutions of fluids, dextrose, and electrolytes or by central vein total nutritional support solutions when symptoms do not subside or recovery rate is slow (consult Chap. 2 for details on the nutrient content and administration of these nutritional support systems).
  2. Less Severe Inflammation. Methodology of the nutritional care plan is that the initial feedings are oral liquid feedings composed of sweetened fruit juices, fruit nectars, gelatin, and skim milk. Then, feedings progress to the chronic phase care plan. The rate of progression depends upon the individual's tolerance.
- Chronic Phase
  1. Nutritional Care Plan. Low-total-fat, low-calorie (if obesity exists), bland diet, as tolerated; designed to reduce discomfort and minimize contraction of the gallbladder
     a. Methodology. Oral feedings
     b. Nutrients Increased. Protein increased from 0.8 g/kg/day to 1.5 to 2 g/kg/day for tissue regeneration; carbohydrate increased to replace fat calories (if there are no caloric restrictions) and to provide energy in order to spare protein (fibrous complex carbohydrates make up the greatest percentage of this increased carbohydrate intake because fiber may decrease transit time and some fibers [*e.g.,* pectin] lower serum cholesterol levels; consequently, the total endogenous supply of cholesterol is reduced); MCT increased if additional calories are needed during severe complications; vitamin and minerals increased, especially A, D, E, and K, for their absorption is curtailed when fat absorption is impaired
     c. Nutrients Decreased. Total fat intake, not just saturated fat, reduced to 40 to 50 g/day because the decrease minimizes gallbladder contractions and adverse symptoms (cholesterol is not lowered, for at present no evidence suggests that lower

intake of exogenous cholesterol will lower biliary cholesterol);
refined carbohydrates limited when calories must be restricted; total calories decreased *gradually* to 1200 to 1800 calories
if obesity exists because without a gradual reduction, cholesterol secretions will be excessive and bile cholesterol saturation increased

  d. Dietary Adaptations

    (1) Consult dietary adaptations for LCT restrictions listed in
Table 8-1

    (2) Limit spicy foods that appear to cause distress

    (3) Limit foods that appear to increase "gas" if distress is evi-
dent (see Table 7-10)

    (4) Limit all foods that add extra calories if obesity exists
(consult Chap. 6)

  e. Meal Plan Modifications

    (1) Advise six small, rather than three large, meals a day

    (2) Introduce foods that may cause discomfort one at a time,
so that individual intolerances can be detected rapidly

2. Behavioral Modifications

  a. Obtain adequate rest

  b. Limit or avoid alcohol

  c. Read labels; many foods have hidden sources of fat

  d. Adjust food preparation methods (*i.e.,* bake and broil foods
instead of frying them)

Liver

Functions

The liver may be called the "central supply" of the human body, for
all the ingested and absorbed nutrients are transported from the small intestines, by way of the portal circulation, to the liver, with the exception
of long-chain fatty acids and fat-soluble vitamins. (These are transported
from the small intestines, by way of the lymph system, to the systemic circulation.) However, even the long-chain fatty acids and fat-soluble vitamins are eventually transported to the liver to be stored, activated, and
used for energy. The liver's major functions in the metabolism of nutrients are as follows:

- For carbohydrates, converts galactose and fructose to glucose,
stores excess glucose in the form of glycogen (glycogenesis), de-
grades glycogen to glucose (glycogenolysis) when glucose is needed
by other tissues for energy, oxidizes glucose to energy

- For protein, converts proteins into glucose (gluconeogenesis); synthesizes plasma proteins such as albumin, globulin, fibrinogen, prothrombin, and transferrin; removes nitrogenous waste products, including ammonia, by producing urea, which is eliminated by the kidneys; synthesizes nonessential amino acids from other amino acids by a process called *transamination*; synthesizes purines and pyrimidines from nitrogen; forms amines by protein decarboxylation

- For fat, synthesizes triglycerides from glycerol and fatty acids, removes excess triglycerides by forming very-low-density lipoproteins (VLDLs) that can transport triglycerides to the adipose tissue for storage, oxidizes fatty acids to ketone acids and energy, synthesizes cholesterol from acetate, synthesizes high-density lipoproteins (HDLs)

- For vitamins, stores vitamins A, D, E, and K and some vitamin C and B-complex vitamins, especially B_{12}; helps transport vitamin A to the eye by binding it to protein; hydroxylates vitamin D at the 25th carbon so that it can be activated in the kidneys

- For minerals, stores iron, copper, zinc, and magnesium

Other functions are to produce and excrete bile to the gallbladder and to detoxify drugs, such as oral contraceptives, morphine, barbiturates, and alcohol.

It is estimated that 10 million Americans can now be considered chronic alcoholics (individuals who consume the equivalent of 16 oz of scotch whiskey/day for over 10 yr). Alcohol addiction leads to progressive liver disease in 10% to 20% of alcoholic clients. The reason that not all chronic alcoholics develop progressive liver disease is unknown, but the progression is thought to be related to the duration and amount of the alcohol intake and to undefined genetic and possibly immunologic factors. Of special note is that recent research by Rubin and Lieber demonstrates that *alcohol, not malnutrition, is the causative factor* in progressive liver disease, although malnutrition may enhance its progression. Malnutrition in the alcoholic client is related to the following factors:

- Substitution of alcohol for nutrient density calories (*i.e.,* 1 g of alcohol yields 7 kcal, or 1 jigger, [1–1½ oz] of 100-proof scotch (50% alcohol) contains approximately 19 g of alcohol, or 133 kcal)

- Inadequate ingestion of all nutrients, due to adverse symptoms such as anorexia, nausea, and vomiting

- Inadequate absorption of all nutrients, due to alcohol toxicity of the small intestine with resultant malabsorption of essential nutrients, especially folic acid and thiamine

- Impaired metabolism of essential nutrients within the hepatocyte, due to alcohol toxicity

- Increased excretion of essential nutrients (*e.g.,* zinc and magnesium)

Common Dysfunctions

Progressive Liver Disease or Hepatic Failure

Description

Progressive liver disease may be acute or chronic, progressing from an impaired fat and protein production and transport to a significant loss of liver cells. Subsequently, this loss of cellular function induces portal hypertension, which ultimately causes shunting of endogenous and exogenous toxic substances into the portal systemic venous collateral circulation and the brain.

Etiologic Risk Factors

Hepatitis A (also called viral hepatitis and formerly called infectious hepatitis)

Hepatitis B (formerly called serum hepatitis)

Non-A, non-B hepatitis (NANBH)

Alcoholic hepatitis

Toxic hepatitis

Drug-induced hepatitis

Alcoholism

Shock

Infections that affect the liver (*e.g.,* Reye's syndrome)

Acute fatty liver of pregnancy

Metabolic disorders (*e.g.,* Wilson's disease, a degenerative disease characterized by abnormal copper metabolism, hemochromatosis [abnormal iron metabolism], and poorly controlled diabetes mellitus)

Energy malnutrition in infancy and early childhood

Characteristics Related to Alcoholism

- Stage I. Increased ingestion of alcohol calories plus nutrient calories may result in obesity, hyperlipidemia, hypertension, or diabetes mellitus.
- Stage II, Hepatomegaly (also called "fatty liver"). Continued chronic ingestion of alcohol results in accelerated ethanol metabolism with an accompanying increased production and decreased disposition of *acetylaldehyde,* a hepatic toxin. An imbalance in metabolism is hypothesized to affect the liver in the following manner:
  1. It depresses mitochondrial functions, including lipid oxidation
  2. It impairs hepatocyte structure, especially the rough endoplasmic reticulum membrane, an organelle responsible for protein synthesis

3. It alters hepatic microtubules, which ultimately reduces the secretion and transport of export proteins (*e.g.*, albumin, transferrin, and clotting factors II, VII, IX, and X); consequently, protein secretion is decreased and protein retention is increased

4. It impairs lipoprotein secretion, which is manifested by engorgement of the Golgi apparatus with VLDL-like particles. Simultaneously, accelerated ethanol metabolism increases hydrogen ion production with an accompanying *increase in triglyceride production.* Subsequently, accumulation of lipid and protein in the liver causes enlargement of the hepatocytes.

- Stage III, Alcoholic Hepatitis. Alcoholic hepatitis is usually chronic in nature, developing over a period of years, while other types of hepatitis are usually acute, developing over a short period of time. However, hepatic inflammation and often hepatomegaly, with accompanying hepatocyte cell necrosis, will also develop in these conditions without effective treatment. If hepatomegaly is not treated — that is, if the individual does not abstain from alcohol — and hepatotoxicity continues, it can induce

  1. Decreased vitamin activity and protein synthesis, which can enhance infection

  2. Increased production of lactic acid, which can enhance hyperuricemia and hypoglycemia

  3. Reduced bilirubin excretion with accompanying jaundice

  4. Hepatocyte inflammation, which leads to cell necrosis and elevation of transaminase enzymes in the serum (*e.g.*, serum glutamic-pyruvic transaminase [SGPT] now called alanine aminotransferase)[ALT]

- Stage IV, Cirrhosis. Cirrhosis is a general term that includes all forms of chronic diffuse liver disease. The characteristics of cirrhosis are

  1. Significant loss of liver cells

  2. Collapse and fibrosis of supporting reticular network with distortion of the vascular bed

  3. Nodular regeneration of the remaining liver cell mass
     The most common types of cirrhosis are Laennec's (alcohol-induced), postnecrotic, biliary, and cardiac or congestive. Laennec's cirrhosis develops, in some individuals, if alcohol consumption continues over a period of years because continued swelling of the cells and "crowding" of other hepatocytes, plus inflammation, lead to excessive necrosis of functioning liver cells, with accompanying *fibrosis* (formation of tough fibrous connective tissue) of supporting tissues and distortion of the vascular bed. Subsequently, deterioration of the liver leads to *portal hypertension* with sustained elevation of venous pressure and *shunting of portal blood into the portal systemic venous collateral circulation.* The last can induce *ascites* (accumulation of fluid in the peritoneal cavity), due

to sodium retention, impaired water excretion, and decreased plasma oncotic pressure as the result of severe *hypoalbuminemia*, which occurs because the liver no longer releases albumin into the serum. Additionally, alcohol toxicity and liver dysfunction often precipitate cardiac and renal dysfunction with accompanying hypertension. Other possible contributors are abnormalities in sympathetic tone and prostaglandin concentrations. Portal hypertension can also induce *esophageal varices* (engorgement of the lower esophageal veins). Of note here is the fact that irritants, such as foods high in roughage, can cause the varices to rupture, resulting in severe hemorrhage. Severe liver dysfunction also causes decreased production of prothrombin, which impairs blood clotting. In addition, it impairs urea synthesis, which causes a subsequent *buildup of ammonia* in the portal systemic venous collateral circulation.

- Stage V, Encephalopathy. Encephalopathy is any degenerative disease of the brain. Ultimately, if ammonia elevation in the systemic blood circulation is not curtailed, it causes central nervous system intoxication with accompanying brain degeneration. This ammonia is produced from endogenous urea and exogenous protein, augmented by intestinal bacteria. Presently, however, substances other than ammonia are thought to be responsible for the brain degeneration that can accompany liver dysfunction. Some of the substances under investigation are elevations of short-chain fatty acids, hypersecretion of glucagon, elevations of mercaptans produced by methionine, and changes in the ratio of aromatic (*e.g.,* tyrosine, phenylalanine, tryptophan, and methionine), and branched-chain (*e.g.,* leucine, isoleucine, and valine) amino acids in the systemic blood and at the blood–brain barrier. (The aromatic amino acids become elevated while the branched-chain amino acids are normal or depressed.) The reason for this change in ratio is thought to be that branched-chain amino acids are metabolized in extrahepatic tissue while aromatic amino acids are extracted in the liver. Subsequently, there is a change in the neurotransmitter system of the central nervous system: serotonin is increased, and norepinephrine is depressed.
- Stage VI, Hepatic Coma and Death. Ultimately, coma and death follow if encephalopathy is left untreated.

Progressive Symptoms of Hepatic Failure*

- Chronic Alcoholism. Weight gain, atherosclerosis, hypertension, and possibly diabetes mellitus

---

* This is only a generalized progression of symptoms; each individual will develop a different set of symptoms at different times throughout the progression of the disease.

- Hepatomegaly. Same as above, or client may begin to have progressive symptoms such as anorexia
- Hepatitis. Anorexia, vomiting, diarrhea, fatigue, abdomen and back pain, headache, weight loss, irritability, depression, jaundice with accompanying dark urine
- Cirrhosis. All the symptoms of hepatitis plus ascites, esophagael varices, reduced liver size, itching, and anemia
- Encephalopathy. Asterixis (flapping tremors of the hands and tongue when extended), fetor hepaticus (liver breath), behavioral changes (lethargy and disorientation)

Drug Therapy*

Drugs are used in liver disease to relieve adverse symptoms. They include diuretics (for treatment of edema), antidiarrheals, potassium chloride (for treatment of hypokalemia), and cholestyramine (for relief of itching). Drugs are also used to relieve the symptoms and possible complications of secondary diseases such as kidney disease, diabetes mellitus (see Chap. 5), and coronary heart disease (see Chap. 3).

Neomycin sulfate and lactulose are used to depress elevated levels of ammonia in systemic blood. Neomycin sulfate (Neomycin) eliminates the bacteria capable of breaking down protein and urea into ammonia. Neomycin enhances the malabsorption syndrome (see Table 7–1). Lactulose (Cephulac) acidifies the colon through bacterial action. This acidification causes ammonia to remain in the colon as the ammonium ion instead of migrating into the systemic blood. Lactulose enhances gaseous distention, leading to flatulence, abdominal discomfort, and diarrhea.

Diet Therapy

Dietary prescriptions or nutritional care plans in liver disease are not static. Instead, they are determined, as in renal disease, by the individual's biochemical and clinical status at any particular time.

- Goals
  1. Improve and maintain nutritional status by curtailing liver degeneration and enhancing tissue regeneration
  2. Control weight gain or loss
  3. Diminish nervous system complications by reducing the ammonia and aromatic amino acid content of the systemic circulation
  4. Other goals listed under goals of diet therapy in gastrointestinal disorders, Chapter 7
- Acute Stage
  For nutritional care plan, see Stage V in Tables 8–3 and 8–4

---

* Drug therapy may be contraindicated in liver disease, since most drugs are detoxified in the liver.

- Chronic Stage
  1. Nutritional Care Plan. Controlled protein, fat, sodium, and fluid diet (see Table 8–3). In chronic alcoholism, treatment by diet will be to no avail if the client continues to drink.
     a. Methodology. Depends upon the stage of the disease (see Tables 8–3 and 8–4)
     b. Nutrients Increased. See Tables 8–3 and 8–4
     c. Nutrients Decreased. See Tables 8–3 and 8–4
     d. Dietary Adaptations
        (1) Milk Group
            (a) Skim milk and dried milk are encouraged to increase calories and protein unless lactose intolerance, prehepatic coma, or ascites evident. If ascites exists, Lonalac (a salt-free milk) should be used.
            (b) Salt-free and fat-free cheeses are encouraged.
        (2) Meat Group. Client should be encouraged to eat foods in this group, especially eggs, for they contain high biologic-value protein. However, if they are not tolerated because of their high aromatic and ammoniogenic amino acid content, low biologic-value proteins such as vegetables (*e.g.*, legumes and nuts) may by substituted (Table 8–5). Client must be monitored, however, for these vegetables may enhance diarrhea and steatorrhea.
        (3) Fruits and Vegetables
            (a) Consumption of canned fruits in heavy syrup or fruit juices with added sugar is encouraged for they enhance caloric intake and spare protein. Fruits are also high in potassium and low in sodium.
            (b) Cooked vegetables with added cream sauces (may also have MCT added) and margarine are also encouraged if fat is not an additional restriction for they enhance calorie, vitamin, and mineral intake.
            (c) Raw fruits and vegetables may be avoided for they enhance diarrhea and satiety, which will ultimately decrease caloric intake.
            (d) All fruits and vegetables must be pureed when esophogeal varices are evident.
        (4) Breads and Cereals
            (a) Whole-wheat products are encouraged because they have a high vitamin B-complex content. Products with a high-fiber content (*e.g.*, added bran) are discouraged for they aggravate esophageal varices and enhance diarrhea and satiety.

(b) Low-protein wheat products must be used when hepatic coma threatens.

(c) Salted breads and instant cereals are limited.

(5) Miscellaneous Foods. Foods such as refined carbohydrates and fats, especially MCT fats, are encouraged because they increase caloric intake and spare protein.

(a) Sugar and modular feedings high in carbohydrate (*e.g.*, Controlyte and Cal Power) should be added to fruit juices, whenever tolerated.

(b) Hard candy, cake, and pie consumption should be encouraged.

(c) Butter and margarines that are salt-free may be added to foods; fried foods are discouraged.

(d) Salty foods and salt at the table should be curtailed. Salt substitutes that contain potassium may be used on the advice of the physician; however, substitutes that contain ammonium ions may not be used (see also Table 3–9 and Appendix VI, Protein, Phosphorus, Sodium, and Potassium Exchange Lists).

e. Meal Plan Modifications

(1) Six to eight meals per day may be better tolerated than three large meals. This plan may also apply when chronic alcoholics are trying to abstain (food may relieve tension). Abstinence is the first priority; weight loss, the second.

(2) During the last stages of the disease, small meals are recommended with the exception of breakfast. Nausea is not as great in the morning; therefore, food may be better tolerated.

2. Behavioral Modifications

(a) Alcohol abstinence

(b) Taste food before salting or use salt substitutes when prescribed.

(c) If hepatitis has been transmitted by a virus, institute the hospital protocol recommended for contagious diseases such as using only disposable dishes, utensils, cups, and trays and disposing of food wastes in the client's room, not in the central dish area.

Nurse's Responsibilities in the Nutritional Care of the Client With Liver Disease

The nurse's first responsibility is to report any evidence of alcoholic intake. The nurse's second responsibility is to enhance food consumption, because food may be the most important therapeutic measure in recovery. Unfortunately, however, clients with liver dysfunctions often find food repugnant. Therefore, in order to enhance consumption, special emphasis must be put on obtaining information on the client's food likes and dislikes and in making mealtime pleasant (*e.g.*, trays should be attractive and atmosphere pleasant). Additionally, consumption may be enhanced if menus are handed out close to mealtime when hunger may be at its peak. A third responsibility is to keep accurate intake and output records so that other members of the health team may adjust treatment, when necessary. Other nursing responsibilities are listed in Chapter 7.

Kidneys

Functions

- Maintain the body's homeostatic environment by filtering blood through the 1 million nephrons located in each kidney; excrete wastes, including excess water, urea, uric acid, creatinine, ammonia, nitrates, sulfates, organic acids, and exogenous toxins found in foodstuffs, into urine; reabsorb nutrients, including glucose, amino acids, electrolytes, and water into the bloodstream, when they are needed by body tissues
- Regulate acid–base balance by regulating bicarbonate reabsorption and hydrogen ion secretion
- Synthesize enzymes (*e.g.*, renin), which regulate blood pressure
- Synthesize hormones (*e.g.*, erythropoietin), which regulate erythroid activity in the bone marrow
- Synthesize glucose from deaminated amino acids
- Maintain calcium–phosphorus homeostasis by activating vitamin D_3 to 1,25-dihydroxycholecalciferol

Terminology Related to Renal Disease

- Nephritis (Bright's Disease). A general term used to indicate any altered kidney function caused by either a diffuse inflammation or a degenerative change
- Glomerulonephritis. Inflammation of the glomeruli
- Nephrotic Syndrome (also called nephrosis or "massive proteinuria.") A stage in renal disease in which physiological changes in the permeability of glomerular capillaries allow filtration of plasma proteins (albumin) into urine, with consequent massive proteinuria, followed by hypoalbuminemia and edema as a result of diminished plasma oncotic pressure.
- Nephrosclerosis. Hardening of the arteries of the kidney
- Pyelonephritis. Inflammation of the kidney and its pelvis caused by bacterial infection (usually *Escherichia coli*)

- Nephrolithiasis. Formation of kidney stones, also called renal calculi, characterized by hypercalciuria (urinary excretion of greater than 300 mg in 24 hr) since approximately two thirds of all kidney stones contain calcium; appears to be induced by increased intestinal absorption of dietary calcium, which may be caused by increased production of 1,25-dihydroxycholecalciferol

Common Symptoms in Renal Disease

Edema; hypertension; hematuria; uremia (toxic condition caused by the retention, in the blood, of nitrogenous substances); oliguria (diminished urine formation) or polyuria (excessive urine volume); anemia; acidosis; pruritus; bone pain; nausea; vomiting; anorexia; diarrhea; weight loss; lethargy; and, in end stage renal disease (ESRD), cardiac arrythmias (related to hyperkalemia) and sometimes coma (an individual may lose more than 85% of renal function before symptoms of uremia and renal failure become apparent)

Renal Failure

Description

Acute renal failure (ARF) refers to sudden, reversible renal shutdown in an individual with a previously adequate renal capacity. Chronic renal failure (CRF) refers to any permanent reduction in renal function.

Etiologic Risk Factors

- Acute Renal Failure. Infection, especially respiratory infections caused by streptococci; allergic reactions to pollens (*e.g.*, poisonous plants and insect stings); shock; burns; septic abortion; surgery in other areas of the body; and drugs
- Chronic Renal Failure. Degenerative changes over time are usually secondary to other diseases such as diabetes mellitus, atherosclerosis, or malignant hypertension

Characteristics

- Acute Renal Failure. A sudden decrease in glomerular filtration rate (GFR)* induces oliguria (diminished urine formation) or anuria

---

* In clinical practice, the GFR is adequately estimated from the endogenous creatinine clearance. The normal value for men is from 140 to 200 liters/day (70 $\pm$14 ml/min/sq m) and for women, 120 to 180 liters/day (60 $\pm$10 ml/min/sq m). Plasma concentration of creatinine varies inversely with the GFR and is therefore a useful index of the GFR if production (related to muscle mass and age) and metabolism (increased uremia) are considered. The upper limit of plasma creatinine concentration in men with normal GFR is 1.2 mg/dl; in women, 1 mg/dl. (Berkow R, Talbott JH [eds]: The Merck Manual, 13th ed, p 675. Rahway, NJ, Merck & Co, 1977)

(complete urinary suppression). Subsequently, the blood urea nitrogen (BUN), serum creatinine, uric acid, and phosphate serum levels may rise rapidly, and acute derangements in electrolyte concentrations can occur. Acute renal failure may last anywhere from hours to 3 to 6 months, after which recovery may begin and physiological changes may be reversed—meaning that polyuria (excessive urinary output) may occur. Polyuria causes excessive sodium and potassium losses; therefore, the individual may have to be monitored as frequently as every hour. Dialysis may be necessary if other treatments fail.

- Chronic Renal Failure. A gradual fibrosis of the glomeruli and afferent arterioles or degenerative changes in the kidney's capillary basement membrane and tubules impair the kidney's ability to filter wastes or reabsorb nutrients.

Drug Therapy

Diuretics, vitamin D, calcium salts (calcium carbonate, lactate, or gluconate), and aluminum or calcium hydroxide antacids may be used. Maalox, Gelusil, and Mylanta should not be used in renal disorders because they contain sodium and magnesium, which may enhance or precipitate hypermagnesemia. Sodium polystyrene sulfonate (Kayexalate) is used to treat hyperkalemia. Kayexalate is a cation exchange resin that enhances potassium excretion; however, it also enhances sodium retention, which may accelerate edema.

Diet Therapy

Dietary prescriptions and nutritional care plans used in renal disease are not static. Instead, they are determined by the individual's biochemical and clinical status at any particular time.

- Goals
    1. Maintain optimal nutritional status
    2. Control tissue catabolism and weight loss
    3. Lessen work load in the diseased kidneys
    4. Help the kidneys maintain homeostasis; that is, replace losses and correct deficits
    5. Lessen adverse symptoms such as anorexia and nausea caused by progressive nephron loss
    6. Retard progression of renal failure
    7. Postpone dialysis initiation
- Acute Phase
    1. Nutritional Care Plans
        a. Methodology. Depends upon the individual's degree of catabolic activity, ability to ingest foods, and medical treatment (*i.e.*, drug therapy, dialysis)

b. Classifications of Nutritional Care Plans

(1) High-Calorie, Minimal-Protein. Protein intake is limited to high biologic value (HBV) proteins. All eight essential amino acids (EAAs) are included, and sometimes histidine and arginine are added. This plan provides sufficient calories for energy needs; thus, gluconeogenesis from tissue protein is minimized. Additionally, endogenous urea is used for tissue synthesis; therefore, BUN levels drop. Low protein intake also reduces phosphorus intake. Solutions or feedings that provide the nutrients allowed on this care plan include

(a) Central Vein Parenteral Solutions. The solution presently being used is Nephramine (5.1% AA) mixed with 1000 ml of D_{70} W (glucose concentration 35%)

   i. Composition. 1500 ml/day provides 26 g of EAA and 2400 kcal; electrolytes, vitamins, and insulin added as needed; kilocalorie-to-protein ratio of 90:1

   ii. Disadvantage. Does not contain arginine, an EAA needed by children

(b) Tube Feeding. The feeding presently being used is Amin-Aid (may also be consumed orally)

   i. Composition. 1000 ml of the formula/day provide 20 g of EAAs and 2000 kcal; electrolytes and vitamins supplied as needed; kilocalorie-to-protein ratio of 100:1

   ii. Disadvantage. High osmolality

(c) Oral Feedings. Based upon the Giordano-Giovanetti diet plan; essential amino acid (EAA) plus histidine supplementation may be instituted if diet is required for a long period of time

   i. Composition. When all foods are consumed, this diet provides 20 g of protein (75% is high biologic protein; therefore, all 8 EAAs are provided) and 2000 to 3000 kcal/day, largely in the form of sugars and fats (see Tables 8–5 through 8–7).

   ii. Disadvantage. Monotonous and very restricted

(2) High-Calorie, High-Protein. Protein content in these solutions and feedings consists of both low biologic value (LBV) proteins (proteins that do not contain all eight EAAs) and HBV proteins. Mixtures of EAA and nonessential amino acids may promote more efficient tissue synthesis than EAAs alone. Additionally, this care plan supplies the quantity of protein needed for positive nitrogen balance during acute uremia, with its superimposed

stress. Solutions or feedings that provide the nutrients allowed on this care plan are

(a) Central Vein Parenteral Solutions. The solutions presently being used are FreAmine II (8.5% AA) and Aminosyn (7%–10% AA), mixed with 600 ml of D_{70} W (glucose concentration of 35%)

    i.   Composition. 1000 ml/day provides approximately 40 g of protein and 1400 kcal; electrolytes, vitamins, and insulin added as needed; kilocalorie-to-protein ratio of 35:1

    ii.   Disadvantage. Dialysis needed more frequently with high nitrogen intake

(b) Oral Feedings. Based upon a diet prescription that provides 1 to 1.5 g of protein/kg IBW/day and 35 kcal/kg IBW/day (for example, this nutritional care plan for a 70-kg male would provide 70 to 105 g of protein and 2450 kcal/day); additionally, fluid usually restricted to 1000 ml/day; sodium to 40 to 120 mEq, or approximately 1000 to 3000 mg/day; and potassium to 60 mEq, or 2340 mg/day

    i.   Disadvantage. Frequent dialysis necessary with this plan

    ii.   See Chapter 2, Tables 8-6 and 8-7, and exchange lists used for controlled protein, phosphorus, sodium and potassium diets (Appendix VI) for additional information on the composition and methodology of administering these nutritional care plans

(3) Diuretic Stage. Protein and calories are no longer restricted. Fluid and electrolyte intake may have to be adjusted as frequently as every hour. Measure or assess for fluid adjustment, daily fluid output.

- Chronic Phase
  1. Nutritional Care Plan. In general the nutritional management of chronic renal failure is based on the following principles: control and regulation of protein intake, assertive maintenance of adequate caloric intake, appropriate vitamin and mineral supplementation, regulation of fluid intake to balance fluid output and insensible water loss, regulation of sodium to balance fluid output, restriction of potassium and phosphate. See Tables 8-5 through 8-7.
     a. Methodology. Oral feedings
     b. Nutrients Increased. See Table 8-6
     c. Nutrients Decreased. See Table 8-7
     d. Dietary Adaptations. See Tables 8-5 through 8-7 and Appendix VI

e. Meal Plan Modifications

(1) Adjust foods to individual dietary prescription. Conversion of the diet prescription into daily menus is accomplished by using exchange lists for meal planning and food preferences. Specific exchange lists have been designed for clients with renal disease. By definition, exchange lists for meal planning are lists of substitute foods with the same basic nutrients as those for which substitution is being made. The nutrients considered in renal disease are protein, phosphorus, potassium, and sodium. Foods within each group may be substituted for each other, but they must not be substituted for a food in another group (see Appendix VI). The caloric content of foods is also considered, as is the fluid content, in most instances (see Appendix VI and Table 8–6).

(2) Divide meals into 6 small, rather than 3 large, meals if adverse symptoms such as nausea are present.

(3) Limit fluid intake at mealtime

(4) Adjust food intake to altered taste sensations if necessary (raised BUN levels often alter taste)

2. Behavioral Modifications

a. Weigh yourself every day to determine if you are exceeding dietary allowances

b. Follow your dietary prescription closely—eat all the foods allowed and avoid all foods not included in the exchange lists

c. Measure foods carefully

d. Drain all foods thoroughly before serving, if fluids and potassium are restricted

e. Cook without salt if sodium is restricted

f. Choose a variety of foods from the allowed list (this will enhance palatability and compliance)

g. Read all food labels, because many foods contain hidden sources of nutrients

h. Write to companies that supply special food products for individuals on restricted diets—many of these foods increase the nutrient density of the diet and enhance palatability. See Suggested Readings or consult a dietitian for information on the use and preparation of these special products.

Nephrolithiasis (Renal Calculi, Kidney Stones)

Etiologic Risk Factors

Immobilization (due to trauma, stroke, paraplegia); geographical area (the Southeast has the highest incidence in the United States); sex and race (highest incidence is in white males); diet (there is a possible association between kidney stones and a high-calcium, high-oxalic-acid, or high-protein diet)

Symptoms

May be asymptomatic or manifest hematuria, urinary tract infection, or pain

Drug Therapy

Thiazide diuretics, because they reduce the renal excretion of calcium; additionally, in certain instances, phosphates, to reduce urinary excretion of calcium; cholestyramine, to limit oxalate absorption

Diet Therapy

1. Nutritional Care Plan. Moderate calcium (600 mg); restricted or moderate phosphorus, high fluid (2400–4000 ml/day) diet; additionally, oxalic acid restricted to 50 mg/day if calcium oxalate stones being formed.
   a. Methodology. Oral feedings
   b. Nutrients Increased. Water and vitamin B_6; when oxalates need to be kept in solution, magnesium given
   c. Nutrients Decreased. Calcium, phosphorus,* and vitamin D (in the form of supplements) are deceased. Exogenous oxalic acid is also decreased when calcium is limited because calcium is necessary to bind oxalates and thus restrict their absorption. Consequently, when calcium is not available, oxalates are absorbed freely and the degree of saturation of the urine, by calcium oxalates, remains unchanged.
   d. Dietary Adaptations
      (1) Limit foods high in calcium such as milk, cheese, and other milk products
      (2) Limit foods high in phosphate such as milk, milk products, eggs, organ meats, and whole grains
      (3) Limit foods high in oxalic acid such as asparagus, spinach, cranberries, plums, tea, cocoa, and coffee
      (4) Drink at least 10 to 12 glasses of water/day unless the local water is hard (hard water contains more calcium)

---

* Extreme reductions of phosphorus are no longer recommended by most clinicians, who believe that when phosphorus intake is decreased, there is a reduction in the urinary excretion of pyrophosphate, an inhibitor of crystal calcium growth and aggregation. In addition, on low-phosphate intake, the serum phosphorus may decrease, thereby stimulating production of 1,25-dihydroxycholecalciferol (active vitamin D_3), which subsequently leads to mild hypercalcemia and hypercalciuria (see calcium intake in Table 8-6).

(5) Increase foods that create an acid urine when alkaline stones are being formed and increase foods that create an alkaline urine when acid stones (*e.g.,* uric acid) are being formed (neutral foods can be used freely in either disorder see List on Acid–Base Formation in Foods)

Acid–Base Formation in Foods

Acid-Forming Foods*

Meat, eggs, fish, poultry, cereal, breads, pasta, rice, cranberry juice, prune juice, and plums

Alkaline-Forming Foods

Milk; fruits (especially dried fruits but not those that are acid forming [*e.g.,* cranberries, prunes, and plums]); and vegetables (especially greens, beans, and peas); breads prepared with baking soda or baking powder

Neutral Foods

Butter, margarine, shortening, oils, sugar, hard candies, gumdrops, honey, and pure starches

   e. Meal Plan Modifications
      (1) Drink fluids with meals and snacks
      (2) Consume foods at snack time that have a high water content, such as melons and tomatoes
   2. Behavioral Modifications. Drink water frequently throughout the day and night (immobilization increases calcium excretion).

Nurse's Responsibilities in the Nutritional Care of the Client With Renal Disease

The nurse's first responsibility to clients on restricted renal nutritional care plans is to prevent malnutrition with subsequent tissue wasting. These clients are often nauseated; in addition, these nutritional care plans are very restrictive, unpalatable for the most part, and difficult to follow. Also, severe complications (*e.g.,* pulmonary edema, cardiac arrythmias) can develop when the client or the individual preparing the food makes the smallest error. Consequently, treatment by diet becomes an added source of tension. The alternative is dialysis, if available, for the diet can be liberalized but not totally unrestricted, in most cases. Another

---

* Salt is sometimes restricted in the acid–ash diet because sodium is alkaline. Baking powder and soda products such as commercial bread products may also be limited.

advantage of dialysis is that the client is in close contact with members of the health team. This closeness should be used to help the client understand his condition and the importance of the diet, encourage his compliance, and reinforce his understanding of difficult concepts. Other responsibilities of the nurse to the client on renal nutritional care plans are listed in Chapter 7.

Table 8–1
Low (25–50g/day) Long-Chain Triglyceride (LCT) Diet

Foods Allowed	Foods Avoided
Milk Group Skim milk and milk products made from skim milk such as cottage cheese, other cheeses, and yogurt Total LCT fat = 0 g/serving	Whole milk and milk products made from whole milk such as cheeses, yogurt, ice cream, and cream sauces; cream also excluded
Fruit Group All plain raw, cooked, or canned fruits except those listed in foods to avoid; use as desserts Total LCT fat = 0 g/serving	Olives and avocados; also exclude any fruits that may cause individual distress, such as those listed in Table 7-10
Vegetable Group All plain raw, cooked, or canned vegetables except those listed in foods to avoid Total LCT fat = 0 g/serving	Vegetables that have butter added and those that have been creamed or fried, unless fat added is MCT oil (see Table 8-2); also exclude vegetables that may cause individual distress, such as those listed in Table 7-10
Bread and Cereal Group Breads, cereals, and pastas made with enriched or whole-grain flours; white or brown rice; adding some fiber to the diet may be beneficial if diarrhea is not present (see Tables 7–6 and 7–7) Total LCT fat = 0 g/serving	Pastry and pastrylike products such as doughnuts, sweet rolls, cookies, pies, and cakes, especially those with nuts, chocolate, or frosting

(continued)

Table 8–1 331

Table 8–1
Low (25–50 g/day) Long-Chain Triglyceride (LCT) Diet (continued)

Foods Allowed	Foods Avoided
Meat Group	
Plain baked, broiled, or roasted meats, such as chicken, veal, beef, lamb; and white fish Total LCT fat = 3–5 g/1 oz serving of lean skinless meat Egg, all but fried; limit all egg consumption to 1/day Total LCT fat = 5 g/egg Legumes such as dried beans or peas; small servings as tolerated Total LCT fat = 3 g/serving	Meat and fish with a high fat content such as ham, beef brisket, spare ribs, bacon, duck, and rib steaks; fried meats and fish; meat products that are highly seasoned such as salami, bologna, pastrami, and frankfurters; meats with added gravy or cream sauces; all nuts; fried eggs; any leguminous vegetable that may cause individual distress such as those listed in Table 7–10
Fat and Sugar Group	
Butter and margarine within the LCT fat restriction Total LCT fat = approximately 5 g/teaspoon Total calories = approximately 45 calories/teaspoon Sugar and sugarlike products such as jelly, syrups, and hard candies within the caloric restriction Total calories = 18 calories/teaspoon sugar Total LCT fat = 0 g/serving	All products that contain oils or shortenings; all cream sauces, gravies, or salad dressings, unless they are made with MCT oil (see Table 8-2) All sugar and products that contain sugar (see Chapt. 6) above the caloric restriction
Beverages	
Skim milk, cereal beverages, coffee, tea, and soft drinks (within the caloric restriction) Total LCT fat = 0 g/serving	Whole milk, buttermilk, milkshakes, chocolate drinks, and alcohol

(Adapted from American Dietetic Association: Handbook of Clinical Dietetics, p E 67. New Haven, Yale University Press, 1981)

Table 8–2
Composition, Advantages, and Disadvantages of MCT (Medium-Chain Triglyceride) Oil

Composition	Advantages	Disadvantages
Composed of glycerol esters of medium-chain (8–10 carbon atoms) fatty acids	Abundant and rapidly digested and absorbed source of energy	Contains fewer calories than LCT, 8.3 kcal vs 9 kcal/g
Predominant acids are caprylic or octanoic acid (C_8) and capric or decanoic acid (C_{10})	Provides 8.3 kcal/g or 116 kcal/tablespoon	Has an unpleasant taste unless added to foods
MCTs liberated from coconut oil by steam hydrolysis	Can be added to foods without sacrificing taste.*	Large amounts of MCT may produce abdominal distention, cramps, nausea, and diarrhea
	Can be transported directly to the liver by the portal vein, bypassing the lymph system	To alleviate symptoms, eat MCT-containing foods more slowly and use smaller amounts, approximately 1 tablespoon, at each meal
	Is easily hydrolyzed despite pancreatic lipase or bile salt deficiencies	May be contraindicated in patients with cirrhosis of the liver and diabetes mellitus (may precipitate ketosis)
	Fecal fat losses may be reduced and steatorrhea alleviated when MCT rather than LCT is consumed	Does not contain linoleic acid (an essential fatty acid)
	Calcium absorption may be enhanced when MCT rather than LCT is consumed	

* Consult suggested readings at the end of this chapter to obtain information on how to incorporate MCT into common foods. Note also that administering pancreatin along with MCT may increase its absorption. (Adapted from American Dietetic Association: Handbook of Clinical Dietetics, p E 65. New Haven, Yale University Press, 1981)

Table 8–3 333

Table 8–3
Calorie, Protein, Carbohydrate, and Fat Intakes Recommended in Progressive Liver Disease

Disease State	Calories	Protein	Carbohydrate	Fat
Stage I, Obesity, with accompanying hyperlipidemia or hypertension	Decreased to obtain IBW (consult Chap. 6)	20% of total caloric intake	58% of total caloric intake (CHO intake division, 48% complex CHO and 10% natural CHO, within total CHO calories)	30% of total caloric intake (fat intake division, 10% saturated fat, 10% monounsaturated fat, and 10% polyunsaturated fatty acids [PUFA]) Cholesterol limited to 300 g if hypercholesterolemia develops
Stage II, Hepatomegaly (also called "fatty liver")	35–40/kcal/kg IBW/day Spares protein	20% of total calories or 2 g/kg IBW/day Repairs degenerated tissue	Same as stage I; however, refined sugar intake will be increased, if fat restriction becomes severe, to maintain caloric intake	25% of total calories (division of fats same as for stage I)
Stage III, Alcoholic Hepatitis, or other types of hepatitis	50 kcal/kg IBW/day or 3000–3500 kcal/day Counteracts catabolism	20% of total kcal, 1.5–2 g/kg IBW/day or 100–120 g/day	50%–60% of total calories or 300–400 g/day (CHO intake division	25%–30% of total calories, depending upon degree of fatty liver

(continued)

Table 8-3
**Calorie, Protein, Carbohydrate, and Fat Intakes
Recommended in Progressive Liver Disease** (continued)

Disease State	Calories	Protein	Carbohydrate	Fat
Stage III, Alcoholic Hepatitis (continued)				
	Liquid feedings in acute stage progressing to solids as condition improves	Regenerates tissue	same as for stages I and II)	Needed for palatability of diet (division of fats same as for stage I)
Stage IV, Cirrhosis	45–50 kcal/kg IBW/day (or present weight without edema) or 2000–5000 kcal/day Enteral feedings or parenteral solutions may be needed to obtain calories if client's appetite is poor; (consult Chap. 2 and Appendix II)	20% of total calories Early stage of disease, 0.8–2 g/kg IBW/day or 56–140 g (division, 60%–75% HBV, 25%–40% LBV protein (see dietary adaptations) Advanced stage, 0–40 g with increases of 10 g as condition improves 35 g of protein lowest level to achieve nitrogen balance Enteral or parenteral feedings may be needed (see stage V)	50%–75% of total calories (division changed from high complex CHO [unless low-protein wheat products are used] to high refined CHO intake High glucose modular feedings may be needed	20%–30% of total calories, depending upon protein allowed MCT oil may be necessary when steatorrhea is evident, but client must be monitored (see Chap. 7 and Table 8-2)

(continued)

Table 8–3 335

Table 8–3
**Calorie, Protein, Carbohydrate, and Fat Intakes
Recommended in Progressive Liver Disease** (continued)

Disease State	Calories	Protein	Carbohydrate	Fat
Stage V, Encephalopathy and Hepatic Coma				
	50 kcal/kg IBW/day Same as stage IV	0–25 g HBV protein Enteral feedings high in branched-chain amino acids and low in aromatic amino acids may be given orally or by tube, if client's appetite is poor (*e.g.,* 1000 ml Hepatic-Aid supplies 1670 kcal, 43.5 g AA, 37 g fat, and 293 g CHO from maltodextrose and sucrose)	Same as for stage IV, except when hepatic coma is induced; then parenteral feedings high in glucose may be indicated (see Chap. 2) High branched-chain amino acid parenteral solutions (*e.g.,* F080, HepatAmine) now being researched	Same as for stage IV except when hepatic coma is induced; then intralipids may be administered to obtain needed calories, depending upon individual condition, because it may aggravate, not alleviate, condition (see Chap. 2)

Table 8–4
Vitamin, Mineral, and Fluid Intake Recommended in Progressive Liver Disease

Disease State	Water-Soluble Vitamins	Fat-Soluble Vitamins	Minerals	Fluids
Stage I				
Obesity, with accompanying hyperlipidemia or hypertension	Hypervitaminosis may occur in alcoholics at this stage who self-medicate with over-the-counter vitamin preparations to "protect" their liver Most prevalent condition is niacin "intoxication"	Same as for water-soluble vitamins Most prevalent condition is hypervitaminosis A	Same as for water-soluble vitamins Most prevalent condition is hemochromotosis (iron overload) in wine-drinking alcoholics In addition, potassium may be lacking if diuretics are taken to relieve hypertension Sodium limited if hypertension is evident (consult Chap. 3)	Unlimited
Stages II and III, *Hepatomegaly and Hepatitis*				
	Supplements of all the water-soluble vitamins are given, with special emphasis on B-complex vitamins, especially folic acid, thiamine, and vitamin B_{12}.	Supplements of all the fat-soluble vitamins (A, D, E, and K) may have to be given owing to poor absorption, activation, or storage They are given orally	Supplements of zinc, magnesium, and phosphorus may be necessary owing to increased excretion Copper and iron may also need to be in-	As desired or in excess if other foods not tolerated

(continued)

Table 8–4 337

Table 8–4
Vitamin, Mineral, and Fluid Intake Recommended in Progressive Liver Disease (continued)

Disease State	Water-Soluble Vitamins	Fat-Soluble Vitamins	Minerals	Fluids
Stages II and III, Hepatomegaly and Hepatitis (continued)				
	They are given orally when possible but parenterally when absorption is poor. All clients with liver disease should receive these preparations, but they are especially important to chronic alcoholics, for alcohol has toxic effects on the intestine (poor absorption of nutrients) and the liver (poor activation and transport of nutrients) All vitamins may have to be added to specialized parenteral solutions	when possible, parenterally when necessary Special emphasis is placed upon vitamin K, for hypoprothrombinemia often is evident	creased owing to poor absorption; however, they may have to be limited if Wilson's disease or hemochromotosis develops In addition, any minerals lost in vomiting have to be replaced	
Stage IV, Cirrhosis				
	Same as for stages II and III	Same as for stages II and III	Same as for stages I to III except that sodium	Depends upon the amount of edema and *(continued)*

Table 8–4
Vitamin, Mineral, and Fluid Intake Recommended in Progressive Liver Disease (continued)

Disease State	Water-Soluble Vitamins	Fat-Soluble Vitamins	Minerals	Fluids
Stage IV, Cirrhosis (continued)			restriction is more severe if ascites is evident Sodium limitation ranges from 10 mEq (250 mg) to 20 mEq (500 mg) or 87 mEq (2000 mg), depending upon the amount of edema and fluid intake Diuretics, if given, should be the kind that spares potassium (*e.g.*, triamterene; see Chap. 3)	renal involvement Fluid limitation ranges from unlimited to 500 ml plus output (see Table 8–7)
Stages V and VI, Encephalopathy and Hepatic Coma	Same as for stages II to IV	Same as for stages II to IV	Same as for stages II to IV except that sodium restriction becomes even more severe Limitation ranges from 10 mEq (250 mg) to	Same as for stage IV

(continued)

Table 8–4 339

Table 8–4
**Vitamin, Mineral, and Fluid Intake Recommended
in Progressive Liver Disease** (continued)

Disease State	Water-Soluble Vitamins	Fat-Soluble Vitamins	Minerals	Fluids
Stages V and VI, Encephalopathy and Hepatic Coma *(continued)*			20 mEq (500 mg), depending upon the degree of liver and kidney impairment Potassium supplements may be necessary if potassium-sparing diuretics are not administered (consult Chap. 3 and discussion of kidney disease)	

Table 8–5
Sample Diet Plans for 20-, 30-, 40-, or 60-g Protein Diets

Foods	20-g Diet	g	30-g Diet	g	40-g Diet	g	60-g Diet	g
Milk	½ c	4	½ c	4	½ c	4	½ c	4
Vegetables								
1 g group	2 servings	2	2 servings	2	2 servings	2	2 servings	2
2 g group			1 serving	2	1 serving	2	1 serving	2
Fruits	3 servings	1.5	3 servings	1.5	3 servings	1.5	4 servings	2
Starches	2 servings	4	3 servings	6	4 servings	8	7 servings	14
Low-protein bread	3 or more servings	1	3 or more servings	1	3 or more servings	1		
Meat	1 serving	7	1 serving*	7	2 servings*	14	4 servings*	28
Egg, large					1 serving	7	1 serving	7
Fats	As desired		As desired		As desired		As desired	
Miscellaneous	Selective		Selective		Selective		Selective	
Total Protein		20 g		31 g		40 g		59 g

* 1 serving of a meat exchange = 1 oz
(Anderson L, Dibble MV, Turkki PR et al: Nutrition in Health and Disease, 17th ed. Philadelphia, JB Lippincott, 1982)

Table 8-6 341

Table 8-6
Nutrients Increased, Rationale for Increase, and Dietary Adaptations in Chronic Renal Failure and the Nephrotic Syndrome

Nutrient Increased	Rationale for Increase	Dietary Adaptations
Caloric Requirements		
Vary substantially with age and activity and are paradoxically increased when protein intake is small. In general, caloric requirements are increased from 30 kcal/kg IBW (normal) to 35–45 kcal/kg IBW in the adult. Total intake is approximately 2000–3000 kcal/day. Children's caloric intake is increased to 1½–2 times their normal requirement. To achieve caloric requirements: (1) Increase carbohydrate intake to at least 200–300 g/day, mostly in the form of refined sugars. However, that carbohydrate intake may be limited to 35% of total calories when hypertriglyceridemia is a complication. (2) Fat contributes 65% of total calories. Increase fat to 70–90 g or more/day, with a polyunsaturated saturated fat ratio greater than 1.5 preferred when hypertriglyceridemia or hypercholesterolemia is a complication.	Increased carbohydrate spares protein for tissue synthesis and regeneration. Additionally, it limits lean tissue catabolism. Consequently, nitrogenous wastes and potassium accumulation in the bloodstream are reduced. Additionally, the end products of carbohydrate plus fat metabolism, carbon dioxide (CO_2) and water do not present a problem in the client with renal dysfunction, for they are expelled via the lungs (CO_2), sweat glands, and feces. It is of clinical significance that overt symptoms of uremia are diminished. Refined sugars are consumed instead of complex carbohydrates because the latter contain low biologic protein (LBV). This type of protein does not contain all 8 essential amino acids (EAAs). *Caution:* high intake of refined sugars increases thirst. Fats contribute energy (calories); thus they also spare protein.	Caloric intake is increased by (1) adding refined sugars such as jelly, honey, sugar, and syrups to beverages, baked goods, and sauces; (2) adding commercial supplements high in calories but low in electrolytes and protein to foods (for example, Hycal, Controlyte, Cal Power, and Polycose); (3) using commercial products that have the LBV protein removed such as d p Low Protein Breads and Wheat Starches and Aproten Pastas (only necessary when protein is restricted); (4) adding fats such as margarines and oils to foods while cooking and at the table.

(continued)

Table 8–6
Nutrients Increased, Rationale for Increase, and Dietary Adaptations in Chronic Renal Failure and the Nephrotic Syndrome (continued)

Nutrient Increased	Rationale for Increase	Dietary Adaptations
Protein Requirements Are increased from daily recommended intakes of 0.8 g/kg IBW in the adult and 1.2–1.5 g/kg IBW in children when the individual is excreting massive quantities of protein (nephrotic syndrome) or when he is on dialysis. Recommended intake is as follows: *Nephrotic syndrome,* adult, 1.2–2 g/kg IBW; children, 2–3 g/kg IBW/day *Hemodialysis,* 1–1.5 g/kg IBW/(dry weight) day for an adult *Peritoneal dialysis,* 1.2–1.5 g/kg IBW/day for an adult	Increased protein is necessary when the client is losing excessive protein in the urine. This will prevent hypoalbuminemia with subsequent edema and malnutrition. Increased protein is necessary when the client is on dialysis because amino acids are water-soluble; consequently, they pass from the serum into the dialysate bath.	Protein intake is increased by (1) adding dried milk and dried or whole eggs to common foods like soups, custards, milkshakes, and meat loaves; (2) adding commercial supplements high in calories and protein to meal plans (for example, Sustacal pudding, Ensure Plus, and Meritene). However, these foods and supplements are also high in sodium. Therefore, when edema is a complication, Lonolac, a salt-free milk, may be used as a protein source.
Vitamin intake Is increased in all chronic renal conditions including those in clients on dialysis. Multivitamin tablets that contain B_1, B_2, B_6, niacin, pantothenate C, and folate are usually necessary to meet these increased needs. However, vitamin A should not be included in the supplement because uremic individuals have elevated vitamin A serum levels.	Increased vitamin intake in the form of supplements is especially necessary when foods that contain high levels of potassium and protein are limited (see Appendix VI, Tables 3–7 and 8–5, and protein dietary adaptations). Uremic toxins may also interfere with vitamin metabolism, especially of B_6.	Foods high in vitamins, such as vegetables, fruits, milk, breads, and meats, are usually limited, for other reasons, when individuals have chronic renal failure; therefore, vitamin requirements cannot be met without supplements.

(continued)

Table 8-6 343

Table 8-6
**Nutrients Increased, Rationale for Increase, and Dietary Adaptations
in Chronic Renal Failure and the Nephrotic Syndrome** (continued)

Nutrient Increased	Rationale for Increase	Dietary Adaptations
Iron Intake Should be increased in most renal conditions even though the client is on dialysis. Oral iron supplements are usually necessary to meet these increased needs. Measurement of serum iron or serum ferritin or assessment of bone marrow iron stores can be a guide to deciding which clients need supplemental iron. The supplement usually advised is ferrous sulfate.	Increased iron is necessary in renal disease because protein foods that contain "heme" iron (meat) are limited; frequent blood sampling, to determine GFR, causes blood loss; formation of erythropoietin (which stimulates erythrocyte production) is impaired, and toxins associated with renal disease shorten the life span of erythrocytes. Of clinical significance are lowered hemoglobin, and hematocrit levels, with resultant anemia.	Iron intake is increased by (1) eating more meat, especially liver (meats contain more "heme" iron, which is more biologically available); (2) drinking citrus juices such as orange juice or lemonade with meat meals (citrus fruits are high in vitamin C, a vitamin known to enhance iron absorption); (3) eating foods that have been fortified with iron, such as cereals and breads. When other nutrients, such as protein, which is available in meats, breads and cereals, are limited, iron supplements will be necessary to meet increased requirements.
Calcium Intake Is increased when phosphorous serum levels rise and calcium serum levels fall (see rationale). Oral calcium supplements are usually necessary to meet these increased needs. The supplements usually recom-	Increased calcium and vitamin D, along with decreased intake of phosphorus, is necessary in renal disorders for the following reasons: As the GFR drops, phosphorus excretion is decreased; therefore,	Meeting increased calcium needs by dietary intake is seldom possible, for foods high in calcium (*i.e.*, milk and milk products) are also high in phosphorus, sodium, and protein, which are usually limited in renal *(continued)*

Table 8-6
Nutrients Increased, Rationale for Increase, and Dietary Adaptations in Chronic Renal Failure and the Nephrotic Syndrome (continued)

Nutrient Increased	Rationale for Increase	Dietary Adaptations
Calcium Intake (continued) mended are calcium carbonate, lactate, or gluconate in dosages ranging from 1 to 3 g/day, except in nephrolithiasis or hyperparathyroidism. Vitamin D intake is increased when calcium serum levels fall (see rationale). Oral vitamin D supplements are usually necessary to meet these increased needs. The supplement usually recommended is Rocaltrol, also known as 1,25-DHCC. Dosage depends upon the calcium serum level (normal, 10 mg/dl) and phosphorus level (normal, 3–4 mg/dl) and the calcium:phosphorus serum ratio. Normal calcium:phosphorus serum ratio is 2:1.	phosphorus serum levels increase and serum calcium levels drop. Consequently, secretion of parathormone (PTH) from the parathyroid gland is increased. This hormone's mode of action is to enhance phosphorus excretion; to enhance reabsorption of calcium from the bone and kidney, to raise serum calcium levels; to enhance the release of active vitamin D_3 (1,25-dihydroxycholecalciferol) from the kidney, which in turn stimulates calcium absorption in the small intestines. In renal insufficiency, however, the hormone's actions are impaired, except for its ability to enhance calcium reabsorption from the bone. Of clinical significance, renal osteodystrophy develops. The disease is essentially of three types: (1) osteomalacia, or bone demineralization; (2) osteitis fibrosa cystica, or dull, aching bone pain caused by excessive PTH action (hormone	disorders. Oral supplementation, therefore, is usually necessary to meet increased requirements. Administer phosphate binders in the form of aluminum-containing antacids (e.g., Amphojel, Basajel) with meals and large snacks or in the form of specialized baked products (see Table 8-7). These phosphate binders will decrease phosphorus absorption and, ultimately, will lower serum phosphorus levels. Meeting increased vitamin D requirements by dietary intake is seldom possible because few foods are high in vitamin D. Sunshine is the best source; however, it is not always available; thus oral supplementation is necessary

(continued)

Table 8–6 345

Table 8–6
Nutrients Increased, Rationale for Increase, and Dietary Adaptations in Chronic Renal Failure and the Nephrotic Syndrome (continued)

Nutrient Increased	Rationale for Increase	Dietary Adaptations
Calcium Intake (continued)	does not shut off until serum calcium and phosphorus ratio is accurate); and (3) metastatic calcification of joints and soft tissue. The last is caused by increased serum phosphorus levels, which prevent decreased PTH action. Consequently, excess calcium is reabsorbed from the bone into the serum and hypercalcemia is induced, if the condition is not controlled by diet therapy, drug therapy, or dialysis.	
Fluid Intake Should be increased when sodium retention is low (*e.g.*, vomiting is excessive) and in other circumstances pertaining to renal disorders (see Table 8–7).	Dehydration may occur if sodium and water losses are excessive. Fluid intake should not be restricted until it is clearly necessary (*e.g.*, client is edematous) in order not to impose further limitation on the kidney's capacity to excrete solutes.	Fluid intake in the form of beverages should be increased from 6 to 8 glasses/day to 9 to 10 glasses/day. Foods that contain a high percentage of water should be increased (*e.g.*, fruits and vegetables), provided other dietary restrictions (*e.g.*, potassium) are not necessary.

Table 8–7
Nutrients Decreased, Rationale for Decrease, and Dietary Adaptations in Chronic Renal Failure and the Nephrotic Syndrome

Nutrient Decreased	Rationale for Decrease	Dietary Adaptations
Phosphorus Intake		
Is decreased to 800–1200 mg/day. This decrease may be accomplished by dietary adaptations, which are difficult when protein needs are high, or by giving oral drugs that sequester phosphorus in the GI tract and prevent its absorption. Oral drugs usually used are listed under dietary adaptations. (see Table 8-6). Recently, however, it has been theorized that the aluminum in dialysis fluid may be responsible for the irreversible dementia experienced by some clients. Consequently, some clinicians prefer using a high fiber diet rather than medications to bind phosphorus in the small intestine.	See Calcium Intake in Table 8-6.	Phosphorus intake is decreased by (1) limiting dairy products, meats, whole grains, chocolate, and nuts; (2) limiting other foods high in phosphorus (see protein, phosphorus, sodium, and potassium exchange lists in Appendix VI); (3) administering aluminum and calcium hydroxide tablets (these are large, unpleasant-tasting tablets; therefore, in order to enhance consumption, they must be broken up and incorporated into foods such as cookies and cakes); (4) increasing fiber intake if low biological protein is not restricted (see Chap. 7 for foods high in fiber).
Protein Intake		
Is decreased in accordance with the individual's GFR at a particular time. Kopple's recommendations for reduction in dietary protein, according to	Protein reduction is not recommended until the GFR drops to 4–10 ml/min because protein enhances tissue synthesis, and exogenous protein prevents tis-	Decreasing dietary protein intake without creating tissue catabolism requires adjusting the protein intake so that high biologic protein (HBV) intake makes up

(continued)

Table 8-7 347

Table 8-7
**Nutrients Decreased, Rationale for Decrease, and Dietary Adaptations
in Chronic Renal Failure and the Nephrotic Syndrome** (continued)

Nutrient Decreased	Rationale for Decrease	Dietary Adaptations
Protein Intake *(continued)* GFR, are as follows (for normal GFR, see p. 322):* GFR of 20–50 ml/min, protein intake up to 90 g/day GFR of 15–20 ml/min, protein intake up to 70 g/day GFR of 10–15 ml/min, protein intake up to 50 g/day GFR of 4–10 ml/min, protein intake up to 40 g/day GFR of less than 4 ml/min, protein intake up to 20 g/day (Giordano-Giovanetti diet) Another assessment tool (recommended by Bergstrom) for regulating exogenous protein intake is measurement of endogenous creatinine clearance. Bergstrom's	sue catabolism with accompanying build-ups of nitrogenous wastes, phosphorus, and potassium in the serum. Protein reduction is recommended when the GFR drops to 4–10 ml/min, however; for when exogenous low biologic proteins (LBV) are limited, it is hypothesized that endogenous urea (nitrogen waste) is recycled to make nonessential amino acids. Of clinical significance, BUN levels drop; thus uremia symptoms are alleviated, tissue catabolism is reduced, and tissue regeneration is increased. The last can only occur, however, when all 8 EAAs plus histidine are supplied by exogenous sources.	75% of the total daily protein intake. HBV proteins are proteins that contain all 8 essential amino acids (EAA). They are found in foods such as eggs, meat, fish, cheese, and milk. Dairy products, however, may have to be limited in renal disease, because they contain high levels of potassium, sodium, and phosphorus (see Appendix VI). However, they may be the only HBV proteins tolerated when the client is nauseated and anorexic. One serving of HBV foodstuffs = 7 g of protein. Low biologic proteins (LBV) are limited to 25% of the total daily protein intake. LBV proteins do not contain all 8 EAAs. They are found in foods such as bread, flour, cereals, and starchy vegetables (*e.g.*, potatoes). One serving of LBV foodstuffs = 2 g of protein. (If the individual finds the 20 g HBV, restricted

*This general recommendation does not apply when the client is on dialysis (see Table 8-6).

(continued)

Table 8–7
Nutrients Decreased, Rationale for Decrease, and Dietary Adaptations in Chronic Renal Failure and the Nephrotic Syndrome (continued)

Nutrient Decreased	Rationale for Decrease	Dietary Adaptations
Protein Intake *(continued)* recommendations are as follows: *Creatinine* *Protein* ml/min g/24 hr >40 unlimited 10–40 60 5–20 40 2–10 15–20 + EAA + histidine <5 dialysis		LBV diet too unpalatable, use commercial products that have the LBV protein removed to increase caloric intake and variety in the diet; see dietary adaptations to increase caloric intakes in Table 8–6).
Sodium and Fluid Intake is determined by an individual's 24-hr urinary output and insensible losses (*e.g.*, from skin), blood pressure, presence of edema, renal function (GFR and creatinine clearance), and dietary intake. Generally, sodium and fluid intake is restricted in chronic renal failure, even though the individual is on dialysis. The exceptions are when the client is in the diuretic stage of ARF, is experiencing excessive vomiting or diarrhea, or is on excessive diuretic therapy. When these	Sodium and fluid intake should remain at normal levels or be increased during diuresis (excessive fluid loss) in order to prevent homeostatic imbalances and dehydration. Usually a client's thirst mechanism is an accurate guide to his fluid balance.	Sodium intake during the diuretic stage of renal disease is based on the mild sodium restriction nutritional care plan (see Table 3–8 and Conversion Table for Sodium-Restricted Diets in Chap. 3, plus protein, phosphorus, sodium, and potassium exchange lists in Appendix VI for *(continued)*

Table 8–7 349

Table 8–7
Nutrients Decreased, Rationale for Decrease, and Dietary Adaptations in Chronic Renal Failure and the Nephrotic Syndrome (continued)

Nutrient Decreased	Rationale for Decrease	Dietary Adaptations
Sodium and Fluid (continued) conditions prevail, the sodium fluid levels may be liberalized. Recommended sodium intake is 84–130 mEq or 2000–3000 mg of sodium/day (see Table 3–8). Recommended fluid intake is 1 ml of fluid for each kilocalorie consumed in food, unless edema or dehydration is apparent. If these disorders occur, further fluid adjustments must be made. Sodium and fluid intake is decreased when the GFR drops to 4–10 ml/min, at which time the client is considered to be approaching end stage renal disease (ESRD). Recommended sodium intake is 40 mEq or approximately 1000 mg/day without dialysis; 65–87 mEq or approximately 1500–2000 mg/day with dialysis (see Chap. 3 and Table 3–8). Recommended or allowed fluids are based upon the following: 1 lb (500 ml) of free	Sodium and fluid reduction is recommended when the GFR drops to approximately 10 ml/min, for at this level the client is excreting very little urine (oliguria) or no urine at all (anuria). Consequently, the kidney is unable to excrete exogenous and endogenous sodium and fluids; therefore, retention of sodium and fluid is enhanced. Of clinical significance, the client develops edema and hypertension, which can precipitate congestive heart failure if he is not controlled by diet therapy, drug therapy, or dialysis. A simplified way to explain this rationale to a client is the following: Blow up a balloon, which represents edema (wet weight); prick the baloon with a pin, which represents dialysis; the	details on sodium dietary adaptations required by this plan). Fluid allowances during the diuretic stage and other stages of renal disease are obtained from (1) beverages and foods that are liquid at room temperature, such as ice cream and gelatin; (2) the water found in solid foods such as lettuce and bread; (3) the water formed from the oxidation of food (called metabolic water). Sodium intake during ESRD is based on the moderate sodium restriction nutritional care plan (see Table 3–8 and Conversion Table plus protein, phosphorus, sodium, and potassium exchange lists in Appendix VI for details on sodium dietary adaptations required by this plan). Salt substitutes cannot be used in renal disease because they contain potassium and ammonia, which may also be restricted (see Table 3–9). Fluid intake during ESRD is obtained from *(continued)*

Table 8-7
Nutrients Decreased, Rationale for Decrease, and Dietary Adaptations in Chronic Renal Failure and the Nephrotic Syndrome (continued)

Nutrient Decreased	Rationale for Decrease	Dietary Adaptations
Sodium and Fluid (continued)		
dietary fluids is allowed to replace insensible fluid losses (fluid lost from the lungs, skin, and GI tract) plus the 24-hr urinary output. Anuric clients (individuals with no urinary output) without dialysis may be limited to 500 ml/day of fluid because fluids in solid foods and metabolic water contribute the amount of fluid lost in insensible losses. Dialysis clients, however, are allowed 1000 ml/day of fluid. This intake is based upon a weight gain of 1 lb (500 ml)/day (known as wet weight gain) or a 2-lb (1000 ml) gain between dialysis (based on a 3-times-a-week dialysis program).	deflated balloon represents dry weight (lean fat and tissue weight).	beverages (approximately 500 ml/day) and fluids found in solid foods and metabolic water (approximately 500 ml/day). This allowance also includes any fluids given to administer drugs. Consequently the client is usually extremely thirsty. To relieve thirst, suggest that he suck on ice cubes (within the fluid allowance) or use mouth sprays to relieve dryness.
Potassium Intake		
Is determined by the individual's 24-hr urinary output, body size, renal function, serum potassium, and frequency of dialysis, if applicable. Generally, potassium intake is restricted in chronic renal failure, even though the client is on dialysis. The exceptions are the same as those that liberalize sodium	Intake of potassium should remain at normal levels or be increased during excessive fluid loss (diuresis) in order to prevent hypokalemia (see Chap. 3 for	Potassium intake is increased by (1) consuming more fruits and vegetables (these foods are recommended because they are low in sodium and protein; *(continued)*

Table 8–7 351

Table 8–7
Nutrients Decreased, Rationale for Decrease, and Dietary Adaptations in Chronic Renal Failure and the Nephrotic Syndrome (continued)

Nutrient Decreased	Rationale for Decrease	Dietary Adaptations
Potassium Intake *(continued)* and fluid intake, namely, the diuretic stage of ARF, excessive vomiting and diarrhea, and diuretic therapy. When these conditions prevail, the potassium intake recommended is 50–150 mEq or 2000–6000 mg/day (see Lists of Signs and Treatment of Hypokalemia and Hyperkalemia, Chap. 3). Potassium intake is decreased when the GFR drops to 4–10 ml/min, at which time the client is considered to be near ESRD. Recommended potassium intake is: 40–65 mEq or approximately 1500–2500 mg with oliguria but without dialysis 40 mEq or 1500 mg with anuria but without dialysis 52 mEq or 2000 mg with hemodialysis 87–130 mEq or 3500–5000 mg with peritoneal dialysis (see list on Hypokalemia and Hyperkalemia in Chap. 3).	signs and treatment of hypokalemia and hyperkalemia). Potassium reduction is recommended when the GFR drops to approximately 10 ml/min, for at this level the client is excreting very little urine (oliguria) or no urine at all (anuria). Consequently, the exogenous potassium consumed and the endogenous potassium that is mobilized when tissue catabolism is excessive increase serum potassium (hyperkalemia). Subsequently, hyperkalemia precipitates cardiac arrhythmias and cardiac arrest if client is not controlled by diet therapy, drug therapy, or dialysis.	therefore, if these nutrients are limited in renal disease, their daily allowance will not be increased by much); (2) other food sources high in potassium are listed in Tables 3–7 and 3–10 and the exchange list for planning controlled protein phosphorus, sodium, and potassium meal plans in Appendix VI. Potassium intake is decreased by (1) limiting intake of fruits and vegetables; (2) leaching fruits and vegetables, that is, by soaking vegetable in a large amount of water, rinsing vegetable thoroughly after soaking, cooking in a large amount of water (leaching also removes water-soluble vitamins); (3) limiting other food sources high in potassium (see Table 3–7 and 3–10 and the exchange list for planning controlled protein, phosphorus, sodium, and potassium meal plans in Appendix VI); (4) limiting potassium intake when protein intake is not limited is difficult. An ion exchange resin [Kayexalate] may have to be administered).

Bibliography

American Dietetic Association: Handbook of Clinical Dietetics. New Haven, Yale University Press, 1981

Anderson L, Dipple MV, Turkki PR et al: Nutrition in Health and Disease, 17th ed. Philadelphia, JB Lippincott, 1982

Bach AC, Babayan VK: Medium-chain triglycerides: An update. Am J Clin Nutr 36:950, 1982

Boeker EA: Metabolism of ethanol. J Am Diet Assoc 76:550, 1980

Burton BT, Hirschman GH: Current concepts of nutritional therapy in chronic renal failure: An update. J Am Diet Assoc 82:359, 1983

Chernoff R, Dean JA: Medical and nutritional aspects of intractable diarrhea. J Am Diet Assoc 76:161, 1980

Greenberger NJ: Gastrointestinal Disorders: A Pathophysiologic Approach, 2nd ed. Chicago, Year Book Medical Publishers, 1981

Hepatic encephalopathy: A unifying hypothesis. Nutr Rev 38:371, 1980

Kerr AA: Nutrition in cystic fibrosis. New Zealand Diet Assoc 36:20, 1982

Kopple JD: Nutritional management of chronic renal failure. Postgrad Med 64:135, 1978

Larter N: Cystic fibrosis. Am J Nurs 81:527, 1981

Levine SE: Nutritional care of patients with renal failure and diabetes. J Am Diet Assoc 81:261, 1982

Lieber CS: The metabolism of alcohol. Sci Am 234:25, 1976

Margie JD, Anderson CF, Nelson RA et al: The Mayo Clinic Renal Diet Book. New York, Golden Press, 1974

Matsuzaki S: Hepatotoxicity of acetaldehyde. Adv Exp Med Biol 126:397, 1978

Mead Johnson and Company: Recipes using MCT oil and Portagen. Evansville, IN 47721

Richards P, Ell S: Nutrition in renal disease. Human Nutrition: Clinical Nutrition 36C:103, 1982

Roe DA: Nutritional concerns in the alcoholic. J Am Diet Assoc 78:17, 1981

Rubin E, Lieber CS: Alcohol-induced hepatic injury in man: Ultrastructural changes. Fed Proc 26:1458, 1967

Spiro AH: Nutritional therapy and liver disease. Clinical Consultations 2:1, 1982

Walser M: Nutritional support in renal failure: Future directions. Lancet 1:340, 1983

Suggested Readings

Bowman F: MCT cookies, cakes, and quick breads: Quality and acceptability. J Am Diet Assoc 62:180, 1973

Howard BD, Morse EH: Muffins and pastry made with medium-chain triglyceride oil. J Am Diet Assoc 62:51, 1973

chapter 9

Special Disorders

In this chapter, nutritional care for certain special disorders is discussed. The etiology, characteristics, and symptoms of these disorders, however, are not elaborated upon because of space limitations.

Nutritional Care of Clients With Burns

Description

Nutritional support of clients with burns is determined by the client's age and sex, the extent of thermal injury, and the accompanying hypermetabolism, which ultimately leads to excessive weight loss and protein wasting. These physiological changes indicate that a nutritional care plan high in calories, protein, electrolytes, vitamins, minerals, and fluids is necessary.

The effectiveness of nutritional therapy is evaluated by weight gain, nitrogen retention, and tissue healing.

Stage I Nutritional Care Plan

The duration depends upon the client and the extent of his burns. The usual time span is 1 to 5 days.

Methodology

Parenteral solutions that contain fluids, electrolytes (sodium and potassium), bicarbonate, glucose, and sometimes amino acids are administered.

Rationale

- Replacement of fluids and electrolytes maintains blood volume and prevents renal shutdown
- Replacement of bicarbonate prevents metabolic acidosis
- Replacement of glucose and amino acids counteracts excessive tissue catabolism

Dietary Adaptations

- If burns are extensive, oral feedings are contraindicated during this stage because paralytic ileus is often a complication
- If burns are not extensive, clear fluids high in potassium and sodium, such as Gatorade, should be encouraged

Stage II Nutritional Care Plan

The plan is instituted approximately 2 to 5 days after thermal injury. Duration extends until burned area is covered with new tissue.

Methodology

Oral feedings high in calories, proteins, vitamins, minerals, electrolytes, and fluids are administered. The level of intake is determined by the extent of thermal injury. Parenteral solutions or enteral supplements may be necessary to augment oral feedings when caloric and nutrient needs are excessive.

Rationale

- *Calories* are increased
  1. To meet the hypermetabolic needs created by extensive release of catabolic hormones (glucagon and norepinephrine) and the subsequent decrease in insulin secretion
  2. To avoid the consequences of protein calorie malnutrition, such as impairment of the immune mechanism, which enhances susceptibility to infection and adversely affects wound healing; and excessive weight loss, which leads to decreased vigor, decreased muscular strength, and, if excessive, death
- *Proteins* are increased
  1. To replace nitrogen lost through tissue catabolism, gluconeogenesis, and exudation of protein from the wound
  2. To enhance synthesis of visceral and circulating proteins, including those found in hemoglobin
  3. To enhance wound healing

- *Vitamins and minerals* are increased
  1. To enhance wound healing (*e.g.*, vitamin C and zinc)
  2. To stabilize homeostatic mechanisms (*e.g.*, sodium and potassium)
  3. To meet increased metabolic demands (*e.g.*, B-complex vitamins)
  4. To reduce anemia (*e.g.*, iron and B-complex vitamins)
- *Fluids* are increased to replace losses in diuresis and exudation from the wound

Caloric and Nutrient Recommendations

Individual nutritional care plans are calculated according to burned surface area (BSA).
- Calories
  Allow
  25 kcal/kg IBW or preburn weight/day + (40 kcal $\times$ % total BSA)
  Or allow
  50–60 kcal/kg IBW/day
  Example, 70-kg male with 30% BSA
  25 kcal $\times$ 70 kg = 1750 kcal + (40 kcal $\times$ 30 = 1200 kcal)
  1750 kcal + 1200 kcal = 2950 kcal total daily kcal requirement
- Protein
  Allow
  1 g protein/kg IBW/day + (3 g protein $\times$ % total BSA)
  Or allow
  2–3 g/kg IBW/day
  Example, 70-kg male with 30% BSA
  1 g protein $\times$ 70 kg + (3 g protein $\times$ 30)
  70 g protein + 90 g protein = 160 g protein total daily protein requirement
- Vitamin daily requirements
  Allow
  5–10 times the RDAs with at least 1 g of vitamin C
- Mineral daily requirements, especially sodium and potassium, determined by output
- Fluid daily requirements determined by output

Dietary Adaptations

- All foods presented to the client must meet his psychological as well as his physiological needs; therefore, foods must be attractive and have flavors that appeal to the client
- Fluids such as fruit juices (high in potassium), tomato juice (high in sodium), or special electrolyte solutions that are flavored and cold should be promoted; and milkshakes (high in protein) should be encouraged (however, milk should be avoided if lactose intolerance is

present or renal calculi are pending); fluid intakes must be monitored constantly in order to prevent overhydration

- Foods with concentrated caloric and nutrient density, such as puddings with fortified dried skim milk powder and cream, and special breads with added wheat germ, should be offered frequently; additionally, complex carbohydrates such as whole wheat breads relieve constipation
- Meat protein should be offered frequently in order to provide heme iron and high biologic protein; also, a citrus fruit, which contains vitamin C, should be added to these meals to enhance the absorption of iron

Feeding Suggestions

- Serve 6 small meals, rather than 3 large meals, per day
- Offer supplements with high caloric and nutrient density (*e.g.*, Sustacal pudding) between meals and at bedtime

Behavioral Suggestions

Encourage moderate exercise; it enhances appetite and fecal evacuation and alleviates calcium excretion

Drug Therapy

Antacids such as Amphojel, Maalox, and Mylanta are used to curtail ulcer development. See Table 7–1 for nutritional implications of antacid therapy. A discussion of the complex drug therapy used in burn treatment is beyond the scope of this book.

Nutritional Care of Clients With Nervous System, Musculoskeletal, and Neuroskeletal Disorders

Present scientific knowledge about the interactions between nutrient intake and brain function is scant. However, recent scientific investigations of amino acids indicate that concentrations of neurotransmitters in the brain may be influenced by diet. It is theorized, therefore, that diet may become a way of changing behavior or of transmitting signals from the brain to other areas of the body. Presently, however, scientific evidence that diet, or any other treatment, can cure certain nervous system disorders is lacking. Unfortunately, individuals with incurable diseases such as epilepsy and multiple sclerosis often read or hear about fad diets and become convinced that certain nutrients, especially megadoses of vitamins, will cure their afflictions. Consequently, members of the health team must be aware of such misleading claims and advise their clients accordingly. Nevertheless, proper nutrition and helpful hints on how to make eating a more pleasant and less fatiguing experience can improve the quality of life and in some cases relieve adverse symptoms.

The nutritional status of individuals with musculoskeletal diseases is usually impaired because fatigue, pain, and stiffness lead to immobilization. Subsequently, the client's ability to procure, prepare, and consume food is curtailed.

Arthritis

Description

Arthritis is a chronic inflammatory disease process that affects the joints.

Classifications

- Rheumatoid Arthritis. A chronic progressive inflammatory tissue disorder that creates pain, stiffness, and swelling
- Osteoarthritis (also called degenerative or hypertrophic arthritis). A joint disorder characterized by degeneration of the articular cartilage and bony outgrowths around the joints
- Gouty arthritis (also called tophic arthritis). A disorder in purine metabolism characterized by an increase in blood levels of uric acid and the deposition of urate crystals as tophi in the small joints and surrounding tissues

Nutritional Care

General Description

Nutritional support of all clients with arthritis involves a well-balanced diet that maintains or obtains ideal weight. Nutritional care plans, however, may have to be adjusted to compensate for adverse symptoms induced by medications (see Table 9–1).* Additionally, in clients with gouty arthritis, intake of purine and fat may have to be limited when an excess of uric acid appears in the blood.

Nutritional Care Plan

- Methodology. Oral feedings; caloric content determined by height, present and ideal body weight, sex, age, and activity level. For clients with gout, a high-carbohydrate, moderate-protein, low-purine,

---

* See tables at the end of this chapter.

low-fat diet with increased fluids and limited alcohol intake may be prescribed, usually during the acute stage of the disorder, to augment drug therapy or when drug therapy is ineffective.

- Rationale
  1. High-caloric intake is often recommended for clients with rheumatoid arthritis; weight loss is usually extensive because food consumption is curtailed by pain, stiffness, and fatigue
  2. Low-caloric intake is often recommended for clients with osteoarthritis and gout; weight gain is usually extensive owing to inactivity—weight-reduction programs, however, must be gradual because rapid weight loss, especially fasting, induces increased serum uric acid levels
  3. Certain protein foods that contain high concentrations of purines (*e.g.*, glandular meats and meat extracts) are limited because purines ultimately produce uric acid—clients with gout appear to produce more uric acid from purines and, also, to have an impaired ability to excrete excessive urates; consequently, uric acid builds up in the serum and eventually urates that are not excreted are deposited in the small joints and tissues
  4. Fats are limited because they impair the excretion of urates
  5. Fluids are increased because they assist the excretion of uric acid and minimize the possibility of calculus (uric acid stone) formation
  6. Alcohol is limited because it enhances the renal retention of urate and weight gain
- Caloric and Nutrient Recommendations
  1. Calories. Reduced or increased to maintain or obtain IBW
  2. Protein. Normal intake usually recommended; in clients with gout, protein is limited to 1 g/kg IBW/day or 60 to 70 g/day
  3. Purines. Limited to 100 to 150 mg/day (normal intake 600–1000 mg/day) in clients with gout during the acute stage and when drugs are ineffective
  4. Carbohydrate. Increased, within total caloric allowance, in clients with gout; fructose intake, however, should be limited because fructose appears to increase uric acid production; in rheumatoid arthritis, refined carbohydrates should be decreased if inflammation has impaired insulin effectiveness
  5. Fat. Limited or increased within the total caloric allowance; limited to 30% to 40% of total caloric intake in clients with gout
  6. Vitamins and Minerals. Normal intake recommended (see RDAs, Appendix IV) unless drug–nutrient interactions decrease nutrient absorption or utilization; supplements are needed when nutrient–drug interactions exist because these drugs are taken over long periods of time, and nutritional status may be impaired without

dietary supplementation (see Table 9-1 for nutrient–drug interactions); however, members of the health team should observe clients for signs of oversupplementation because individuals with these disorders are often vulnerable to false claims that megadoses of vitamins or minerals (especially calcium) will be curative

7. Fluids. Normal intake; in gout, intake as high as 4000 ml/day may be recommended

- Dietary Adaptations
  1. Serve foods with concentrated caloric and nutrient density frequently to individuals with weight loss that is due to fatigue and pain
  2. Serve low-caloric foods such as fruits and vegetables to individuals with excessive weight gain
  3. When uric acid levels are high in gout clients
     a. Limit intake of foods with high purine concentrations such as glandular meat, meat extracts, fish, dried legumes, and lentils
     b. Increase intake of eggs, cheese, and skim milk to provide adequate protein
     c. Limit foods with high fat content such as ice cream, rich desserts, and fried food
     d. Increase fluid intake, especially fruit juice, because it maintains an alkaline urine that prevents crystallization of the urates into stones; exceptions are cranberry, plum, and prune juices, which produce an acid urine
     e. Limit alcohol intake
  5. Other dietary adaptations may be necessary when certain medications are taken over long periods of time; for instance, low-sodium or diabetic diets may be prescribed when steroids (see Table 7-1) are used to reduce inflammation (consult related chapters for further dietary adaptation suggestions)
- Feeding Suggestions
  1. Six small meals, rather than 3 large meals, per day should be served to relieve fatigue at mealtime
  2. Help clients with finger and hand joint disorders obtain self-feeding devices that will make food preparation and consumption easier; consultation with the occupational therapist may be helpful

Drug Therapy

Anti-inflammatory medications (see Table 9–1), including steroid agents (see Table 7–1), may be prescribed. In clients with gouty arthritis, medications that reduce serum levels of uric acid (*e.g.*, allopurinol) are administered (see Table 9–1).

Down's Syndrome (Mongolism)

Description

Down's syndrome is a congenital form of mental deficiency, accompanied by physical deformities, related to a chromosomal abnormality.

Nutritional Care

General Description

Nutritional support of clients with Down's syndrome usually involves a well-balanced diet that will promote growth. Caloric and nutrient intake is determined by the individual's height, present and ideal body weight, age, sex, and activity level. Overweight is often a problem in these clients; the caloric content of the diet usually has to be limited.

Nutritional Care Plan

- Methodology. Oral feedings. If weight loss is necessary, caloric intake is adjusted to produce a loss of 1 to 2 lb weekly (reduction in calories of 500–1,000 kcal/day); the caloric level, however, must be sufficient to enhance growth (consult Chap. 6 and the RDAs in Appendix IV).
- Rationale
  1. Children with Down's syndrome are frequently shorter and heavier than the general population
  2. They are also less active, owing to hypotonia; consequently, if they consume the same caloric intake as other children of their age, obesity may be induced
- Caloric and Nutrient Recommendations
  1. Calories. Reduced (see Methodology)
  2. Protein. Allow 1 to 1.5 g/kg IBW/day, depending upon the age of the child (see RDAs, Appendix IV).
  3. Carbohydrate
     a. Reduce intake of refined sugars. Parents of children with this affliction often have a tendency to provide foods in this category (*e.g.*, cakes and cookies) in excess because they are easier to chew and can be used to keep children quiet and reward good behavior.
     b. Increase intake of complex carbohydrates and natural sugars (*e.g.*, whole-grain cereals and raw fruits) for they add texture, satiety, and fiber (relieves constipation, which is a common adverse symptom; prune juice given in the morning will also relieve constipation).
  4. Fat. Reduce intake to 30% of total caloric requirements.

5. Vitamins and Minerals. Supplements are often necessary. Supplements of calcium and vitamin D are used frequently because milk is often limited to reduce mucus formation and thereby avoid an excessive nasal discharge. Iron supplements are used if meat is difficult to chew. Vitamin C supplements are indicated when drooling is excessive, because citrus fruits enhance the condition. However, oversupplementation and the use of "health foods" are often prevalent because many parents of these children are looking for a cure and are particularly vulnerable to claims that vitamins alleviate all medical disorders.

6. Fluids. Increased intake is recommended to replace fluids lost in spilling or drooling. Additionally, increased fluids may alleviate constipation and urinary infections.

- Dietary Adaptations*
  1. Foods with concentrated calories and nutrients (*e.g.,* cream, margarine, wheat germ, and milk powder added to foods) may be necessary when the child's oral cavity is impaired, when he tires easily while eating (owing to flaccid muscles), or when he refuses a variety of foods.
  2. Obese children, however, should be introduced to foods that have texture but few calories (*e.g.,* raw carrot sticks and fresh fruits).
  3. Strained foods should be limited when the child is capable of handling solid foods. Introduce solid foods gradually so that the child is excited by his new skill, not frustrated by failure.
  4. Fluids, especially fruit juices, should be encouraged unless the child drools excessively.

- Feeding Suggestions*
  1. Self-feeding skills can be enhanced, in children developmentally ready to acquire the skill, by obtaining dishes that will not tip over, easy-to-handle cups, and utensils that can be handled easily (*e.g.,* shorter spoons).
  2. Drooling can be controlled by placing a hand under the jaw and pushing the mouth closed.
  3. Tongue sucking can often be alleviated by introducing solid foods with texture, since these foods promote the development of oral motor skills. Additionally, if the tongue projects outward, insert the feeding spoon toward the center of the tongue, with a slight downward pressure, rather than at the tip of the tongue.

---

* These dietary adaptions and feeding suggestions may also be helpful when caring for a child with *cerebral palsy*. Additionally, in this disorder, allow only small amounts of food and fluid at a time so that the muscles can relax between bites and food can be swallowed.

4. Mouth breathing, caused by heavy nasal secretions, may mean the child needs a longer eating period in order to consume adequate quantities of food; never rush such a child.

5. Sucking difficulties caused by a narrow palate can be alleviated, while bottle feeding, by holding the child upright and supporting the head slightly downward, not backward.

6. Hoarding food in the mouth can be alleviated by closing the child's mouth and not permitting him to eat more food until he has swallowed what is in his mouth.

7. Throwing of food can often be curtailed if the child is allowed to socialize during mealtime with other children of his own age.

Drug Therapy

Drug therapy should be individualized to secondary complications such as constipation (see Table 7–1).

Epilepsy

Description

Epilepsy is recurrent paroxysmal disturbance of nervous system function, often associated with impairment of consciousness with or without convulsive movement. It results from abnormal electrical activity of the brain.

Nutritional Care

General Description

Nutritional support of clients with epilepsy usually involves a well-balanced normal diet used in conjunction with drug therapy (see Table 9–1). Both stimulants (*e.g.,* coffee and cola drinks with caffeine) and alcohol, including beer, are restricted.

Occasionally, drug therapy is not tolerated or therapy is ineffective. In these cases, the ketogenic nutritional care plan is recommended. This plan is designed to produce ketosis by reversing the usual dietary fat:carbohydrate ratio. Generally, the regimen is more effective in children. It is rarely used alone; in most cases it is prescribed in conjunction with drug therapy.

Ketogenic Nutritional Care Plan

• Methodology. No solid foods are given for a period of 2 to 3 days. Allowed liquids are broth, tea, and 6 to 8 oz of orange juice/day. The client then progresses to solid oral feedings that have a high long-chain triglyceride (LCT) fat content and a decreased carbohydrate content. The fat:carbohydrate ratio is altered gradually, so that adverse symptoms such as nausea, vomiting, and diarrhea do not develop. The effective ratio (that which reduces or eliminates seizures) is 3:1 or 4:1. An alternate plan is to use medium-chain triglyceride (MCT) oil to increase the fat content of the diet rather than the LCT content of the diet. The advantage this plan confers is that the carbohydrate and protein content of the diet can be increased (see caloric and nutrient recommendations).

- Rationale
  1. A 2-to-3-day fast creates a weight loss of approximately 10%, which subsequently increases the amount of ketone bodies in the plasma and urine.
  2. Increased ketone bodies in the plasma mediate a direct action on cerebral excitability, which ultimately lessens or eliminates seizures. A child's brain has a greater capacity to oxidize ketone bodies; consequently, the diet is more effective in the young.
  3. MCTs are absorbed and utilized more rapidly; thus they enhance a more rapid induction of ketosis.
- Caloric and Nutrient Recommendations*
  1. Calories. In children, determined by growth and activity requirements; in adults, determined by height, present weight (reduced or increased to obtain IBW), sex, age, and activity level (see Chap. 6, IBW charts in Appendix I, and RDA recommendations in Appendix IV).
  2. Remaining Nutrient Recommendations. To illustrate the remaining nutrient recommendations, observe the following example for an 1800-kcal diet prescription (if the MCT regimen is used, the kilocalorie distribution recommended is 60% fat in the form of MCT oil, 10% fat in the form of LCT, 10% protein, and 20% carbohydrate).
     a. Protein. Reduce intake to 7% of total kilocalories/day (normal intake is 12%–20%)
        7% of 1800 kcal = 126 kcal ÷ 4 = 32 g protein/day
     b. Carbohydrate. Reduce intake gradually, to 7% of total kilocalories/day (normal intake is 50%–60%; see protein, above)
     c. Fat. Increase intake to 80%–90% of total kilocalories/day (normal intake is 30%–40%).
        86% of 1800 = 1548 kcal ÷ 9 kcal/g =
        172 g fat/day

---

* Nutrient recommendations are adapted from Krause, Thiele, and Pemberton and Gastineau (see Bibliography at the end of this chapter).

3. Vitamins and Minerals. Supplements are often necessary. Vitamin D and calcium supplements are recommended because milk is limited when the amount of protein allowed is decreased. Additionally, the availability of these nutrients is decreased by the drugs used for treatment of seizures (see Table 9–1). Iron supplements recommended because meat is limited when protein allowances are decreased. Water-soluble vitamin supplements, especially folic acid, B_{12}, and B_6, are recommended because the availability of these nutrients is decreased by drug therapy (see Table 9–1). Supplements must be prescribed by the physician; excesses of these nutrients may compromise the effectiveness of drug therapy.

4. Fluids. Intake may be reduced because dehydration seems to reduce seizures. Fluid limitations, however, should never be instituted unless the client is under constant medical supervision.

• Dietary Adaptations
   1. To determine the amount of protein, carbohydrate, and fat in various foods, consult diabetic exchange lists (see Appendix V)
   2. If the LCT plan is used
      a. Add whipped cream or cream to desserts such as Knox gelatin (a carbohydrate-free gelatin that can have sugar-free flavorings added)
      b. Add cream, butter, or margarines to casseroles
      c. Use additional oils or margarines in cooking
   3. If the MCT plan is used, add MCT oil to skim milk, fruit juices, casseroles, salad dressings, and sandwich spreads (see Table 8–2 and Chap. 8 for a more detailed discussion of the chemical composition and use of MCT oil).

• Feeding Suggestions
   1. Serve MCT oil with sufficient quantities of other foods, especially orange juice, to reduce nausea.
   2. Serve food containing the LCT or MCT addition slowly
   3. Serve 6 small, rather than 3 large, meals a day because high intake of dietary fats can cause adverse symptoms

Drug Therapy

Anti-epileptic drugs commonly administered are phenytoin (Dilantin), phenobarbital, primidone (Mysoline), ethosuximide (Zarontin), and carbamazepine (Tegretol) (see Table 9–1 for nutritional implications). Additionally, drugs that lower cholesterol may be necessary because serum cholesterol levels often become elevated, owing to the high fat content of the diet (see Table 3–11).

Multiple Sclerosis

Description

Multiple sclerosis (MS) is a disease of the central nervous system characterized by a localized inflammatory response that results in or is caused by destruction of myelin. Symptoms include weakness and incoordination.

Nutritional Care

General Description

The role of diet in MS either as a preventive measure or as a part of management of the disease is very controversial. Many dietary hypotheses have been put forth, including a gluten-free diet, low-saturated-fat–high-polyunsaturated- (linoleic fatty acid) fat diet, natural-food diet, and megavitamin therapy. The most promising regimen involves increasing dietary linoleic acid, because individuals with MS often have low levels of linoleic acid. The effectiveness of this treatment, however, is still unproven; consequently, the only nutritional care plan that is scientifically sound, at present, is a well-balanced diet that maintains or obtains IBW or relieves complications.

Nutritional Care Plan

- Methodology. Oral feedings that contain all the nutrients essential for the individual's height, sex, age, and weight, with added fiber and fluids. If the condition is being aggravated by overweight, the caloric intake should be adjusted to enhance a weight loss of 1 to 2 lb per week. Consult the RDAs in Appendix IV and Chapter 6 for more information on individual nutrient and caloric requirements and medically approved ways of losing weight. If dysphagia develops as the disease progresses, gastrostomy tube feedings may be indicated. Consult Chapter 2 for the composition and administration of tube feedings.
- Rationale
  1. A well-balanced diet enhances physiological and psychological functions; malnutrition encourages more rapid deterioration.
  2. Fiber and fluids added to the diet relieve adverse symptoms such as constipation and urinary infections.
  3. Obesity enhances inactivity and fatigue.
- Caloric and Nutrient Recommendations
  1. Calories. Adjust to maintain or obtain IBW
  2. Protein, Polyunsaturated Fats, Vitamins, and Minerals. Provide according to normal individual requirements

3. Carbohydrates. Increase complex carbohydrates such as whole wheat products; decrease refined carbohydrates such as granulated sugar

4. Fluids. Increase water intake (see rationale)

- Dietary Adaptations

  1. Provide foods that contain nutrient-dense calories without creating obesity and fatigue (*e.g.,* meat patties [bran may be added here also] and strawberries [easy to chew])

  2. Provide foods that alleviate constipation (*e.g.,* whole-wheat cereals with bran added and vegetables and fruits that can be chewed easily)

  3. Increase intake of fluids for they alleviate urinary infections and constipation; citrus fruit juices provide the vitamin C needed to alleviate or heal decubitus ulcers

- Feeding Suggestions

  1. Help the individual obtain commercial devices that alleviate or eliminate neck tremors experienced while eating (*e.g.,* a neck collar or brace)

  2. Help the client obtain commercial devices that may diminish incoordination in the upper extremities (*e.g.,* weighted bracelets and utensils); this will enhance food consumption and lessen fatigue

  3. Serve 6 small meals rather than 3 large meals, because the 3-meal schedule increases fatigue and decreases nutrient consumption

Drug Therapy

Drug therapy includes antispasticity agents, such as Baclofen (see Table 9–1), as well as bulk formers such as Metamucil and softeners such as Colace (see Table 7–2).

Hyperkinesis

Description

Hyperkinesis is a behavior syndrome in which there is moderate to severe distractability, developmentally inappropriate inattention, hyperactivity, emotional lability, and impulsiveness.

Nutritional Care

General Description

Nutritional support for a child who has excessive gross motor activity involves a well-balanced high-caloric diet fed in small, frequent servings.

Other nutritional treatments that have been advocated are megavitamin therapy and the Feingold diet. The Feingold diet limits or excludes all foods that contain salicylates (*e.g.,* oranges, apples, tomatoes), artificial flavors and colors, and the preservative butylated hydroxytoluene (BHT). It is claimed that these limitations will alter unacceptable hyperkinetic behavior. Other scientific investigations, including double-blind studies, however, have not verified these claims. If parents of children with hyperkinesis wish to try this means of treatment as an alternative to drug therapy, supplements of vitamin C, calcium, and vitamin B_2 must be administered because this diet limits foods that contain these nutrients. Additionally, it limits commercially prepared carbohydrate foods that spare protein for growth requirements; home-baked breads and other carbohydrates must be provided.

Psychologically this diet may be beneficial, for Dr. Feingold advocates consumption of only home-cooked foods, such as cookies that the parent bakes with the child. Such family projects may establish a closer relationship between parents and child with resultant improved behavior.

Nutritional Care Plan

- Methodology. Oral feedings that are high in calories and other nutrients (*e.g.,* protein and B vitamins)
- Rationale
  1. Increased caloric intake is required to furnish the energy needed for excessive gross motor activity
  2. Protein and other macronutrients are needed to prevent growth retardation and weight loss related to drug therapy (see Table 9–1)
- Caloric and Nutrient Recommendations
  1. Calories. Increased to maintain or obtain IBW and height
  2. Protein, carbohydrates, and fats. Increased to furnish caloric requirements for growth
  3. Vitamins and minerals. Increased to furnish the coenzymes (*e.g.,* B-complex vitamins) and cofactors needed to release exogenous energy for increased metabolic requirements
  4. Fluids. Normal intake is recommended because excessive intake will decrease intake of nutrient-dense solid food
- Dietary Adaptations
  1. Feed foods that contain concentrated calories (*e.g.,* puddings that are made with added cream, margarine, and dried milk powder)
  2. Limit foods that dull the appetite and provide calories without contributing other nutrients (*e.g.,* Popsicles and candies)
- Feeding Suggestions
  1. Feed small, nutrient-dense meals frequently
  2. Involve the child in food preparation to stimulate the appetite

Drug Therapy

Central nervous system stimulants such as dextroamphetamine (Dexedrine), methylphenidate (Ritalin), pemoline (Cylert), and sometimes caffeine are used (see Table 9–1 for nutritional implications).

Paraplegia

Description

Paraplegia is paralysis of the lower extremities.

Nutritional Care

General Description

Providing nutritional support for paraplegics immediately after the initial injury without using parenteral solutions or tube feedings is difficult because clients may lose up to 15% of their usual weight. The reason for this weight loss is anorexia caused by depression or medications used to control pain. Additionally, food refusal may be used as a means of hastening death. Consult Chapter 2 for details on the nutrient content and administration of parenteral solutions.

After this initial stage, however, nutritional alterations are often instituted

1. To alleviate the formation of renal stones (immobilization enhances calcium excretion)
2. To maintain or obtain IBW. Caloric intake, immediately following injury, may have to be increased because sepsis or decubitus ulcers increase needs, oral food consumption may be impaired by depression or drug therapy, or physical therapy may be so intensive that caloric intake will need to be increased to meet energy requirements. Following the initial injury, however, caloric intake may need to be decreased; when immobilization decreases activity, energy requirements are reduced.
3. To augment bowel training. Constipation is often an adverse symptom of paraplegia because spinal cord injury impairs gastrointestinal muscle tone, and immobilization reduces activities that enhance excretion.

Nutritional Care Plans That Alleviate Renal Stones

See Neprolithiasis and List of Acid–Base Formation in Foods in Chapter 8.

Nutritional Care Plans That Maintain or Obtain IBW

See Nutritional Care Plans for obesity in Chapter 6.

Nutritional Care Plans That Alleviate Constipation

See Nutritional Care Plans for constipation in Chapter 7 plus Tables 7–6 and 7–7. A high-fiber diet should be monitored frequently because excessive fiber can cause fecal impaction. Additionally, foods that contain excessive sugar must be avoided or osmotic diarrhea will ultimately develop.

Drug Therapy

Laxatives may be administered to relieve constipation (see Table 7–1). Additionally, drugs used to alleviate renal calculi may be indicated (consult Chap. 8).

Parkinson's Disease

Description

Parkinson's disease is a degenerative disease of the nervous system in which low concentrations of dopamine are found in the brain. It is characterized by masklike facies, tremor of the resting muscles, and other signs.

Nutritional Care

General Description

Nutritional support of clients with Parkinson's disease involves a well-balanced diet that is limited in protein and pyridoxine in order to augment drug therapy (see Table 9–1).

Nutritional Care Plan

- Methodology. Oral feedings that are well balanced but contain limited amounts of protein and pyridoxine
  1. Protein intake limited to 0.5 g/kg/day or about 35 g/day of high biologic value (HBV) protein; see Table 8–5; the RDA for protein is 0.8 g/kg/day or about 44 g to 56 g/day. The protein intake of most Americans, however, ranges from 70 g to 110 g/day.
  2. Pyridoxine (vitamin B_6) intake is limited to below 10 mg to 25 mg/day. The RDA for pyridoxine is 2 to 2.2 mg/day with a high protein intake (100 g), and 1.25 to 1.5 mg/day with a low protein intake (30 g). Normal intake is usually in excess of the RDA, since pyridoxine is found in many protein foods.
- Rationale. The most common drug used in the treatment of Parkinson's disease is levodopa (Larodopa), which interacts with protein and pyridoxine in the following manner.

1. Levodopa is an amino acid; therefore, other amino acids compete with it for absorption from the intestine and passage across the blood–brain barrier. Consequently, if other amino acids, from protein foods, are available in excess, the therapeutic effect of the drug is impaired.

2. Levodopa is converted to dopamine in the plasma, gut, liver, and kidneys by the enzyme dopa decarboxylase, which utilizes pyridoxine as a cofactor. Consequently, if pyridoxine is available in excess, levodopa will be converted before it reaches the brain, and the therapeutic effect of the drug will be diminished.

- Caloric and Nutrient Recommendations
  1. Calories. Reduced or increased to maintain or obtain IBW
  2. Protein. See Methodology
  3. Carbohydrate. Increased within caloric allowance so that protein can be utilized for tissue synthesis rather than for energy. Additionally, complex carbohydrates are increased to alleviate constipation.
  4. Fat. See Carbohydrate
  5. Vitamins and Minerals. Normal intake except for vitamin B_6 (see Methodology). If vitamin supplements are necessary for other medical reasons or if a variety of foods is not consumed, however, a commercial supplement that contains B-complex vitamins (without vitamin B_6) plus vitamin C should be administered (*e.g.*, Larobec).
  6. Fluids. Normal to increased intake to alleviate constipation and dry mouth enhanced by medications

- Dietary Adaptations
  1. Limit intake of low biologic value (LBV) protein foods (*e.g.*, pastas, breads, and rice) so that HBV protein foods (*e.g.*, milk, meat, and eggs) can make up the protein allowance (35 g/day)
  2. Limit intake of foods high in pyridoxine (*e.g.*, yeast, wheat germ, pork, liver, whole-grain cereals, legumes, potatoes, bananas, and oatmeal). Milk, eggs, and most fruits and vegetables may be consumed, however, for they contain only small amounts of pyridoxine.
  3. Increase fiber and fluid intake to alleviate constipation
  4. Limit or avoid alcohol because it impairs drug effectiveness

- Feeding Suggestions
  1. Serve 6 small meals, rather than 3 large meals, per day
  2. Never rush the individual; allow him to chew small bites until all food is consumed
  3. If dysphagia develops, soften foods in the blender to enhance swallowing (see Table 3–19)

Drug Therapy

Drugs that increase the amount or effectiveness of dopamine in the brain are used such as levodopa (see Table 9–1)

Mental Illness

Nutritional Care

General Description

Nutritional support of individuals with mental illnesses must fulfill psychological as well as physiological needs. Food represents security, love, pleasure, and relief from stress; accepting or refusing food is also a way to exert control over one's own life.

It is important for members of the health team caring for individuals with mental illnesses to present nourishment in a pleasant, patient, and understanding manner.

Nutritional Care Plan

See Table 9–2.

Drug Therapy

Antipsychotic medications, antidepressants, and tranquilizers are used (see Table 9–1 for nutritional implications).

Nurses' Responsibilities in the Nutritional Care of Clients With Special Disorders

Oral Nutritional Care Plan

Initiate Good Care

Procure instructions from trained professionals, including rationales for treatment by diet (*e.g.*, relief from adverse symptoms) and dietary adaptation suggestions immediately following diagnosis. Compliance is often enhanced if the client knows that the nutritional care plan has been designed to help him function more effectively for a longer period of time. This knowledge is especially important if the client might be vulnerable to claims for "miracle cures," which may include unfounded nutrient recommendations. In addition to professional advice, when the client is receptive, procure advice from individuals who have learned to cope with similar conditions.

Participate in Care

1. Weigh client upon admittance to the clinic or out-client clinic. Weigh frequently, for increased weight can often enhance fatigue and adverse symptoms such as pain. If weight is gained, report the increase to other health-team members (*e.g.*, the physician).
2. Motivate and encourage the client to feed himself, whenever feasible. Enhance this motivation by contacting the occupational therapist, who can often suggest commercial devices that facilitate feeding when muscles and nerves are impaired.
3. Observe
   a. Food consumption (*e.g.*, what foods is the client still eliminating even though he says they no longer distress him [*e.g.*, red tomato] or what foods should he be able to manage with commercial devices [*e.g.*, peas]?)
   b. Behavior while eating (*e.g.*, does he still eat compulsively or hoard food?)
   c. Mental status before and after meals (*e.g.*, is client depressed because he feels like a baby when he needs assistance?)
   d. Physiological status after meals (*e.g.*, has the lack of fiber in the diet enhanced constipation?)
   e. Reactions to medications (*e.g.*, if aspirin is not taken with the meal, the client may have adverse GI tract symptoms such as abdominal pain between meals)
   f. Compliance with the dietary regimen (*e.g.*, is client still refusing to eat because he feels he does not deserve food?)
4. Enhance compliance with the new nutritional care plan by making sure the atmosphere is pleasant (*e.g.*, soft music in the dining area) and foods are palatable.
5. Collect urine or stool specimens when indicated.
6. Record fluid intake and output. This is especially important if the client is likely to avoid liquids because he is afraid he will spill them or drool.

Coordinate Care

The overall responsibility of the nurse is to help clients function as effectively as possible for as long as possible. She can accomplish this by obtaining, observing, and reporting subjective as well as objective information to other members of the health team in meetings she has organized.

Since optimal nutritional status is an important factor in enhancing maximum function, the nurse should report subjective or objective information that may affect nutritional status.

- *Subjective information* to be reported includes what the client reveals about appetite, usual eating and drinking habits, pain while trying to manipulate utensils, and any other observations listed above under Participate in Care that will influence nutritional status
- *Objective information* to be reported includes present weight, weight gain or loss, fluid intake and output recordings, and any new laboratory findings that may affect nutritional status or indicate that a new nutritional care plan should be instituted.
- *Clinical signs* to be reported include signs of general malnutrition (*e.g.,* mouth or tongue changes), decubitus ulcers, inability to use hands effectively while eating, and depression or hyperactivity during mealtime, which may indicate that nutritional treatment should be adjusted

Reinforce and Follow Up Care

1. Empathize with the client. Many of the dietary adjustments, designed to relieve symptoms and enhance maximum functioning, will have to be followed for a lifetime. Help the client make his diet as palatable as possible. Accomplish this goal by assisting him when he must select food. *Assure him he is not alone.* Seek advice and consultation from others with the same condition whenever possible.

2. Compliment a client who tries new foods, although he may associate them with adverse effects. Also compliment a client who tries new devices that will facilitate self-feeding, even though he may not be successful the first time.

3. Obtain a working knowledge about the rationales behind dietary treatments in these disorders. Rationales can be obtained from information in this book, in advanced nutritional care books, and in most hospital diet manuals. Be medically up to date—know what nutritional care plans are obsolete, what care plans have been substituted, why the substitutions have been made, and what nutritional "cures" are unfounded. Additionally, be familiar with what special organizations are doing (*e.g.,* the National Multiple Sclerosis Society) and where they are located so that you can direct the client to them for additional help.

Enteral and Parenteral Care Plans

The nurse's responsibilities to clients with special disorders (*e.g.,* burns), who require these specialized care plans are the same as those for any individual receiving these care plans. Consult Chapter 2 for details on responsibilities.

Table 9–1
Effects of Medications for Special Disorders on Nutritional Status

Medication	Mechanism of Action	Adverse Side-Effects With Nutritional Implications	Dietary Suggestions
Anticonvulsants			
Grand mal seizures Phenytoin (Dilantin) Phenobarbital Primidone (Mysoline) Carbamazepine (Tegretol) *Petit mal seizures* Ethosuximide (Zarontin) Clonazepam (Clonopin) Trimethadione (Tridione)	Modify the ability of the brain tissue to respond to seizure-provoking stimuli	Induce nausea, vomiting, diarrhea, and decreased sensitivity to taste; all these effects enhance anorexia with subsequent weight loss and possible growth retardation in children Induce vitamin D catabolism or block hydroxylation, which may lead to poor calcium absorption and ultimately to osteomalacia and rickets Decrease serum folate levels, which may lead to megaloblastic anemia Inhibit vitamin K synthesis, which may lead to hemorrhage and anemia Decrease serum levels of vitamin B_6 and cerebral spinal fluid levels of B_{12}, which may lead to mental or neurological disorders (each drug's action may vary slightly)	Individualize diet to enhance palatablity and ultimately caloric and nutrient consumption Increase intake of vitamin D–fortified milk and cheeses Give supplements of vitamin D and calcium when advised by physician Increase intake of fruits and vegetables; they are good sources of folacin Give supplements of vitamins K, B_6, and B_{12} when advised by physician

Table 9–1 375

Table 9–1
Effects of Medications for Special Disorders on Nutritional Status (continued)

Medication	Mechanism of Action	Adverse Side-Effects With Nutritional Implications	Dietary Suggestions
Antipasticity Drugs			
Baclofen (Lioresal)	Inhibit both monosynaptic and polysynaptic reflexes at the spinal level to relax muscles and relieve spasticity	Induce nausea, constipation, or diarrhea and dry mouth; all these effects enhance anorexia with subsequent weight loss	Individualize diet to enhance palatability and ultimately caloric and nutrient consumption To relieve dry mouth, suck hard candies, chew sugar-free gum, or increase fluid intake When spasticity is relieved, the individual may have less trouble consuming food, and weight gain may be induced
Central Nervous System Stimulants Used in Hyperkinesis			
Dextroamphetamine (Dexedrine) Methylphenidate (Ritalin) Pemoline (Cylert)	Formerly thought to create a paradoxical tranquilizing phenomenon when given to hyperactive children, now thought that hyperactive children only give the clinical impression of being hyperaroused and that in actuality they often exhibit physiological signs of low arousal.	Induce insomnia and nervousness, which increase caloric and nutrient needs Induce anorexia, which enhances the weight loss due to increased activity If these effects persist, child's height and weight may not reach the full potential	Give drugs in morning and at lunch, if necessary, not at night Give medication with meals Increase caloric and nutrient intake by giving foods that have a high concentration of calories and nutrients such as

(continued)

Table 9–1
Effects of Medications for Special Disorders on Nutritional Status (continued)

Medication	Mechanism of Action	Adverse Side-Effects With Nutritional Implications	Dietary Suggestions
Central Nervous System Stimulants Used in Hyperkinesis (continued)			
	If this is true, it follows that the stimulants activate the hyperkinetic child in the same way that they activate adults, resulting in an increased attention span (see discussion of hyperkinesis in text)		milkshakes with added skim milk powder and ice cream and puddings with added cream Give frequent snacks that enhance nutrient density, such as peanuts and popcorn with added butter Involve child in food preparation to enhance food consumption
Antiparkinsonism Drugs			
Levodopa (Larodopa)	Levodopa, an amino acid, is a precursor of dopamine that can cross the blood–brain barrier, where it presumably is converted into dopamine	Induces nausea, anorexia, vomiting, dry mouth, dysphagia, bitter taste, and diarrhea; all these effects enhance weight loss	Individualize diet to enhance palatability and ultimately caloric and nutrient consumption Give foods that are easy to chew and consume so client does not tire before meal is finished Give drug with food or immediately following meals to decrease adverse symptoms such as nausea

(continued)

Table 9–1 377

Table 9–1
Effects of Medications for Special Disorders on Nutritional Status (continued)

Medication	Mechanism of Action	Adverse Side-Effects With Nutritional Implications	Dietary Suggestions
Antiparkinsonism Drugs (continued)			
		Increase secretion of sodium and potassium	Maintain normal levels of sodium and potassium by giving foods that have high amounts of these minerals (See Chap. 3)
		Vitamin B_6 is a cofactor for dopa decarboxylase, an enzyme that enhances the extracellular conversion of levodopa, therefore, it must be limited so more of the drug reaches the brain	Maintain dietary intake of vitamin B_6 to achieve normal levels. Give supplements that do not contain this vitamin (*e.g.,* Larobec)
			Exogenous protein limited to 35 g high biologic (*e.g.,* meat, milk, and eggs)/day
Bromocriptine mesylate (Parlodel)	A dopamine receptor agonist which activates postsynaptic dopamine receptors	Protein is limited because it competes with levodopa, an amino acid, for absorption and transport across the blood–brain barrier	
		Same as for levodopa except that constipation may be induced	Same as for levodopa
			Increase fluid and fiber intake if constipation is present
Levodopa and carbidopa (Sinemet)	Carbidopa inhibits decarboxylation of peripheral levodopa, which enhances the amount of levodopa available for transfer to the brain	Same as for levodopa except that nausea and vomiting are often minimized	Same as for levodopa except that food consumption may be enhanced by lessened adverse effects
		Pyridoxine's effect on peripheral decarboxylation of levodopa is lessened	Dietary intake of pyridoxine may be increased and supplements

(continued)

Table 9–1
Effects of Medications for Special Disorders on Nutritional Status (continued)

Medication	Mechanism of Action	Adverse Side-Effects With Nutritional Implications	Dietary Suggestions
Antiparkinsonism Drugs (continued)			may be given Additionally, because more levodopa is available for the brain, protein intake may be increased but client must be monitored closely
Antidepressants			
Tricyclic agents (TCADs) Amitriptyline hydrochloride (Elavil, Endep) Imipramine pamoate (Tofranil)	May enhance the activity of nor-epinephrine by blocking its reuptake into the storage granules of nerve endings May potentiate 5 hydroxytryptamine (5 HT, serotonin) by blocking its reuptake or its metabolism	Induce dry mouth, constipation, or diarrhea and metallic taste, effects that may enhance anorexia with resultant weight loss Also, induce hyperphagia, which may enhance weight gain Enhance CNS depressant effects of alcohol	Allow client to suck on hard candies and chew sugar-free gum to relieve dry mouth and metallic taste Increase fiber and fluids if constipation is evident Decrease fibrous foods when diarrhea is evident Increase or decrease caloric intake to obtain or maintain IBW Avoid alcohol

(continued)

Table 9–1 379

Table 9–1
Effects of Medications for Special Disorders on Nutritional Status (continued)

Medication	Mechanism of Action	Adverse Side-Effects With Nutritional Implications	Dietary Suggestions
Antidepressants (continued)			
Monamine oxidase inhibitors (MAOIs) Isocarboxazid (Marplan) Phenelzine sulfate (Nardil) Tranylcypromine sulfate (Parnate)	MAO enzyme system regulates amines (norepinephrine, dopamine, and 5 HT), which are chemical transmitters of electrical impulses that maintain homeostasis. MAOIs block this action, with a resultant increase in norepinephrine and an increase in tyramine levels. The former reaction lessens depression, but the latter, if excessive, can cause a hypertensive crisis.	Induce headaches, diarrhea, high blood pressure, and even death if intake is excessive or if there is concomitant high intake of foods that contain natural sources of amines	Foods with naturally high amounts of tyramine are restricted Dairy products: yogurt and aged cheeses (*e.g.,* cheddar, brie, and mozzarella) Alcoholic beverages: beer, ale, and wine (*e.g.,* chianti and sherry) Meats: chicken livers and dried fish (*e.g.,* herring and cod) Vegetables: Italian broad beans Others: vanilla, chocolate, yeast, and soy sauce
Antipsychotics			
Phenothiazines Chlorpromazine hydrochloride (Thorazine) Prochlorperazine edisylate (Compazine)	May exert an effect on the neurotransmitters dopamine, norepinephrine, and serotonin and on their ultimate activities in neural transmission	Induce hyperphagia with accompanying weight gain Induce dry mouth (feels like cotton)	Reduce caloric intake to a level that will maintain or obtain IBW Give client hard candies to suck or sugar-free gum to chew

(continued)

Table 9–1
Effects of Medications for Special Disorders on Nutritional Status (continued)

Medication	Mechanism of Action	Adverse Side-Effects With Nutritional Implications	Dietary Suggestions
Antipsychotics (continued)			
		Induce constipation	Increase intake of fiber and fluids
		May limit B_{12} and xylose (a carbohydrate) absorption	Supplements of B_{12} may be necessary
			Increase intake of other carbohydrates if weight is not excessive
Lithiums Lithium carbonate (Lithonate, Lithotabs)	May replace intracellular sodium, thereby stabilizing the axonal membrane, decreasing the amplitude of the action potential, and reducing CNS activity	Induce diarrhea, vomiting, and nausea	Give drug after meals to lessen GI tract irritations
		Induce hyperphagia	Reduce caloric intake to a level that will maintain or obtain IBW
		Lithium can replace sodium, and the absence of sodium can induce toxicity	Maintain a normal sodium intake
		Induce polyuria with resultant thirst	Increase fluid intake if polyuria is excessive
		Alcohol can induce toxicity	Limit alcohol intake
Ataractics (Tranquilizers)			
Chlordiazepoxide hydrochloride (Librium) Diazepam (Valium)	Depress CNS stimulation, which clinically lessens learned avoidance responses or	Induce dry mouth	Give client hard candy to suck or sugar-free gum to chew and increase fluid intake

(continued)

Table 9–1 381

Table 9–1
Effects of Medications for Special Disorders on Nutritional Status (continued)

Medication	Mechanism of Action	Adverse Side-Effects With Nutritional Implications	Dietary Suggestions
Ataractics (Tranquilizers) *(continued)*			
	diminishes anticipatory responses to external or imagined danger and unpleasant situations	Induce constipation Induce hyperphagia with resultant weight gain Induce fatigue and inactivity, which enhances weight gain Alcohol may enhance toxicity	Increase fluids and liquids Reduce caloric intake to a level that will maintain or obtain IBW Encourage moderate activity Limit alcohol intake
Anti-inflammatory Salicylates (Aspirin)			
APC tablets, Bayer aspirin Enteric-coated aspirin (Ecotrin)	Inhibit certain factors believed to be involved in the inflammatory process, namely, leucocyte migration, the release or activity of lysosomal enzymes that cause inflammation, and prostaglandin synthesis (by inhibiting prostaglandin synthetase); consequently, pain is relieved, as prostaglandins appear to enhance pain at the inflammation site by sensitizing nerve endings	Decrease uptake of vitamin C in leukocytes Impair the protein-binding ability of folate Inhibit protein synthesis Stimulate carbohydrate utilization (aspirin has an insulinlike effect that can lead to hypoglycemic episodes)	Increase intake of vitamin C; supplements may be needed if citrus juices irritate GI mucosa Give folate supplements Increase protein intake to ensure proper cell growth and replace losses during hemorrhage Carbohydrate intake may need to be increased along with protein

(continued)

Table 9–1
Effects of Medications for Special Disorders on Nutritional Status (continued)

Medication	Mechanism of Action	Adverse Side-Effects With Nutritional Implications	Dietary Suggestions
Anti-inflammatory Salicylates (Aspirin) (continued)			
		Inhibit prothrombin synthesis and platelet function (effect on vitamin K is not established)	Vitamin K supplements may be recommended by some physicians
		Induce gastric irritation, namely, epigastric pain, nausea, ulcers, and sometimes severe GI hemorrhage, which may lead to hypovolemia with resultant cardiovascular collapse and possibly death	Give frequent small bland meals that have limited amounts of acidic foods such as citrus juices (see Chap. 7 for other foods limited on a bland diet)
			Iron supplements may be necessary in severe hemorrhage
			Give aspirin tablets in the middle of the meal
			Give antacids after the meal if advised by the physician (see Table 7-1)
Nonsteroidal Anti-inflammatory Agents			
Indomethacin (Indocin) Ibuprofen (Motrin) Naproxen (Naprosyn) Fenoprofen (Nalfon) Tolmetin (Tolectin)	Mode of action similar to that of aspirin	Induce GI irritation similar to that induced by aspirin	Give drugs with meals or milk
			Give antacids after meals when advised by the physician (see Table 7-1)
Phenylbutazone (Butazolidin)	Pyrazoline-derivative drugs (*e. g.,* Butazolidin) increase the renal		Limit sodium intake when pyrazolone-derivative drugs

(continued)

Table 9-1
Effects of Medications for Special Disorders on Nutritional Status (continued)

Medication	Mechanism of Action	Adverse Side-Effects With Nutritional Implications	Dietary Suggestions
Nonsteroidal Anti-inflammatory Agents *(continued)*			
Oxyphenbutazone (Tandearil)	tubular reabsorption of sodium, which ultimately leads to water retention		have been prescribed (see Chap. 3 for sodium restrictions)
Steroid Anti-inflammatory Agents (see Table 7-1)			
Anti-inflammatory Agents Used in Gout			
Indomethacin (Indocin) Phenylbutazone (Butazolidin) Oxyphenbutazone (Tandearil) Colchicine (Colchicine)	Decrease the inflammatory response to deposited urate crystals by inhibiting leukocyte phagocytosis	Induce GI irritation similar to that induced by aspirin	Give drugs with meals or milk Give antacids after meals when advised by the physician (see Table 7-1)
		Colchicine decreases the absorption of fat, carotene, sodium, potassium, vitamin B_{12}, lactose, nitrogen, and cholesterol	Clients who are on colchicine should be monitored closely for symptoms that may be related to nutrient deficiencies (*e.g.*, hypokalemia); if symptoms develop, foods high in the nutrient should be increased or supplements should be given
Uricosuric Agents Used in Gout			
Probenecid (Benemid) Sulfinpyrazone (Anturane)	Inhibit the renal tubular reabsorption of urate, thus increas-	Induce anorexia, nausea, vomiting, and diarrhea or	Individualize diet to enhance palatability

(continued)

Table 9-1 383

Table 9-1
Effects of Medications for Special Disorders on Nutritional Status (continued)

Medication	Mechanism of Action	Adverse Side-Effects With Nutritional Implications	Dietary Suggestions
Uricosuric Agents Used in Gout (continued)			
	ing the urinary excretion of uric acid and decreasing serum urate levels	constipation	Give drug with food or milk
			Give antacids after meals when advised by the physician (see Table 7-1)
			Increase fiber and fluids when constipation exists and decrease fiber when diarrhea exists (see Chap. 7)
		Induce uric acid renal stone formation in some instances	Increase fluid intake to prevent renal stone formation
			Give an alkaline ash diet to maintain an alkaline urine (see Chap. 8)
			Limit foods high in purine and total fat (see dietary adaptations in gouty arthritis)
Xanthine Oxidase Inhibitors Used in Gout			
Allopurinol (Zyloprim, Lopurin)	Inhibit xanthine oxidase, the enzyme needed for the formation of uric acid, by competing with uric acid precursors for the active site of the enzyme; consequently, serum urate levels are reduced	Same as with uricosuric agents	Same as for uricosuric agents

Table 9–2 385

Table 9-2
Feeding Alterations Encountered in the Mentally Ill

Feeding Alterations	Feeding Suggestions That May Alleviate Alterations
Depression Often causes disinterest in food	Serve colorful food in light, pleasant, nonthreatening atmosphere
Overactivity May have difficulty sitting still long enough to consume adequate amounts of food	Serve 6 small, rather than 3 large, meals per day; nutrient-dense supplements may be necessary between meals, but tube feedings should be avoided whenever possible
Delusions May develop fears and suspicions about food, such as fear of not being fed again (hoards food), fear of being poisoned (refuses to eat), and aversions to a food because of its color (*e.g.*, a red tomato may be associated with blood or death), smell, or taste	Nurses (without uniforms) eating the same food as these individuals may relieve some anxieties such as fear of being poisoned; additionally, serving foods in the "whole" form, such as plain meat and unpeeled fruits, rather than mixed dishes, may relieve anxieties Hoarding of foods should be discouraged because unrefrigerated foods can precipitate bacterial illnesses; foods that obviously cause distress should be removed until individual can cope
Guilt Complexes May refuse food as a means of punishment	Serve foods frequently that have concentrated caloric and nutrient value, such as casseroles and puddings with added dried skim milk powder; additionally, evaluate person carefully to see if eating alone or with others enhances food consumption

(continued)

Table 9–2
Feeding Alterations Encountered in the Mentally Ill (continued)

Feeding Alterations	Feeding Suggestions That May Alleviate Alterations
Emotional Insecurity, Anxiety or Compulsion	
May overeat to relieve anxiety	Serve low-calorie foods such as fruits and vegetables often but serve them in a dining area so that the individual, as he begins to cope, becomes aware of his eating behavior
	If weight-reduction programs are introduced to enhance the client's self-image, they must be introduced *slowly* to prevent increased frustration
	If the person accepts the program, reinforcement must always be positive (*e.g.*, small monetary payments may be offered or increased privileges may be allowed); never negative (*e.g.*, punishment for noncompliance must never be employed)
Medications	See Table 9–1
May increase or decrease appetite; additionally, some foods may have to be eliminated because they cause adverse reactions when consumed with medications	
Shock Therapy	
May have increased caloric requirements	Serve 6 small, rather than 3 large, meals a day that have concentrated caloric and nutrient value. Supplements such as Sustacal pudding may be used between meals

Bibliography

Ainsley BM, Blackburn GL: Nutritional needs of a paraplegic patient. JAMA 248:2180, 1982

American Dietetic Association: Handbook of Clinical Dietetics. New Haven, Yale University Press, 1981

Anderson L, Dipple MV, Turkki PR et al: Nutrition in Health and Disease, 17th ed. Philadelphia, JB Lippincott, 1982

Bollet AJ: Diagnostic and therapeutic aids in gout and hyperuricemia. Med Times 109:23, 1981

Bollet AJ: Nonsteroidal anti-inflammatory drugs: Part I. Med Times 110:31, 1982

Calvert SD, Vivian VM, Calvert GP: Dietary adequacy, feeding practices, and eating behavior of children with Down's syndrome. J Am Diet Assoc 69:152, 1976

Fernstrom JD: Effects of the diet on brain neurotransmitters. Metabolism 26:207, 1977

Harris FA: Treatment with a position feedback-controlled head stabilizer. Am J Phys Med 58:169, 1979

Howard RB, Herbold NH: Nutrition in Clinical Care. New York, McGraw–Hill, 1978

Howe PS: Basic Nutrition in Health and Disease. Philadelphia, WB Saunders, 1971

Kaplan PE, Gandhavadi B, Richards L et al: Calcium balance in paraplegic patients: Influence of injury duration and ambulation. Arch Phys Med Rehabil 59:447, 1978

Krause MV, Mahan LK: Food, Nutrition and Diet Therapy, 6th ed. Philadelphia, WB Saunders, 1979

Lasser JL, Brush MK: An improved ketogenic diet for treatment of epilepsy. J Am Diet Assoc 62:281, 1973

Olson WH: Diet and multiple sclerosis. Postgrad Med 59:219, 1976

Pemberton CM, Gastineau CF (eds): Mayo Clinic Diet Manual. Philadelphia, WB Saunders, 1981

Pipes PL, Holm VA: Feeding children with Down's syndrome. J Am Diet Assoc 77:277, 1980

Polednak AP, Auliffe J: Obesity in an institutionalised adult mentally retarded population. J Ment Defic Res 20:9, 1976

Roe DA: Drug–nutrient interactions. Med Times 109:66, 1981

Rotatori AF, Rotatori L: Behavioral weight reduction for the mentally retarded. J Am Diet Assoc 75:46, 1979

Scheinberg LC, Abissi C: Multiple sclerosis: Diagnosable and treatable. Med Times 109:38s, 1981

Schneitzer L: Rehabilitation of patients with multiple sclerosis. Arch Phys Med Rehabil 59:430, 1978

Schulman EA: Diagnosis and treatment of epilepsy. Med Times 110:39, 1982

Signore JM: Ketogenic diet containing medium-chain triglycerides. J Am Diet Assoc 62:285, 1973

Springer NS, Fricke NL: Nutrition and drug therapy for persons with developmental disabilities. J Ment Defic 80:317, 1975

Sudarsky L: Problems in the management of Parkinson's disease. Med Times 109:31, 1981

Thiele VF: Clinical Nutrition, 2nd ed. St Louis, CV Mosby, 1980

Wender EH: Hyperactivity and the food additive free diet. Fla Med Assoc 66:466, 1979

Weiner MB, Pepper GA, Kuhn–Weisman G et al: Clinical Pharmacology and Therapeutics in Nursing. New York, McGraw–Hill, 1979

Young RR: Step therapy for Parkinson's disease. Patient Care 14:74, 1980

chapter 10

Pregnancy and Lactation

Terminology

Gravida. A pregnant woman

Parity. The state of a woman regarding the number of live or stillborn infants she has delivered

Gestation. The 40-week period from conception to birth, divided into three trimesters: weeks 1 to 13 (first trimester), weeks 14 to 27 (second trimester), weeks 28 to 40 (third trimester)

Prenatal Period. The time from conception through the early fetal period, weeks 1 to 20; and the late fetal period, weeks 21 to 40

Perinatal period. The late fetal period and the neonatal period (time that surrounds birth, and the first 28 days)

Lactation. The period during which the mother secretes milk

Neonatal Period. The first 28 days after birth

Postneonatal Period. From 29 days after birth to 1 year

Full-term Infant (or appropriate for gestational age [AGA]). An infant born at 40 weeks, weighing approximately 3300 g

Low-Birth-Weight Infant. A general term for all infants weighing 2500 g or less, regardless of the cause (*e.g.*, impaired intrauterine growth or gestation of less than 37 wk)

Growth. An increase in physical size of the body as a whole or an increase in any of its parts, as associated with an increase in cell number or cell size

Development. The acquisition of function associated with cell differentiation and maturation of individual organ systems

Growth and Development. An individual's growth pattern as determined by genetic, hormonal, environmental, and behavioral factors that interact with one another

Maternal Factors in High-Risk Pregnancy

Age under 17 years or over 35 years

First pregnancy or high parity

Frequent pregnancies (3 pregnancies within 2 yr)

Small stature

Preconceptional weight below standard for height (85% of standard or below) or above standard for height (120% of standard or more)

Inadequate weight gain (less than 1 kg/month) or excessive weight gain (more than 3 kg/month) during pregnancy

Poor preconceptional or gestational nutritional status

Prior obstetrical complications

Presence of infection before or during pregnancy

Presence of chronic disease (*e.g.*, diabetes mellitus)

Hemoglobin below 11 g/dl; or hematocrit below 33%

Low level of education

Unfavorable social environment

Poverty

Cigarette smoking

Excessive ingestion of caffeine, nonfood substances (pica), alcohol, addictive drugs, medications that pass the placenta (Table 10–1).*

Nutritional Care Plans During Pregnancy

Goals

Provide sufficient calories, high biologic protein, vitamins, minerals, and fluids to meet the nutritional needs of the synergistic response to pregnancy of the mother, the fetus, and the placenta (Table 10–2)

Provide nutrient-dense caloric foods that will enhance lean tissue synthesis rather than adipose tissue or inappropriate fluid weight gain

Provide sufficient calories and nutrients to reach the recommended gestational weight gain (22–27 lb) in the recommended weight gain pattern (*i.e.*, increased weight gain during the last two trimesters)

Provide a nutritional care plan that will enable the mother to reach and maintain optimal nutritional status so that she may have a safe and successful pregnancy, may give birth to an infant that has reached

---

* See tables at the end of this chapter.

its maximum physical and mental potential, and may have sufficient energy to breast feed and care for an infant

Provide nutritional care plans that will alleviate or reduce adverse symptoms (*e.g.*, nausea and vomiting)

Provide nutritional care plans that will augment medical treatment of complications during pregnancy (*e.g.*, gestational diabetes)

Motivate the mother, over the long term, to develop good lifelong eating habits that can and will be passed on to her child

General Factors
Interview Chart (Components With Special Significance)

- Age. Determines calories and recommended nutrient intake needed to reach or maintain optimal nutritional status, enhance tissue synthesis, and reach recommended weight gain (see Table 10–2)

- Ethnic and Religious Background. Determines what foods are customarily most desirable and those that will not be consumed; also may uncover bizarre eating habits

- Socioeconomic Factors (*e.g.*, education, occupation, income, number of other children, marital status). Interaction of these factors determines which foods can be procured, the amount of food that can be procured, the mother's ability to prepare purchased foods (fast foods *vs.* traditional foods), and the number of calories needed to meet the mother's activity as well as pregnancy needs

- Obstetrical History. Helps determine nutrient needs, because frequent pregnancies and multiple births can deplete nutrient stores

- Medical History. Mothers with chronic diseases (*e.g.*, hypertension) will need nutritional care plans that reflect their pregnancy as well as their primary disease; additionally, mothers with a history of discomfort during pregnancy (*e.g.*, vomiting) will need special dietary suggestions to help alleviate their distress

- Mental Status. Mothers experiencing psychological stress during pregnancy will need additional calories and nutrients to meet their stress needs as well as pregnancy needs (see Tables 1–2 and 2–1).

- Medications. Dosage may have to be adjusted to increased caloric and nutrient needs (*e.g.*, insulin) during pregnancy; some medications may even have to be discontinued during pregnancy, making further dietary adaptations necessary (see Table 10–1)

- Allergies. Determine the need for dietary substitutions or dietary supplements; for example, if the pregnant woman will not or cannot consume milk, she will need to use substitutes (*e.g.*, cheese) or take supplements to meet her calcium needs

- Appetite. Although the usual advice during pregnancy is "eat to appetite," special dietary adjustments are indicated when the mother's preconceptional weight is 20% above ideal body weight (although low-calorie diets are not advocated) or when the mother has adverse symptoms such as frequent vomiting. Additionally, excessive cigarette smoking or excessive consumption of alcohol or caffeine will decrease appetite. Consequently, caloric and nutrient needs will be impaired and need adjusting.

Nutritional Assessment Data

It is important to identify caloric or nutrient deficiencies, inadequacies, or excesses at the intake, absorption, transport, or storage level in the mother that may influence the quality and quantity of nutrients transferred in the placenta. Assessment of these data plus proper nutritional treatment may prevent impaired intrauterine fetal growth or development.

- Diet History. Obtain a 24-hour recall or food frequency intake analysis (see Table 1–10 and chart of Food Preference Questionnaire in Chap. 1); compare findings with the Basic Four Food Groups or Daily Food Guide recommendations (see Tables 1–5 to 1–8 and the Daily Food Guide Recommendations for Pregnancy and Lactation [Table 10–3] plus the Recommended Dietary Allowances Before and During Pregnancy and Lactation [see Table 10–2])

  Additional factors that should be considered when obtaining a diet history for a pregnant woman are

  1. How often food is eaten
  2. Where food is eaten
  3. How much and what types of foods are procured
  4. How foods are prepared (*e.g.*, are fat and bread added in the frying process?)
  5. Type of and how often are foods and other substances that do not contain nutrient density (*e.g.*, alcohol, clay, and laundry starch) consumed
  6. What foods or smells seem to precipitate discomfort
  7. What foods are limited for various reasons (*e.g.*, meat)

- Anthropometric Measurements
  1. Weight and Height
     a. Obtain Mother's Preconceptional Weight. Determined by asking the woman about her weight before conception. Mothers whose preconceptional weight is estimated at 10% below or 20% above their ideal body weight (IBW) for height and age are considered to have poor nutritional status. Consequently, their chances of delivering a high-risk infant are elevated.
     b. Obtain Mother's Present Weight. Determined by weighing the mother on the first visit. To obtain accurate weights, use a beam scale. Mother should be dressed in light clothing with

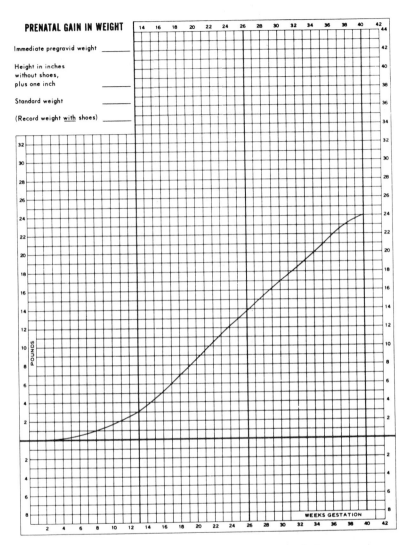

Figure 10–1 Recommended normal weight gain pattern during pregnancy. (U.S.) Department of Health, Education and Welfare, Social and Rehabilitation Service, Children's Bureau).

1-inch-heel shoes. Record weight so that follow-up weights can be compared to initial weight.

c. Estimate IBW. Determined by measuring and weighing the mother and comparing her height and weight with recommended standard height and weight charts (*e.g.,* Metropolitan Life Insurance Company Height and Weight Charts and Build and Blood Pressure Study Average Weights, see Appendix I) or by estimating a mother's IBW for height (see Chaps. 1 and 6).

d. Estimate Mother's Pattern of Weight Gain. Determined by following progression from the initial visit through subsequent visits and then comparing the weight gain to the recommended weight gains set up by the American College of Obstetricians and Gynecologists. This recommended pattern is as follows:

(1) First Trimester: 2- to 4-lb weight gain (Fig. 10–1). Desired components of weight gain during this period of gestation are listed in Table 10–4.

(2) Second and Third Trimesters: 0.8- to 0.9-lb weight gain per week until gestation period terminates (Fig. 10–1). Desired components of weight gain during this period of gestation are listed in Table 10–4. Weight gain of less than 1 kg/month or more than 3 kg/month during this period may induce early labor or the birth of a baby that is too small or too large. Rapid weight gain, especially wet (water) weight gain, after 20 weeks of gestation may indicate preeclampsia.

(3) Total Weight Gain at Termination of Pregnancy (normal gestational period, 40 wk): 22 to 27 lb (Fig. 10–1). Desired components of weight gain throughout the entire gestational period are listed in Tables 10–4 and 10–5.

2. Triceps Skinfold and Mid-arm Muscle Circumference

If height and weight measurements indicate that the client's nutritional status is poor, determine the extent of adipose tissue depletion or excess (triceps skinfold) or of lean tissue depletion (mid-arm muscle circumference). Consult Chapter 1 and Appendix III for the methodology and standards used in these ad-

Table 10–5
Components of Average Weight Gain by the Termination of Normal Pregnancy

Component	Weight (lb)
Average full-term baby	7.5
Placenta	1.0
Amniotic and body fluids	2.0
Enlarged uterus	2.0
Enlarged breasts	2.0
Blood volume	4.0 (1500 ml)
Maternal fat storage	3.5–8.0
Total pregnancy weight gain	22–27

vanced assessment procedures. To estimate treatment effectiveness (*e.g.*, caloric and nutrient increases or decreases), obtain these measurements periodically throughout pregnancy.

- Physiological and Biochemical Data
  1. Vital Signs
     a. Blood Pressure. Blood pressure readings raised above 120/80 may indicate that pregnancy-induced hypertension (PIH), with resultant adverse symptoms of preeclampsia, may be pending. Improving nutritional status by increasing caloric and protein intake early in pregnancy is thought, but not proven, to be beneficial in the prevention of this complication.
     b. Temperature. Temperatures raised above 98.6°F may indicate infection. Fever or infection in the mother increases basal metabolic rate and protein requirements. Consequently, the flow of essential nutrients through the placenta to the fetus may be reduced. Ultimately, intrauterine growth may be impaired if the mother's infection does not abate, and caloric and nutrient intake is not increased.
  2. Laboratory Data. Laboratory values during normal gestation should not be compared to standards applied to nonpregnant women. Failure to take pregnancy into account may cause over- or underestimation of deficiency disorders. For instance, blood level concentrations of a number of substances—glucose, calcium, albumin, trace minerals (*e.g.*, iron and zinc), most amino acids, and nearly all water-soluble vitamins—decline during normal gestation. However, blood concentrations of other substances—triglycerides, free fatty acids, fat-soluble vitamins (*e.g.*, vitamins A and E) and alpha and beta globulins—rise. In many instances the reasons for these alterations are not known. Adjusting these levels by dietary adaptations or supplementation may not be advisable because these physiological adaptations may be beneficial to the mother or infant. However, frank caloric or nutrient deficiencies may induce maternal or infant complications.
     a. Blood Analysis
        (1) Hemoglobin and Hematocrit. Anemia is prevalent during gestation owing to an increased maternal blood volume and fetal nutrient requirements. To determine if a mother has anemia, compare her blood levels to the guidelines for estimating deficient and acceptable hemoglobin and hematocrit levels presented in Table 10–6. The amount and type of nutrient increases and supplements prescribed depend upon the type of anemia diagnosed and the extent of the nutrient deficiency. See Anemia under High-Risk Pregnancy Complications for dietary suggestions and supplementation recommendations for the treatment of specific anemias. If advanced laboratory tests, such as of

transferrin levels, are needed to confirm the severity of the deficiency, consult Chapter 1 and Table 1–12 for the procedures, normal values, advantages, and disadvantages of these advanced tests.

(2) Leukocytes. Leukocyte counts may be an index of fetal nutritional status. Consult Chapter 1 for the nutritional implications when white blood cell levels are too high or too low.

(3) Fasting Blood Sugar. High levels may indicate gestational or overt diabetes mellitus. Consequently, the quantity, composition, and time of macronutrient ingestion may need to be altered. Additionally, medications (*e.g.*, insulin) may need to be initiated, or dosage may need to be adjusted. Failure to adjust diet and medication intake in the mother may cause excessive fetal growth or hypoglycemia in the infant at birth. Consult Gestational Diabetes in this chapter and Chapter 5 for diagnosis and dietary treatment.

(4) Albumin. Low levels may indicate poor nutritional status (see Chap. 1), but normal gestational levels should be taken into consideration before dietary adjustments are implemented. Failure to improve albumin levels may induce early delivery or the birth of a low-birth-weight infant.

b. Urinary Analysis

(1) Acetone and Glucose. High levels may indicate the mother has gestational or overt diabetes mellitus. See Fasting Blood Sugar, above, for diagnosis, treatment, and adverse fetal effects. See Gestational Diabetes in this chapter.

(2) Protein (Albumin). Increased levels of protein in the urine during midpregnancy (20 wk) may indicate preeclampsia in the mother. Caloric and protein intake may need to be increased. Failure to treat this complication may induce early delivery, the birth of a low-birth-weight infant, or fetal and maternal death.

- Clinical Evaluations. Clinical signs of excessive weight gain as a result of increased wet (water) weight (edema) may indicate mother is preeclampsic. Low weight gain may indicate maternal and fetal malnutrition. Consult Table 1–9 for the nutritional implications of other clinical signs that may appear during pregnancy.

Specific Factors

Low-Risk Pregnancies

- Nutritional Care Plan
  1. Methodology. Oral feedings

2. Nutrients Increased. Table 10–7
3. Nutrients Decreased

   At present, there are no routine caloric or nutrient restrictions during pregnancy. In the past, calories were restricted if the mother was overweight; however, this is no longer recommended because it seems more beneficial to the fetus to have the mother follow the recommended weight gain pattern. Instead of caloric restrictions, it is now recommended that the mother increase her level of moderate exercise in order to prevent excessive weight gain. In the past, sodium (Na) or salt (NaCl) was also restricted because excess sodium intake was believed to enhance fluid retention with resultant edema and preeclampsia. Recently, however, evidence has suggested that increased sodium retention during pregnancy is a normal physiological adjustment, and severe restrictions are hazardous. Consequently, sodium is not restricted unless severe edema develops, in which case reduced sodium intake may be recommended; however, the total intake should never be lower than 2 g daily. See Table 3–8 for dietary adaptations required to reduce sodium intake to this level.

   The increased need for sodium during pregnancy is related to the increased (50%) glomerular filtration rate (GFR) during early pregnancy, which ultimately promotes sodium loss, and the increased production of progesterone, which retards the absorption of filtered sodium through the renal tubules. Consequently, the only physiological mechanism that conserves sodium and counterbalances the sodium-depleting tendency of progesterone and the increased GFR is the renin–angiotension–aldosterone–antidiuretic system. Clinicians claim, therefore, that sodium restriction during pregnancy may intensify the action of this system, to ensure positive sodium balance. Such intensification may cause this system to be excessively stressed, which could induce hyponatremia. The clinical signs of maternal hyponatremia are essentially those of a combination of water intoxication and peripheral vascular collapse (*e.g.*, thirst, low blood pressure, weakness, cool clammy skin, and possible convulsions). The adverse effects of this low blood volume on the infant involve poor nutrient flow through the placenta, which impairs fetal growth and development. The most recent recommendation for the treatment of mild edema during pregnancy is to rest with the feet elevated rather than to take diuretics or restrict sodium below the recommended intake.

4. Dietary Adaptations Consult Tables 10–3 and 10–7 for detailed changes in the quantity and quality of foods required during pregnancy. Additional dietary adaptation recommendations are
   a. "Eat to appetite." This is not a license to overeat or to indulge in excessive intake of "empty calorie" food, only a recommendation to enhance adequate weight gain and nutrient intake.

b. Add dried skim milk powder to mixed dishes (*e.g.*, meat loaves or desserts) if whole plain milk is not desired or tolerated. Additionally, if lactose cannot be tolerated, add cheeses (they contain a very low lactose content) to casseroles and sauces or eat as snacks in order to obtain calcium and protein requirements.

c. Limit caffeine intake to less than 444 mg/day (the amount recommended by the March of Dimes Birth Defects Foundation). See Table 10–8 for the caffeine content of common beverages. The rationale for limiting caffeine during pregnancy is that it curtails the appetite; increases GI motility, which subsequently decreases the maternal absorption of essential nutrients; increases nervous tension; and increases hydrochloric acid production, which may induce vomiting and nausea.

d. Abstain from or restrict alcohol intake to no more than 1 oz of absolute alcohol daily. The rationale for limiting alcohol during pregnancy is that alcohol can pass through the placenta and induce fetal alcohol syndrome (FAS). This syndrome may be related to impaired cell differentiation during blastogenesis; maternal malnutrition (including zinc, folic acid, and magnesium deficiency); or dehydration of some of the developing fetal brain cells, since alcohol may be a dehydrating agent. Additionally, the fetus lacks the enzyme alcohol dehydrogenase, which metabolizes alcohol. Consequently, the toxic effects of alcohol are intensified. Signs of FAS observed in the infant are intrauterine growth retardation with poor catch-up weight gain, small head circumference, prominent ears, abnormalities of the face such as ptosis (drooping of the eyelids), strabismus (cross-eyedness), and a wide mouth. Other

Table 10–8
Caffeine Content of Common Beverages

Beverage	Caffeine Content
Brewed coffee	85 mg/150 ml*
Instant coffee	60 mg/150 ml
Brewed black tea	50 mg/150 ml
Brewed green tea	30 mg/150 ml
Instant tea	30 mg/150 ml
Decaffeinated coffee	3 mg/150 ml
Cola drinks, including some diet colas	32–65 mg/12 oz
Cocoa	6–142 mg/150 ml

* Based on 150-ml average beverage cup size (Reprinted with permission. Stephenson PE: Physiologic and psychotropic effects of caffeine on man. J Am Diet Assoc 71: 241, 1977)

manifestations are mental retardation, irritability, hyperactivity (a withdrawal symptom), and a high mortality rate.

5. Meal Plan Modifications

   a. Eat 6 small, rather than 3 large, meals per day. This modification may alleviate or prevent common adverse symptoms such as nausea or vomiting.

   b. Drink lots of fluids daily with or between meals.

- Behavioral Modifications

   1. Exercise moderately each day to enhance excretion.

   2. Abstain from or limit cigarette smoking, because it curtails appetite; it may narrow blood vessels in the heart, which would reduce oxygen delivery to the fetus; it narrows blood vessels in the maternal GI tract, which subsequently decreases absorption of essential nutrients; it may reduce the utilization of calories in the fetus, which impairs weight gain; and cigarette smoke contains toxic substances (*e.g.*, carbon monoxide), which may directly affect the fetus. The overall consequence of excessive smoking during pregnancy is the delivery of a low-birth-weight infant.

   3. Consult the physician before taking any medications during pregnancy (see Table 10–1). Caffeine and alcohol are also considered drugs.

Dietary Adaptations for Common Discomforts of Pregnancy

See Table 10–9.

High-Risk Pregnancies

Adolescents

- Description. Clients under 14 to 18 years of age or those who conceive shortly (less than 3–4 yr) after menarche

- Characteristics. Usually under or over IBW for age and height, in poor nutritional status, and not yet at full stature; may consume large quantities of non-nutritive foods (*e.g.*, alcohol) or may be addicted to drugs; may have social and emotional problems that impair procurement, preparation, and consumption of nutrient-dense food

- Nutritional Care Plan

   1. Nutrients Increased. All those increased in nonrisk pregnancies (see Tables 10–2 and 10–7); additionally, all nutrient increases necessary to promote proper growth and development of adolescent mother (see Table 10–2); in order to estimate individual total caloric and nutrient requirements, add the recommended

increments for pregnancy in the older woman to the RDAs appropriate for the adolescent's age

2. Nutrients Decreased. Refined carbohydrates; substitute complex carbohydrates in order to meet caloric needs and spare protein

3. Dietary Adaptations
   a. All those advised during nonrisk pregnancies (see Tables 10–3 and 10–7)
   b. Limit intake of foods that are highly processed, refined, or fried but do not restrict completely (to accommodate peer pressure)
   c. Introduce foods into the diet that are nutrient-dense and help the client procure and prepare these foods

4. Meal Plan Modifications
   a. Encourage client not to skip meals
   b. Encourage client to limit snacking if it interferes with meals but do not insist on avoiding all snacking (encourage the use of nutrient-dense snacks, [*e.g.*, peanuts *vs.* candy bars])

- Behavioral Modifications. Same as those recommended for nonrisk pregnancies

Vegetarians

- Description. Individuals who limit intake of all or certain animal foods
- Characteristics. Usually at or below IBW for age and height; anemia, especially pernicious anemia (B_{12} deficiency); osteoporosis (protein, calcium, and vitamin D deficiency); ocular symptoms (*e.g.*, eyestrain and eye fatigue or itching from a riboflavin deficiency); psychological or philosophical commitments to oneself (*e.g.*, improved physiological or emotional well-being) or to others (*e.g.*, religious organizations)
- Classifications
  1. Lacto-ovo-vegetarians. Exclude meat, poultry, and fish from their diet but include eggs and dairy products
  2. Lacto-vegetarians. Exclude meat, poultry, fish, and eggs from their diets but include dairy products
  3. Vegans. Exclude all foods of animal origin from their diet including meat, poultry, fish, eggs, and dairy products, such as milk, ice cream, and cheese
- Nutritional Care Plan
  1. Nutrients Increased. Depends upon what foods of animal origin are excluded and the individual's ability to procure and prepare foods that complement one another (*e.g.*, grains should be eaten with soybeans in order to obtain all eight essential amino acids). If properly prepared meals are eaten, a vegan may need only a

vitamin B$_{12}$ supplement. However, if she does not prepare meals with caution, she may lack many essential nutrients such as calcium, zinc, iron, protein, and riboflavin.

2. Nutrients Decreased. None, unless intake of complex carbohydrates (fiber) is so excessive that they decrease caloric intake or impair other nutrient absorption (*e.g.,* iron and calcium)

3. Dietary Adaptations for Lacto-ovo-vegetarians*

   a. Consume at least 4 glasses of milk

   b. Consume 4 servings of eggs, dried beans, peas, or soybean curd (Tofu), or nuts

   c. Consume 5 servings of fruits and vegetables, including those rich in vitamin C (citrus fruits) and vitamin A (yellow vegetables)

   d. Consume 6 servings of whole-grain or enriched cereal products

   e. Consume 3 servings of fats or oils (serving, 1 teaspoon)

4. Dietary Adaptations for Vegans*

   a. Consume 4 glasses of fortified soy milk

   b. If eggs are avoided, consume 3 servings of dried beans and peas

5. Meal Plan Modifications. Eat small meals frequently in order to obtain the caloric requirements necessary for proper weight gain and protein conservation.

- Behavioral Modifications. Excessive exercise such as jogging may have to be limited if weight gain is impaired.

Hyperemesis Gravidarum (Pernicious Vomiting)

- Description. The uncontrollable vomiting of pregnancy
- Characteristics. Dehydration; electrolyte imbalances (*e.g.,* hypochloremia and hypokalemia); abnormal metabolism, including ketonemia; excessive weight reduction (a loss of more than 5% of total weight); and laboratory or clinical signs of vitamin and mineral deficiencies
- Nutritional Care Plan
  1. Methodology

     a. Phase I. If vomiting is severe enough to require hospitalization, parenteral solutions containing glucose, fluids, and electrolytes are usually infused. Vitamins and minerals may also be added to the solutions to replace stores.

---

* Counselors are advised to make dietary suggestions within a client's dietary pattern, in order to ensure acceptance. Do not try to force the client to eat meat and meat products, even though they are high in essential nutrients. Additionally, if nutrient intake appears to be low, supplements should be recommended.

   b. Phase II. If vomiting subsides, parenteral feedings may be augmented with oral liquid feedings (*e.g.,* ginger ale, broth, and gelatin) as long as the liquids are tolerated by the client.

   c. Phase III. If vomiting begins to subside and client begins to gain weight (usually around the third month, if not before), client is introduced to semisolid or solid foods that are palatable and usually tolerated by clients with mild nausea (see Table 10–9).

2. Nutrients Increased. Complex carbohydrates and fats to supply calories needed to reach proper weight gain and conserve protein, protein to replace and synthesize new lean tissue, all vitamins and minerals necessary for proper growth and metabolism, and water to replace losses

3. Nutrients Decreased. None

4. Dietary Adaptations

   a. See vomiting and nausea, Table 10–9

   b. Include foods that have concentrated caloric and nutrient density (*e.g.,* casseroles with added cheese and dried milk powder)

   c. Limit intake of sweet foods, which may enhance nausea

   d. Include enteral supplements such as Sustacal pudding if traditional foods are not supplying enough calories and nutrients for a proper pattern of weight gain (see Fig. 10-1)

5. Meal Plan Modifications

   a. Eat 6 small, rather than 3 large, meals a day

   b. Consume foods when nausea is least severe

- Behavioral Modifications

   1. Decrease exercise if proper weight gain is not being reached

   2. Seek psychological consultation

Obesity

- Description. Preconceptional weight of 20% above IBW for age and height or pregnancy weight gain of more than 3 kg (6–7 lb) per month. Weight loss during pregnancy is not recommended because it may precipitate dehydration or ketosis, which may lead to neuropsychological damage to the fetus. Client is advised to achieve the customary weight gain but not to exceed the upper limits (27 lb) (see Figure 10–1, Tables 10–4 and 10–5). Weight loss after pregnancy is recommended (see Chap. 6).

- Nutritional Care Plan

   1. Nutrients Increased. Complex carbohydrates (fiber) if they increase satiety

   2. Nutrients Decreased. Macronutrients that provide empty calories

3. Dietary Adaptations. See Chapter 6 for dietary suggestions that enhance weight reduction—use discretion (see p. 402)
4. Meal Plan Modifications. Limit snacking if it enhances caloric intake
- Behavioral Modifications. Increase moderate exercise

Gestational Diabetes

- Description. Glucose intolerance occurring during pregnancy and reverting to normal following delivery; however, 20% to 30% of these women develop traditional diabetes within 5 years.
- Characteristics. Carbohydrate intolerance, manifested as higher plasma glucose values, an enhanced insulin response, and a decreased tissue sensitivity to insulin, especially after 15 weeks' gestation, is a feature of normal pregnancy. Clients who have an increased response to this normal stress of pregnancy, such as fasting venous blood sugar levels of 105 mg/dl or 3-hour postprandial venous blood sugar levels of 145 mg/dl after a 100-g oral glucose challenge, are diagnosed as having gestational diabetes. At present, gestational diabetes is believed to be caused by the following sequence of events during pregnancy: Maternal glucose (the preferential source of energy for the fetus) passes through the placenta along with amino acids, but free fatty acids and insulin do not. This increased demand for glucose by the fetus causes many swings in maternal glucose levels, ranging from hypoglycemia during the first trimester or during the night to hyperglycemia and ketonemia, especially when maternal insulin sensitivity increases. This sensitivity is related to the increased production of other hormones such as human placental lactogen during pregnancy that antagonize insulin action. If left untreated, the infant produces more insulin to compensate for the levels of glucose passing through the placenta. Subsequently, this leads to an increased production of triglycerides and glycogen in the fetus. Glycogen increases the infant's size, which makes delivery more difficult. At birth the infant's glycogen supply diminishes, but his insulin levels remain high; consequently, he becomes hypoglycemic. In addition, the metabolic imbalance of hypoglycemia and hyperinsulinemia increases the infant's oxygen needs, often inducing the respiratory system syndrome.
- Signs and Symptoms. Hyperglycemia, ketonemia, ketonuria, and glycosuria (glycosuria is not a good criterion for the diagnosis of gestational diabetes because the GFR is increased by 50% during pregnancy); clinical signs include overweight (see Chap. 5 for other signs and symptoms)
- Drug Therapy. Oral hypoglycemic agents or insulin may or may not be prescribed, depending upon the severity of the condition. If insulin is prescribed, it is usually a mixture of regular and long-acting insulin, given before breakfast and dinner.

- Nutritional Care Plan
  1. Goals. Maintain fasting blood glucose levels below 100 mg/dl and postprandial glucose levels below 120 mg/dl (see Chap. 5 for additional goals)
  2. Nutrients Increased. Caloric intake is adjusted according to individual's age, preconceptional weight, height, activity, and stage of gestation. Caloric levels must never be less than 35 kcal/kg, however, or fetal growth and maternal metabolic needs will be impaired. Complex carbohydrates, especially as soluble fibers (*e.g.*, guar), are increased because they are believed to prevent ketosis. Some clinicians also increase intake of vitamin B_6 (both of these dietary suggestions are experimental).
  3. Nutrients Decreased. See Chapter 5
  4. Dietary Adaptations
     a. Macronutrient intake is adjusted according to laboratory analysis and drug therapy, if applicable; usual division is protein 12% to 24%, carbohydrate 45% to 55%, and fat 25% to 35%, with saturated fat limited to 12% to 18% of total intake (see Chap. 5 for the variety of foods that can be used)
     b. Limit all foods that induce nausea or ketosis will be enhanced
     c. Limit all foods and nonfoodstuffs that should be avoided during nonrisk pregnancies
     d. Follow dietary adaptations advised for insulin-dependent or noninsulin-dependent diabetics, depending upon the treatment needed to obtain optimal blood glucose levels (see Chap. 5)
  5. Meal Plan Modifications. Meals are usually divided into 3 meals plus 3 snacks. The carbohydrate division is as follows: 25% at breakfast (save some for midmorning snack); 30% at lunch (save some for midafternoon snack); 30% at dinner; 15% at bedtime in order to prevent hypoglycemia during the evening. Strict adherence is necessary if insulin is required. If insulin dose is mixed and split, carbohydrate division may be adjusted (see Chap. 5).
- Behavioral Modifications
  1. See Modifications for nonrisk pregnancies
  2. See Modifications for diabetes mellitus (Chap. 5)

Pregnancy-Induced Hypertension (PIH) (Hypertension Gestosis)

- Description. A syndrome characterized by hypertension, proteinuria, and edema
- Characteristics. A systolic blood pressure of 140 mm Hg or a dia-

stolic blood pressure of 90 mm Hg, or both, obtained on two separate occasions, 6 hours apart. It should be noted however, that blood pressure usually goes down during the second trimester of pregnancy; thus even a normal blood pressure (120/80) may indicate hypertension. Additional characteristics are edema and abnormal excretion of protein (500 mg–5 g) in a 24-hour urine sample. These signs occur because there is a decrease in the intravascular volume (hypovolemia), due to peripheral vasoconstriction, which leads to a decreased flow of nutrients through the placental circulation to the fetal circulation. The latter impairs fetal intrauterine growth and development, which can precipitate an early delivery or fetal mortality.

- Classifications
    1. Preeclampsia. Hypertension with proteinuria or edema (wet weight gain), appearing after the 20th week of pregnancy
    2. Eclampsia. The occurrence of one or more convulsions in a client with the criteria for the diagnosis of preeclampsia. (In the past, *toxemia* was the term used to denote hypertension in pregnancy. This term, which literally means "poison in the blood," is becoming obsolete)
- Symptoms. Rapid wet weight gain (greater than 2 lb/wk in the 20th wk), dizziness, headache, visual disturbances, upper abdominal pain, anorexia, nausea, vomiting, and eventually convulsions if the condition is not treated (edema related to hypertension should not be confused with uncomplicated edema of the lower extremities, which is a fairly common occurrence during pregnancy and is not indicative of preeclampsia).
- Drug Therapy. Drugs administered, if any, depend upon the total clinical picture. They are usually given only to clients with chronic hypertension (see Chap. 3). In this condition, the drug of choice is usually methyldopa (Aldomet). Diuretics are advised only when there is pulmonary edema or coronary heart failure; they are not recommended as routine treatment.
- Nutritional Care Plan
    1. Methodology. Acute phase, parenteral solutions; chronic phase, oral feedings
    2. Nutrients Increased. At present, what nutrient increases affect the progression of pregnancy-induced hypertension are not known; however, some clinicians believe that a well-balanced diet somewhat high in protein (75–80 g) plus a high intake of calcium may alleviate the condition. Caloric intake should also be increased to spare protein, especially when dry weight gain is low.
    3. Nutrients Decreased. Sodium and water when pulmonary edema is a complication; otherwise, sodium intake remains above 2 g/day (see sodium intake in nonrisk pregnancies)

4. Dietary Adaptations
   a. Increase intake of a variety of nutrient-dense foods (see nonrisk dietary adaptations and Tables 10-3 and 10-7)
   b. Increase intake of high biologic protein foods (*e.g.*, meat, eggs, fish, poultry, and dairy products; note that the last is also high in calcium)
   c. Restrict intake of non-nutritive foods not recommended in nonrisk pregnancies
5. Meal Plan Modifications. See vegetarian modifications
- Behavioral Modifications
  1. Seek prenatal medical care during the first trimester
  2. Rest in the left lateral position, which prevents compression of the vena cava, resulting in increased cardiac output, and prevents compression of uterine blood flow

Cardiac Disease

Nutritional care plans should be adjusted to meet the nutritional requirements of the mother and fetus without aggravating the cardiac condition. See nutritional care plan recommendations for nonrisk pregnancy and those recommended for cardiovascular diseases (Chap. 3).

Anemia

- Description. A blood disorder in which there is a deficiency of red blood cells or of hemoglobin (see Table 10-6 for evaluation of anemia in pregnancy)
- Classifications and Characteristics
  1. Nutritional Anemia. Small (microcytic) and pale (hypochromic) red blood cells, low hemoglobin levels; induced in pregnancy by increased maternal blood levels; for example, iron-deficiency anemia (anemia due to a lack of iron stores in the body)
  2. Megaloblastic Anemia. An increased number of megaloblasts (large [macrocytic], oval, immature nucleated red blood cells) and very low serum folacin levels; induced in pregnancy by inadequate folacin intake, vomiting, and increased maternal and fetal tissue synthesis
  3. Pernicious Anemia. A form of megaloblastic anemia caused by malabsorption of vitamin B_{12} due to a lack of intrinsic factor, or poor intake of vitamin B_{12} induced in pregnant women who practice vegan dietary regimens.
- Symptoms
  1. Nutritional Anemia. Fatigue, weakness, anorexia, pallor, gaseous indigestion, diarrhea, brittle spoon-shaped nails, and bizarre appetite (pica) in pregnancy

2. Megaloblastic Anemia. Diarrhea, sore tongue, irritability, forgetfulness, anorexia, headache, weakness, tiredness, and dyspnea.

3. Pernicious Anemia. Anorexia, weight loss, weakness, constipation, numbness or tingling of the extremities, poor muscular coordination and memory, hallucinations, and evidence of peripheral nerve degeneration

- Nutritional Care Plan

   1. Nutritional Anemia. A well-balanced diet containing foods that are good sources of heme iron, protein, copper, vitamin B_6, vitamin B_2, and vitamin C (see Tables 10–3 and 10–7 for foods that are good sources of these nutrients). Reduce intake of fiber, tea, and coffee, which may decrease iron absorption. If foods cannot supply the necessary iron required during pregnancy, it is recommended that the diet be supplemented with 30 mg to 60 mg of elemental iron, daily, in the form of ferrous salts (*e.g.,* ferrous sulfate and ferrous fumarate). Supplements should be given only on the advice of the physician, however, because iron supplementation may augment nausea, constipation, and vomiting, and it may impair zinc absorption.

   2. Folic Acid Deficiency Megaloblastic Anemia. A well-balanced diet that contains foods that are good sources of folic acid and vitamin C (see Tables 10–3 and 10–7). If foods cannot supply the necessary folic acid required during pregnancy, it is recommended that the diet be supplemented with 400 μg to 800 μg of folacin daily.

   3. Pernicious Anemia. Supplementation of vitamin B_{12}, given intramuscularly. Additional dietary alterations may be necessary to relieve adverse symptoms (*e.g.,* weight loss).

Nutritional Care Plan During Labor

Initial Stages

In the initial stages of labor, some clinicians allow clear liquids that contain carbohydrates such as ginger ale, Jell-O, or tea with sugar. Others recommend that all foods be withheld after labor begins.

Advanced Stages

All foods are avoided in order to reduce vomiting and prevent aspiration. If extreme thirst develops, however, the mother may be allowed to suck ice cubes. In the event of a complicated, prolonged labor, parenteral solutions of glucose, electrolytes, and fluids may be infused in order to prevent dehydration or electrolyte imbalance.

Nutritional Care Plan for Lactation

Nutrients Increased

Calories

The recommended caloric increase for the nursing mother, during the first 3 months of lactation, is 500 exogenous calories (from foods) and 200 to 300 endogenous calories (from maternal fat stores) daily (see Table 10–2). This recommendation is based on the premise that each 100 ml of breast milk supplies 67 to 77 calories. The conversion of food energy to milk energy is 80% to 90% efficient; 80 to 95 calories are necessary to produce 100 ml of milk. The average daily production of milk, 850 ml, represents 600 infant calories, which requires an expenditure of 750 maternal calories. If lactation continues beyond 3 months or if the mother's weight falls below IBW for height and age, the mother's exogenous energy allowance should be increased.

Carbohydrates

Carbohydrates are increased to supply caloric requirements and to spare protein. Foods that supply complex carbohydrates (*e.g.*, whole-grain products) should be the predominant source of the additional carbohydrate intake.

Fats

Fats are increased to supply caloric requirements and to spare protein. Polyunsaturated fats contain linoleic acid, an essential fatty acid, and should be the predominant source of the additional fat intake. Vegetable oils supply polyunsaturated fats.

Protein

The recommended protein increase for the nursing mother is 20 g/day. This recommendation is based on the premise that each 100 ml of human milk contains 1.2 g of protein. Thus, 850 ml of milk, daily, would yield 10 g protein. The conversion of dietary protein to milk protein is 70% efficient, with individual variations; the recommended allowance for lactation is an additional 20 g protein, daily. This increase is required not only for transformation into human milk but also to synthesize the hormones needed for milk production (prolactin) and milk release (oxytocin). Foods that supply high biologic value protein (*e.g.*, milk and meat) should be the predominant source of the additional protein intake.

Calcium

The recommended calcium increase for the nursing mother is 400 mg/day. This recommendation is based on the premise that human milk contains 25 to 30 mg/dl of calcium or approximately 250 mg in an average daily production of 850 ml. This increase is required not only for transmission into human milk but also to maintain maternal stores.

Iron

The recommended iron intake of 18 mg/day is the same for nursing mothers as for nonpregnant females. The reason is the absence of menstruation during the first months of lactation. If lactation continues over a long period of time, however, or if the maternal stores are low, a supplement of 30 mg to 60 mg of elemental iron is recommended. This recommended intake of iron is essential to replace maternal and infant stores (see Tables 10–3 and 10–7 for dietary adaptations that increase iron intake).

Vitamins and Minerals

Additional vitamin and mineral increases recommended for the nursing mother are listed in Table 10–2. It should be noted, however, that concentrations of water-soluble vitamins and sodium in milk generally correlate with maternal levels in plasma and with maternal dietary intake. Thus, these nutrients can be raised in milk by increasing maternal intake. However, the levels of fat-soluble vitamins, fluoride, and zinc transmitted in human milk are relatively unaffected by maternal intake. An exception may be vitamin D, which has reportedly been found in a water-soluble form in human milk. Increased intake of vitamins and minerals is essential not only for transmission into milk but also to help metabolize the increased intake of carbohydrates, fats, and protein.

Fluids

The recommended fluid intake for the nursing mother is 2 to 3 quarts/day (2000–3000 ml). This increase is essential to provide adequate milk volume and prevent maternal dehydration.

Nutrients Decreased

No nutrients should be decreased.

Dietary Adaptations

- Eat a well-balanced diet that has a variety of foods daily. This practice will enhance the adequacy of essential nutrients (see Tables 10–2 and 10–3).

- Consume at least 2 to 3 quarts of milk daily, including 1 quart of milk in liquid form or mixed with foods (see Tables 10–3 and 10–7 and Sample One-Day Menu for a Lactating Mother).

Sample One-Day Menu for a Lactating Mother

Breakfast

Orange juice
Shredded wheat cereal with milk
Poached egg on whole-wheat toast
Light coffee (½ milk, ½ coffee) if desired

Midmorning

Milk

Lunch

Cream of tomato soup (made with milk)
Tunafish salad sandwich on whole-wheat toast
Vanilla ice cream with peaches (½ cup)
Fruit juice

Midafternoon

Milk or fruit juice

Dinner

Creamed chicken on a bed of rice
Sweet peas with margarine
Cranberry fruit salad
Small roll with margarine
Lemon snow pudding
Light tea (½ milk, ½ tea) if desired

Bedtime

Milk

- Restrict intake of caffeine and alcohol; they are transmitted in breast milk and may cause adverse effects in the infant (see Tables 10–8 and 10–10, and List of Drugs Excreted in Human Milk). Limit intake of any foods that cause maternal or infant GI distress, such as strongly flavored vegetables (*e.g.,* cabbage) or spicy food (*e.g.,* chili).

Drugs Excreted in Human Milk*

Alcohol
Allergens
Ambenonium chloride (Mytelase)
Aminophylline (theophylline with ethylenediamine)

Drugs Excreted in Human Milk* (continued)

Amphetamines

Amphetamine salts (Benzedrine and numerous other trade names)

Dextroamphetamine salts (Dexedrine and numerous other trade names)

Analgesics (nonnarcotic)

Acetaminophen (numerous trade names, including Amdil, Anelix, Apamide, Elixodyne, Febrolin, Fendon, Lestemp, Lyteca Syrup, Metalid, Nacetyl, Nebs, Tempra, Tylenol)

Aspirin

Dextropropoxyphene (Darvon)
Pehnacetin
Sodium salicylate

Analgesics (narcotic)

Mefenamic acid (Ponstel)
Methadone (Adanon, Althose syrup, Dolophine)
Morphine (trace)
Heroin

Anesthetics

Chloroform
Cyclopropane
Ether

Antibiotics and chemotherapeutics

Chloramphenicol (Chloromycetin)
Cycloserine (Seromycin)
Erythromycin
Flabayl
Furadantin
Isoniazid (more than twenty trade names)
Mandelic acid
Neomycin (Mycifradin, Neobiotic)
Nitrofurantoins
Novobiocin (Albamycin, Cathomycin)
Para-aminosalicylic acid and salts (numerous trade names)
Penicillin G
Streptomycin
Sulfonamides (breast concentration may exceed maternal plasma level; this represents a small oral dose for infant)
Sulfamethoxazole (Ganthanol)
Sulfadimethoxine (Madribon)
Tetracycline

Antihistamines (most pass into milk)

Brompheniramine (Dimetane)
Diphenhydramine (Benadryl)
Methdilazine (Tacaryl)

Drugs Excreted in Human Milk* (continued)

Atropine

Barbiturates

    Amobarbital (Amytal)
    Methohexital (Brevital)
    Phenobarbital (Luminal)
    Secobarbital (Seconal)
    Thiopental (Pentohal)

Bromides

Caffeine

Chloral hydrate

Cortisone

Ergot

Estrogens

Ethinamate (Valmid)

Ethyl biscoumacetate (Tromexan)

Cyclophosphamide (Cytoxan)

DDT (chlorophenothane)

Dicumarol (bishydroxycoumarin, Melitoxin)

Ephedrine

Hexachlorobenzene

Imipramine hydrochloride (Tofranil)

Iodides including ^{131}I

Iopanoic acid (Telepaque)

Laxatives and cathartics

    Aloin
    Calomel (mild mercurous chloride)
    Cascara
    Danthron (Dionone, Dorbane, Istizin)
    Rhubarb (said either not to pass or, conversely, to purge infant)

Levopropoxyphene (Novrad)

Mephenoxalone (Trepidone)

Methimazole (Tapazole)

Methocarbamol (Robaxin)

Metals, salts, minerals

    Arsenic
    Calcium
    Chloride
    Copper
    Iodides
    Lead
    Magnesium

Drugs Excreted in Human Milk* (continued)

Mercurous chloride (see Calomel)
Mercury
Phosphate
Potassium
Sodium
Sulfur
Nicotine
Papaverine
Phenylbutazone (Butazolidin)
Phenytoin (diphenylhydantoin, Dilantin)
Propylthiouracil
Pseudoephedrine (Sudafed)
Pyrimethamine (Daraprim)
Quinidine
Quinine
Reserpine (many trade names)
Salicylates
Scopolamine (hyoscine)
Sodium chloride
Thiazides
Thiouracil
Thyroid
Tolbutamide
Tranquilizers
 Chlorpromazine (Thorazine)
 Hydroxyzine (Atarax, Vistaril)
 Phenaglycodol (Ultran)
 Trifluoperazine (Stelazine)
Vitamins
 A, B_1, B_{12}, D, C, E, K
 Folic acid
 Niacin
 Pantothenic acid
 Riboflavin
 Thiamine

* Synonyms and combinations may be found in Billups NF (ed): American Drug Index. Philadelphia, JB Lippincott Company, 1983. Concentrations may be found in Knowles JA: Excretion of drugs in milk—A review. J Pediatr 66:1068, 1965 and Arena JM: Contamination of the ideal food. Nutrition Today 5:8, 1970

Meal Plan Modifications

- Eat 6 meals per day in order to ensure an adequate supply of calories.
- Drink fluids often in order to enhance milk volume.

Behavioral Modifications

See Table 10–11 for behavioral and environmental factors that enhance or inhibit lactation.

Nurses' Responsibilities in the Nutritional Care of Pregnant and Lactating Mothers

Initiate Good Care

Motivation to improve undesirable eating and behavioral patterns is higher during pregnancy and lactation than at any other time during the life cycle. Consequently, it is the responsibility of the health team to initiate good eating patterns throughout the prenatal and perinatal periods. The nurse has a special responsibility here for she may be the first health-team member the mother contacts, reports information to, and discusses lifestyle with, including eating patterns. Therefore, the nurse should listen well and direct the client toward proper medical and nutritional assistance, which includes visiting a physician and dietitian, if available. If a dietitian is not available, however, it becomes the nurse's responsibility to institute good nutritional care. This does not mean handing out sheets of paper that explain the Basic Four Food Groups, for example, and telling the client to follow the information at home. Instead, it means that the nurse in this position (*e.g.,* obstetrician's office or outclient clinic), must acquire a good working knowledge of nutrition so that she can explain not only what foods and how much food is recommended during pregnancy and lactation but also how the client can apply this information to daily menus within her individual lifestyle. Teaching a client proper eating habits, however, has no value if the individual financially or educationally is unable to procure or prepare the recommended foods. The nurse can close this gap in the following manner: introduce the mother to community programs that will offer her assistance. Explain the requirements and help her fill out the application if she qualifies. Local and federal programs that offer this assistance are federal welfare programs; federal food stamp programs; federally funded women, infant, and children programs; and education programs in home management sponsored by federal- and state-funded cooperative extension programs.

Participate in Care

- Weigh client on the first visit. Additionally, obtain preconceptional weight and compare that to standard IBW for height and age. Weigh at each follow-up visit. Record findings and report any excessive deviations in weight to the physician.
- Motivate and encourage the mother to practice dietary habits that will enable her to gain weight in the recommended pattern (See Fig. 10–1 and Tables 10–4, and 10–5). Still any fears that the recommended weight gain (22–27 lb) will create life-long obesity.
- Monitor and assess the effectiveness of nutritional interventions in nonrisk and high-risk pregnancies.
- Provide information early in prenatal care about the nutritional components contained in breast milk and prepared formulas (see Chap. 11). Allow the mother to assess this information gradually so that she will be fully prepared to practice the method of feeding she desires to institute at birth. In order to provide this information, the nurse must continuously remain up to date on rapidly developing scientific advances in various infant feeding methods.
- Be available to help the mother when she feeds the infant for the first time. This is especially important when the mother is breast feeding because if she becomes anxious or upset, the milk may not be released, and she will become very apprehensive. However, if she is comfortable and relaxed, she will look forward to the next feeding.
- Collect urine and blood specimens when indicated.

Coordinate Care

Obtain, observe, and report subjective as well as objective information to other members of the health team, in organized meetings when possible.

- Subjective information to be reported includes any information the client reveals about appetite, usual eating and drinking habits, and any foods or smells that cause discomfort, such as vomiting. If possible, any information the client reveals about consumption of alcohol or number of cigarettes smoked should also be reported because these two habits are believed not only to decrease appetite but also to induce other adverse effects that impair intrauterine growth.
- Objective information to be monitored and reported includes structural data; present weight and any excessive deviation in weight; laboratory data (hemoglobin and hematocrit, blood sugar, albumin, and protein levels in the urine); and clinical signs (*e.g.*, fever, pallor, fatigue, or overall edema). If any of these findings, such as raised blood sugar levels, indicate that the mother may be developing

complications that would put her in the high-risk pregnancy category, she should be provided with advanced medical and nutritional care so that medical and nutritional care plans can be adjusted according to her needs.

Reinforce and Follow Up Care

- Empathize with the client. Assure clients who have mild or advanced complications that they are not alone. Relate information that will assure them they can have a normal pregnancy if they follow medical and nutritional advice. Explain why some of the complications have developed, when applicable, because explanations often still fears and enhance compliance.

- Encourage client discussions about nutritional care plans during monthly visits. Compliment good nutritional habits such as the limitation of refined carbohydrates, and tactfully suggest improved food habits when indicated.

- Obtain a working knowledge on the rationales for increased caloric and nutrient needs during pregnancy and lactation and dietary practices that provide these requirements. Rationales can be obtained from information in this book, in advanced nutritional care books, government publications, and most hospital diet manuals. Relate information on nutrient needs during lactation to the client, slowly, throughout the prenatal period so that she will be familiar with eating patterns and foods that will supply her needs. This knowledge will give her the confidence that she is providing her baby with all the nutrients he needs for proper growth and development. Additionally, be familiar with the work special organizations are doing (*e.g.,* La Leche League—see Bibliography) and where they are located so that you can direct the mother to them for additional help and advice.

Table 10–1 417

Table 10–1
Drugs Reported to Affect the Fetus

Drug	Effect		
	Morphologic	Functional	Delayed
Analgesics			
Narcotics		Withdrawal syndrome	?
Salicylates	↑ Minor anomalies	↓ Hyperbilirubinemia	
		Platelet dysfunction	
		↓ Factor XII	
Anesthetics			
General		Depression	
Local		Depression	
		Bradycardia	
		Acidosis	
		Methemoglobinemia	
Antimicrobials			
Sulfonamides		Kernicterus	
Nitrofurantoin		Hemolysis	
Tetracyclines	Teeth staining		
	Enamel hypoplasia		
Streptomycin		8th nerve damage	Deafness
Isoniazide		Encephalopathy	
Anticonvulsants			
Phenytoin	Cleft lip and palate	Coagulation defects	?
			(continued)

Table 10–1
Drugs Reported to Affect the Fetus (continued)

Drug	Morphologic	Functional	Delayed
		Effect	
Anticonvulsants *(continued)*			
Phenobarbital		Coagulation defects Enzymes induction	?
Barbiturates		Addiction Enzymes induction ↓ Sucking	
Anticoagulants			
Coumarin		↓ Prothrombin time Hemorrhages	
Diuretics			
Thiazides		Thrombocytopenia Hyponatremia ? Electrolyte imbalance	? ?
Antihypertensives			
Reserpine		Nasal stuffiness	
Cancer Chemotherapeutic Drugs			
Methotrexate Chlorambucil	Malformation of head Unilateral absence of kidney and ureter		

(continued)

Table 10–1 419

Table 10–1
Drugs Reported to Affect the Fetus (continued)

Drug	Effect		
	Morphologic	Functional	Delayed
Immunosuppressants			
Azathioprine	?	?	?
Psychopharmacologic Drugs			
Phenothiazine		?	Behavioral changes
Chlorpromazine	? (Eyes)	Extrapyramidal dysfunction	
Imipramine	? Limb defects		
Lithium	?	Toxicity	
Diazepam	?	? Temperature	
Antithyroids			
Potassium iodide	Goiter	↓ Thyroxine synthesis	
Propylthiouracil	Goiter	Hypothyroidism	
I₁₃₁			? Malignant changes
Antidiabetics			
Tolbutamide	Anomalies	Thrombocytopenia	?
Chlorpropamide	Anomalies	Severe hypoglycemia	?
Cyclamates		?	?
Saccharin		?	?
Hormones			
Cortisone	Cleft palate ?	? Hemorrhages	
		? Hypoglycemia	

(continued)

Table 10–1
Drugs Reported to Affect the Fetus (continued)

Drug	Effect		
	Morphologic	Functional	Delayed
Hormones *(continued)*			
Prednisolone	Ancephaly ? Low birth weight ?	Normal adrenal activity ? Hemorrhages ? Hypoglycemia Normal adrenal activity	
Androgens	Masculinization female		
Progestins	Masculinization female		
Diethylstilbestrol	Clitoris hypertrophy		Adenocarcinoma vagina (adolescence)
Smoking			
	Low birth weight ↑ Stillborn		Smaller at 1 year of age
Alcohol			
Chronic intake Acute administration	Intrauterine growth failure	Fetal alcohol syndrome Withdrawal symptoms	Developmental delay ?
Pollutants and Pesticides			
Mercury		Severe neurologic defects	Severe handicaps Mental retardation

(continued)

Table 10–1 421

Table 10–1
Drugs Reported to Affect the Fetus (continued)

Drug	Effect		
	Morphologic	Functional	Delayed
Pollutants and Pesticides (*continued*)			
Lead	Low birth weight	↑ Abortions Anemia	
DDT and metabolites		Enzyme induction	
Parathion	? Teratogen		
Fungicides	?	?	
Herbicides	?	?	
Miscellaneous			
Atropine		Tachycardia	
Tubocurarine	? Arthrogryposis Multiplex congenita	Muscular paralysis	?
LSD	? Minor limb deformities		
Chloroquine		Deafness	

(Adapted from Avery GB [ed]: Neonatology: Pathophysiology and Management of the Newborn, 2nd ed. Philadelphia, JB Lippincott, 1981)

Table 10-2
Recommended Dietary Allowances Before and During Pregnancy and Lactation

Nutrient	11–14 Years	15–18 Years	19–22 Years	23–50 Years	Pregnancy	Lactation
Energy (kcal)	2200	2100	2100	2000	+300	+500
Protein (g)	46	46	44	44	+30	+20
Vitamin A, RE	800	800	800	800	+200	+400
IU	4000	4000	4000	4000	+1000	+2000
Vitamin D (µg)	10	10	7.5	5	+5	+5
Vitamin E (mgα TE)	8	8	8	8	+2	+3
Ascorbic acid (mg)	50	60	60	60	+20	+40
Thiamine (mg)	1.1	1.1	1.1	1.0	+0.4	+0.5
Riboflavin (mg)	1.3	1.3	1.3	1.2	+0.3	+0.5
Niacin (mg equiv)	15	14	14	13	+2	+5
Vitamin B_6 (mg)	1.8	2.0	2.0	2.0	+0.6	+0.5
Folacin (µg)	400	400	400	400	+400	+100
Vitamin B_{12} (µg)	3.0	3.0	3.0	3.0	+1.0	+1.0
Calcium (mg)	1200	1200	800	800	+400	+400
Phosphorus (mg)	1200	1200	800	800	+400	+400
Magnesium (mg)	300	300	300	300	+150	+150
Iron (mg)	18	18	18	18	*	*
Zinc (mg)	15	15	15	15	+5	+10
Iodine (µg)	150	150	150	150	+25	+50

* Supplemental iron, 30–60 mg, daily, is recommended.
(Food and Nutrition Board, National Academy of Sciences: Recommended Dietary Allowances, 9th ed. Washington, DC, National Research Council, 1980)

Table 10–3 423

Table 10-3
Daily Food Guide for Pregnancy and Lactation

Food Group	Amounts	
	Pregnancy	Lactation
Protein Foods		
Animal protein foods also supply iron, riboflavin, niacin, B_6, B_{12}, phosphorus, zinc, and iodine	two 3-oz servings	two 3-oz servings
Vegetable protein (dried peas, beans, nuts, seeds) foods also supply iron, thiamine, folacin, B_6, E, phosphorus, magnesium, and zinc; should include at least 1 serving of legumes	Serving size varies; plan with nutritionist	
Milk and Milk Products*		
Supply calcium, phosphorus, vitamin D, riboflavin, A, E, B_6, B_{12}, magnesium, zinc, and protein	4 servings Serving equals 8 oz of milk or its equivalent	4–5 servings
Grain Products		
Supply thiamine, niacin, riboflavin, iron, phosphorus, zinc, magnesium (whole grains provide more magnesium and zinc and should be encouraged), and fiber	4 servings Serving equals 1 slice of enriched bread or ½ cup of enriched macaroni, rice, or hot cereal	4 servings
Vitamin C-Rich Fruits and Vegetables		
Supply ascorbic acid; when fresh, supply fiber	1 serving Serving equals approximately ½ cup of fruit or ¾ cup of vegetables	1 serving

(continued)

Table 10–3
Daily Food Guide for Pregnancy and Lactation (continued)

Food Group	Amounts	
	Pregnancy	Lactation
Leafy Green Vegetables Supply folacin, vitamins A, E, B$_6$, riboflavin, iron, magnesium, and fiber	2 servings	2 servings
	Serving equals approximately 1 cup raw or ¾ cup cooked	
Other Fruits and Vegetables Include yellow fruits and vegetables, which supply large amounts of vitamin A as well as B complex, E, magnesium, phosphorus, zinc, and fiber	1 serving	1 serving
	Serving equals approximately ½ cup	

* Vitamin D is necessary for the utilization of calcium. Milk is fortified with vitamin D; most other sources of calcium are not. A supplement to ensure an adequate vitamin D intake may be necessary if milk is not consumed.
(Reprinted with permission from Howard RB, Herbold NH: Nutrition in Clinical Care. New York, McGraw–Hill, 1982)

Table 10-4 425

Table 10-4
Components of the Average Weight Gained During Normal Pregnancy

Component	Amount (g) Gained at			
	10 wk	20 wk	30 wk	40 wk
Total gain of body weight	650	4000	8500	12500
Fetus	5	300	1500	3300
Placenta	20	170	430	650
Amniotic fluid	30	250	600	800
Increase of				
Uterus	135	585	819	900
Mammary gland	34	180	360	405
Maternal blood	100	600	1300	1250
Total (rounded)	320	2100	5000	7300
Weight not accounted for by above	330	1900	3500	5200

(Committee on Maternal Nutrition, Food and Nutrition Board, National Research Council, National Academy of Sciences: Maternal nutrition and the course of pregnancy. Washington, DC, US Government Printing Office, 1970)

Table 10–6
Guidelines for Laboratory Evaluation of Anemia in Pregnancy

	Hemoglobin (g/100 ml)	Hematocrit (Packed Cell Vol %)	Serum Iron (μg/100 ml)	Transferrin Saturation (%)	Serum Folacin (ng/ml)*	Serum B$_{12}$ (pg/ml)[†]
Pregnancy						
Deficient	<9.5	<30	<40	<15	<2.0	<100
Marginal	9.5–10.9	30–32	40	15	2.1–5.9	100
Acceptable	>11.0	>33	>40	>15	>6.0	>100
Nonpregnant woman, normal values	>12.0	36–50	>50	>15	6.0–25.0	>100

* Nanograms per milliliter
[†] Picograms per milliliter
(Adapted from U.S. Department of HEW: Ten State Nutrition Survey, 1968–1970, DHEW Pub (HSM) 72-8130. Atlanta, Center for Disease Control, 1972)

Table 10-7 427

Table 10–7
Recommended Caloric and Nutrient Increases, Rationales, and Dietary Adaptations During Pregnancy

Nutrient	Normal	Pregnancy Increase	Rationale for Increased Intake in Pregnancy	Dietary Adaptations
Energy	2000–2200 kcal	+300 If activity levels remain high throughout pregnancy, caloric needs may be increased. Inadequate intake is less than 18 kcal/lb.	Increased intake helps meet the gross energy cost of 75,000 kcal for a 40-week gestation period. Increased calories are needed for the raised maternal basal metabolism rate, to spare protein for tissue synthesis, and to provide the energy needed for maternal organ growth, maternal fat storage, placenta development, and fetal growth. Insufficient intake can impair weight gain, which will ultimately reduce maternal fat stores, which may impair lactation performance and infant growth; induce hypovolemia, which can decrease gestational length (*e.g.*, premature infant); or induce infant mal-	The addition of two 8-oz glasses of whole milk provides 160 kcal/glass or a total of 320 kcal/day. All additional calories should be obtained from foods that have nutrient density such as complex carbohydrates or fats (*e.g.*, whole-grain breads or peanuts), not empty caloric foods (*e.g.*, candies or potato chips). See Table 10–3 for other dietary suggestions that will help meet caloric requirements.

(continued)

Table 10–7
Recommended Caloric and Nutrient Increases, Rationales, and Dietary Adaptations During Pregnancy (continued)

Nutrient	Normal	Pregnancy Increase	Rationale for Increased Intake in Pregnancy	Dietary Adaptations
Energy (continued)			nutrition → ↓ blood volume → ↓ cardiac output → ↓ placenta flow → ↓ maternal nutrient transfer to fetus → ↓ intrauterine growth rate in the fetus.	
Protein	44–46 g	+ 30 Energy intake should not fall below 18 kcal/lb/day in order to ensure that protein is used for tissue synthesis, not energy.	Increased intake helps meet gross protein needs of 925 g for a 40-week gestation period. Proteins needed during gestation for maternal tissue growth (e.g., breast and uterus); placental growth; fetal tissue growth; amniotic fluid; increased maternal circulating blood volume; and maternal storage reserves of nitrogen for labor, delivery, and the physiological demands of lactation. Insufficient intake may induce maternal edema with resultant preeclampsia maternal anemia, maternal in-	Of the daily protein requirement, ⅔ should be acquired from high biologic protein foods (e.g., milk, cheese, eggs, fish, poultry, and meat). The addition of two 8 oz glasses of milk or its equivalent (see calcium) provides 9 g of protein/glass or a total of 18 g/day. ⅓ of the daily protein may be acquired from low biologic protein foods (e.g., whole grains, dried beans, nuts, and seeds).

(continued)

Table 10–7 429

Table 10–7
Recommended Caloric and Nutrient Increases, Rationales, and Dietary Adaptations During Pregnancy (continued)

Nutrient	Normal	Pregnancy Increase	Rationale for Increased Intake in Pregnancy	Dietary Adaptations
Protein *(continued)*			fection, poor uterus muscle tone, fetal nutritional anemia, reduced fetal stature, and impaired fetal intrauterine growth.	
Fat-Soluble Vitamins				
Vitamin A, retinol	4000 IU* 800 RE†	+1000 IU +200 RE Excess dietary supplements may be toxic. Acquire increased requirements from foods.	Increased intake raises maternal vitamin A levels. Consequently, more vitamin A is transmitted to the fetus, which is essential for fetal cell development, tissue growth, tooth formation, bone growth, and storage for neonatal needs.	Increase intake of natural preformed vitamin A foods such as liver, butter, cream, whole milk, or cheeses. Increase intake of carotene, a precursor of vitamin A, in foods such as dark green leafy vegetables and yellow vegetables and fruits.
Vitamin D, chole-calciferol	400 IU 10 µg	+5 Supplements of vitamin D may enhance hypercalcemia in the fetus and premature closure of the fontanelle. Ac-	Increased amounts from foods and supplements of ultraviolet light facilitate greater maternal calcium absorption. Consequently, less calcium is reabsorbed from	Exposure to a few minutes of ultraviolet light a day is advised. The addition of two 8-oz glasses of fortified vitamin D milk a day

(continued)

Table 10–7
Recommended Caloric and Nutrient Increases, Rationales, and Dietary Adaptations During Pregnancy (continued)

Nutrient	Normal	Pregnancy Increase	Rationale for Increased Intake in Pregnancy	Dietary Adaptations
Fat-Soluble Vitamins (continued)				
		quire requirements from foods or ultraviolet light, if possible. Excess dietary supplements may be toxic. See vitamin A.	maternal bones, and more calcium is available for mineralization of fetal bones and cells. Insufficient intake may precipitate osteomalacia in the mother, neonatal hypocalcemia, or congenital rickets.	provides 5 µg of vitamin D daily. Dietary supplements should be taken only on the advice of a physician.
Vitamin E, tocopherol	8 TE‡	+2 TE	Escalated caloric requirements increase tocopheral needs in the mother and fetus. It is essential for tissue growth and cell-wall integrity. Insufficient intake may precipitate fetal red blood hemolysis.	Increase intake of vegetable oils, wheat germ, if desired, green leafy vegetables, meat, eggs, and whole milk.
Water-Soluble Vitamins				
Vitamin C, ascorbic acid	50–60 mg Supplements are not advised in most cases if adequate amounts are acquired from foods. Excesses may precipi-	+20 mg Insufficient intake may precipitate maternal abortion or congenital anomalies.	Increased intake is needed because maternal blood levels fall during pregnancy. Subsequently, fetal blood levels exceed maternal levels by 50%–100%. It is essential	Increase intake of citrus fruits (*e.g.*, oranges, grapefruits, lemons, limes, and tangerines). Addition of 1 glass of juice daily provides

(continued)

Table 10–7 431

Table 10–7
Recommended Caloric and Nutrient Increases, Rationales, and Dietary Adaptations During Pregnancy (continued)

Nutrient	Normal	Pregnancy Increase	Rationale for Increased Intake in Pregnancy	Dietary Adaptations
Water-Soluble Vitamins (continued)				
	tate congenital anomalies or conditioned scurvy.		for collagen synthesis and the intracellular cement substance in connective tissue, vascular tissues, and teeth in the fetus. It enhances maternal iron absorption.	100–120 mg of ascorbic acid. Other good sources are strawberries, tomatoes, green peppers, broccoli, and potatoes.
Vitamin B₁, thiamine	1.0–1.1 mg	+0.4 mg	Escalated energy intake increases requirements. It is essential as a coenzyme in energy metabolism, and also essential for RNA and DNA synthesis. Insufficient intake may precipitate maternal and fetal beriberi.	Increase intake of pork, beef, liver, whole or enriched grains, and yeast.
Vitamin B₂, riboflavin	1.2–1.3 mg	+0.3 mg	Escalated energy and protein intake increases requirements. It is essential as a coenzyme in energy and protein metabolism. Insufficient intake may impair fetal growth.	The addition of two 8-oz glasses of milk each day provides 0.41 mg of riboflavin/glass or a total of 0.82 mg/day. Other good sources are liver and enriched grains.

(continued)

Table 10–7
Recommended Caloric and Nutrient Increases, Rationales, and Dietary Adaptations During Pregnancy (continued)

Nutrient	Normal	Pregnancy Increase	Rationale for Increased Intake in Pregnancy	Dietary Adaptations
Water-Soluble Vitamins (continued)				
Vitamin B_3, niacin	13–15 mg	+2 mg	Escalated energy and protein intake increases requirements. It is necessary for the metabolism of carbohydrates, proteins, fats, and alcohol.	Increase intake of foods (60 mg of tryptophan, an essential amino acid, equals 1 mg of niacin) such as meats and poultry. Other good sources of niacin are peanuts, beans, peas, enriched grains, and corn.
Vitamin B_6, pyridoxine	1.8–2.0 mg	+0.6 mg	Escalated protein intake increases requirements. It is necessary for absorption, deamination, and transamination of amino acids and aids in the conversion of tryptophan to niacin. It aids hemoglobin production in the fetus and mother and may help relieve nausea in pregnancy.	Increased intake of protein foods such as meat, egg yolk, and liver will supply the increased requirements. Other good pyridoxine sources are yeast, wheat germ, legumes, and bananas.

(continued)

Table 10–7 433

Table 10–7
Recommended Caloric and Nutrient Increases, Rationales, and Dietary Adaptations During Pregnancy (continued)

Nutrient	Normal	Pregnancy Increase	Rationale for Increased Intake in Pregnancy	Dietary Adaptations
Water-Soluble Vitamins *(continued)*				
Folacin	400 μg	+400 μg	Increased intake is required because folacin is an essential coenzyme in purine and pyrimidine metabolism. Requirements also increase when there is rapid cell division, which occurs in pregnancy and during fetal growth. It is essential for maturation of RBCs in the mother and fetus. Insufficient intake may precipitate maternal megaloblastic anemia, premature labor, or abortion. Fetal adverse effects due to deficiency may be growth retardation (?) or fetal malformation (?).	Increase intake of organ meats, beef, eggs, dark green leafy vegetables, dried beans, nuts, and cereals, especially those fortified with folacin. Some physicians advise a dietary supplement of 400 μg if dietary intake is low or if other factors such as chronic hemolytic anemia, multiple pregnancy, or anticonvulsant drug therapy are involved.
Vitamin B$_{12}$, cyanocobalamin	3.0 μg	+1.0 μg	Increased intake is required for fetal growth. It is essential for carbohydrate protein and fat metabolism, for myelin synthesis in fetus, and for DNA production in	Increase intake of animal foods such as organ meats, eggs, milk, and cheese. Most plant foods contain only minute quantities *(continued)*

Table 10–7
Recommended Caloric and Nutrient Increases, Rationales, and Dietary Adaptations During Pregnancy (continued)

Nutrient	Normal	Pregnancy Increase	Rationale for Increased Intake in Pregnancy	Dietary Adaptations
Water-Soluble Vitamins (continued)				
			mother and fetus. It aids RBC formation in mother and fetus. Insufficient intake may precipitate maternal and fetal pernicious anemia.	of vitamins B_{12}; consequently, vegetarian mothers will need vitamin B_{12} supplements.
Minerals				
Calcium	800–1200 mg	+400 mg Excessive intake above this level may precipitate calcification of soft tissue (?).	Increased intake is necessary for enhanced calcification of the fetal skeleton, especially during the third trimester. However, calcium may also be stored during the first and second trimesters. Also it is essential for fetal tooth formation and to maintain maternal calcium stores. Insufficient intake may precipitate maternal osteomalacia or congenital rickets in the infant. Fortunately, calcium absorption doubles during	Increased intake of milk or dairy products. Addition of two 8-oz glasses of whole milk or its equivalent (see below) provides 288 mg calcium/glass or a total of 576 mg of calcium/day. Foods that can be used as substitutes for milk (containing similar quantities of protein and calcium) during pregnancy are

(continued)

Table 10–7 435

Table 10–7
Recommended Caloric and Nutrient Increases, Rationales, and Dietary Adaptations During Pregnancy (continued)

Nutrient	Normal	Pregnancy Increase	Rationale for Increased Intake in Pregnancy	Dietary Adaptations
Minerals *(continued)*				
			pregnancy, but vitamin D is needed to enhance this absorption.	1⅓ oz cheddar cheese; 1⅓ cups cottage cheese (protein tripled); 1½ cups ice cream (calories increased); ½ cup undiluted evaporated milk; 1 cup yogurt; 3 oz or 6 tbsp dried milk powder; 16 oz cream cheese (calories increased). Other foods high in calcium are 1 large orange (96 mg); 1 stalk raw broccoli (105 mg); ½ cup cooked collards (152 mg).
Phosphorus	800–1200 mg	+400 mg	In conjunction with calcium, phosphorus intake is increased to enhance fetal bone and tooth mineralization. Escalated energy intake	The addition of two 8-oz glasses of whole milk/day will provide the phosphorus requirement. Other

(continued)

Table 10–7
Recommended Caloric and Nutrient Increases, Rationales, and Dietary Adaptations During Pregnancy (continued)

Nutrient	Normal	Pregnancy Increase	Rationale for Increased Intake in Pregnancy	Dietary Adaptations
***Minerals* (continued)**				
			also increases requirements. It is essential for carbohydrate and fat metabolism. It is an essential component of stored energy (*e.g.*, ATP), a constituent of all body cells, and cell membrane integrity. Insufficient intake may impair fetal growth and skeletal formation.	good sources of phosphorus are meat, egg yolk, whole grains, and nuts. Obtaining phosphorus requirements by consuming highly preserved foods or sodas is not advised because the natural calcium-to-phosphorus ratio will be imbalanced.
Magnesium	300 mg	+ 150 mg	In conjunction with calcium and phosphorus, magnesium intake is increased to enhance mineralization of the fetal skeleton. Escalated energy intake increases requirements. Magnesium is a cofactor in enzymatic reactions that produce energy from carbohydrate, protein,	Increase intake of green vegetables (part of the chlorophyll molecule) nuts, cereal grains, and seafood.

(continued)

Table 10–7 437

Table 10–7
Recommended Caloric and Nutrient Increases, Rationales, and Dietary Adaptations During Pregnancy (continued)

Nutrient	Normal	Pregnancy Increase	Rationale for Increased Intake in Pregnancy	Dietary Adaptations
Minerals *(continued)*				
Iron	18 mg	Supplements of iron, 30–60 mg, daily, is recommended. Mothers should be instructed that the number of stools and color (tarry to black) may be altered when iron supplements are taken. Supplements may also irritate the GI tract. Take with meals to minimize irritation.	and fat. Insufficient intake can impair fetal growth and skeletal formation. Increased intake is necessary to augment increased blood cell production in the expanded maternal circulating blood volume. Also, it is essential for iron storage in the fetal liver. Insufficient intake may precipitate maternal nutritional anemia or postnatal nutritional anemia in the infant. Fortunately, the rate of iron absorption is increased in pregnancy and the absence of menstruation decreases iron losses.	Increase intake of liver and meats, which are excellent sources of readily absorbable heme iron. Other reasonably good sources of nonheme iron are whole enriched grains, dark green leafy vegetables, nuts, legumes, and dried fruits. Consuming foods high in vitamin C along with foods high in iron enhances iron absorption. Cooking in iron skillets also increases the iron content of the

(continued)

Table 10–7
Recommended Caloric and Nutrient Increases, Rationales, and Dietary Adaptations During Pregnancy (continued)

Minerals (continued)

Nutrient	Normal	Pregnancy Increase	Rationale for Increased Intake in Pregnancy	Dietary Adaptations
				diet. Ferrous supplements, 30–60 mg, daily, may be advised during the second and third trimester if dietary intake is low. However, these supplements may aggravate adverse GI symptoms such as constipation and indigestion and decrease zinc absorption. Limit coffee and tea intakes. These beverages inhibit iron absorption.
Zinc	15 mg	+ 5 mg	Increased intake is essential for fetal and placental growth. It is a constituent of enzymes involved in RNA and DNA synthesis and also important in reproductive	Increase intake of animal foods such as meat, liver, eggs, seafood, and milk. Plant foods are poor sources of zinc; thus

(continued)

Table 10–7 439

Table 10–7
**Recommended Caloric and Nutrient Increases, Rationales,
and Dietary Adaptations During Pregnancy** (continued)

Nutrient	Normal	Pregnancy Increase	Rationale for Increased Intake in Pregnancy	Dietary Adaptations
Minerals (continued)				
			organs. Insufficient intake may induce maternal atonic bleeding and prolonged labor. Adverse effects in the infant, due to deficiency, may include growth retardation and congenital anomalies.	vegetarian mothers may need supplements. However, supplements may decrease copper and calcium absorption.
Iodine	150 μg	+ 25 μg	Increased intake is necessary to meet metabolic needs. Iodine is essential for thyroxine production, which is escalated when basal metabolic rates rise. Insufficient intake may precipitate goiter in the mother or cretinism in the infant.	Use iodized salt.
Fluids				
	1 ml/kcal or approximately two liters/day	+ 300 ml to complement 300 kcal increase	Increased intake is essential for expanding maternal and fetal extracellular and intra-	Increase intake of all fluids daily. 6–8 glasses of water are recommended/day.

(continued)

Table 10-7
Recommended Caloric and Nutrient Increases, Rationales, and Dietary Adaptations During Pregnancy (continued)

Nutrient	Normal	Pregnancy Increase	Rationale for Increased Intake in Pregnancy	Dietary Adaptations
Fluids (continued)			cellular fluid needs, including expanded maternal blood volume. Also it enhances maternal and fetal waste elimination. Insufficient intake precipitates maternal dehydration and hypovolemia. Adverse effects in the fetus, due to deficiency, may include dehydration and malnutrition (See hypovolemia under energy requirements).	They may be drunk in the form of fruit juices or water. Sodas, tea, and coffee should be limited because of the caffeine content. The addition of two 8-oz glasses of milk provides 240 ml/glass or a total of 480 ml/day.

* IU = international units
† RE = retinol equivalents
‡ TE = tocopherol equivalents

Table 10–9 441

Table 10-9
Rationales and Dietary Adaptations for Common Physiological Discomforts of Pregnancy

Physiological Disorder	Rationale for Disorder	Dietary Adaptations
Vomiting and nausea	Hormonal imbalances Increased satiety, which may be escalated by decreased HCl production; consequently, food remains longer in the stomach—this may enhance regurgitation Decreased cardiac sphincter contraction, which may allow stomach contents to reflux back into the esophagus Disturbed carbohydrate metabolism Vitamin deficiencies Immunologic interactions between mother and fetus Anxiety Rejection of pregnancy	Eat a few crackers or dry cereal before rising Arise slowly Drink fruit juices after the meal Avoid coffee or tea at breakfast Eat 5 or 6 small meals, rather than 3 large meals, which helps keep a small amount of food in the stomach at all times Eat dry foods at meals (*e.g.*, toast without margarine) Drink fluids between meals rather than with meals Drink skim milk instead of whole milk Avoid spicy, fatty, or fried foods Consume concentrated caloric and nutrient-dense foods when nausea is decreased (*e.g.*, bland casseroles with added cheese and milk) Avoid cooking foods with strong odors Practice good oral hygiene to prevent bleeding gums and tooth decay (caries), especially when vomiting is excessive Consult a physician if vomiting is frequent and profuse

(continued)

Table 10-9
Rationales and Dietary Adaptations for Common Physiological Discomforts of Pregnancy (continued)

Physiological Disorder	Rationale for Disorder	Dietary Adaptations
Constipation	Pressure exerted by the expanded uterus on the colon and rectum impairs excretion	Increase fiber intake (*e.g.*, raw fruits and vegetables and whole grains or add a teaspoon of bran to cereals in the morning)
	Increased progesterone production relaxes the muscles of the GI tract, reducing motility	
	Insufficient fiber in the diet	
	Poor defecation habits (*i.e.*, not allowing time for defecation)	Arise early and drink a cup of hot water with lemon or a glass of prune juice
		Allow time to defecate before continuing with daily activities
	Insufficient fluid intake	Consume at least 8–10 glasses of water or its equivalent daily
	Skipping meals, especially breakfast	Eat 3 meals a day at regular times
	Exercise limited	Exercise moderately every day with physician's permission
	Iron supplementation	Limit iron supplements to every other day rather than every day
		Increase intake of foods that contain heme iron (*e.g.*, meats) on alternate days

(continued)

Table 10–9 443

Table 10–9
Rationales and Dietary Adaptations for Common Physiological Discomforts of Pregnancy (continued)

Physiological Disorder	Rationale for Disorder	Dietary Adaptations
Heartburn	Decreased gastric motility and pressure of the uterus against the stomach may cause stomach contents to be regurgitated into the esophagus Decreased cardiac sphincter contraction may allow stomach contents to reflux into the esophagus	Eat 5–6 small meals rather than 3 large meals daily Avoid fried foods, spicy foods, coffee, and rich desserts Abstain from alcohol and cigarettes Do not take antacids; they may disturb acid-base balance and impair vitamin B complex and phosphorus absorption Consume yogurt or buttermilk rather than whole milk Avoid bending or lying down after a meal Wear loose clothing not tight, restricting garments
Leg cramps (cramping of the gastrocnemius muscle, usually at night)	Neuromuscular irritability that may be caused by a low serum calcium and high serum phosphate concentration	Limit intake of foods high in phosphorus but low in calcium (*e.g.*, sodas, meats, and highly preserved foods) Limitation of milk, although high in phosphorus, may not be advisable, however, for it is also high in calcium; the alternative to limited milk ingestion may be supplements of aluminum hydroxide (binds phosphorus), or calcium lactate or carbonate, if prescribed by the physician

(continued)

Table 10-9
Rationales and Dietary Adaptations for Common Physiological Discomforts of Pregnancy (continued)

Physiological Disorder	Rationale for Disorder	Dietary Adaptations
Pica (An unusual craving for and consumption of nonfood substances [*e.g.*, clay eating (geophagia), laundry starch, cigarette ashes, dirt, newspapers, or ice-chewing (pagophagia)])	Iron or calcium deficiency? Social acceptance or expectations in some cultures Relieves tension Relieves hunger pains Appetite stimulant Unusual beliefs about childbirth, such as baby will slideout more easily, prevents birthmarks, baby will be lighter in color	Encourage ingestion of concentrated nutrient-dense foods because escalated intakes of non-nutritive foods will impair appetite Set up and conduct nutritional education programs that will present the adverse maternal and infant effects that may develop from the ingestion of non-nutritive foodstuffs (*e.g*, maternal and infant anemia, malabsorption of essential nutrients) Supplements of iron may be needed to relieve anemia Increase fluid intake and nutrient dense fibrous foods (*e.g.*, salads) for they enhance defecation, and chances of fecal impaction are increased when substances like clay or laundry starch are consumed in excess Monitor for signs of diarrhea and vomiting, because chances of parasitic infections or toxicities are increased with increased ingestion of non-nutritive foodstuffs Increase fluid intake if adverse symptoms such as diarrhea develop

Table 10–10 445

Table 10–10
Adverse Effects Induced in Infants When Common Medications Are Transmitted in Breast Milk

Medication Category	Adverse Effects in Infants
Analgesics	
Aspirin	Relatively safe in small doses
	Chronic aspirin therapy for arthritis, however, may cause a combined platelet and prothrombin deficiency with resultant neonate bleeding; infant may need prophylactic treatment at birth with parenteral vitamin K_1 (Konakion)
Antimicrobials	
Cephalexin (Keflex), cephalothin (Keflin), oxacillin (Prostaphlin)	Not excreted in human milk, thus relatively safe
Penicillin G, benzathine (Bicillin)	Penicillin is relatively safe but may cause candidal diarrhea and thrush in the nursing infant; additionally, the infant may become sensitized to penicillin
Sulfisoxazole (Gantrisin)	Sulfa drugs should not be taken by a nursing mother during the first month of lactation; infant may develop neonatal jaundice
Anticonvulsants	
Phenobarbital (Luminal), primidone (Mysoline), phenytoin (Dilantin)	May act as a sedative in nursing infants, which would decrease the sucking reflex
Antihistamines	
Diphenhydramine (Benadryl), trimeprazine (Temaril)	Relatively safe during lactation but in large doses may diminish the milk supply or sedate infant
Tranquilizers	
Diazepam (Valium)	May cause drowsiness, lethargy, and jaundice in the infant, especially with high doses; sedative effect may decrease milk intake with a resultant reduced infant growth rate

(continued)

Table 10–10
**Adverse Effects Induced in Infants When Common
Medications Are Transmitted in Breast Milk** (continued)

Medication Category	Adverse Effects in Infants
Antidiabetics	
Insulin	Safe because, like all proteins, is destroyed (digested) in the infant's GI tract
Oral Agents (acetohexamide [Dymelor], chlorpropamide [Diabinese], tolbutamide [Orinase])	May cause neonatal jaundice and hypoglycemia
Anticoagulants	
Heparin	Not excreted in human milk
Warfarin (Coumadin), dicumarol	Warfarin and dicumarol are relatively safe but infant prothrombin times should be monitored; infant should be given vitamin K_1 when indicated
Cardiovascular Drugs	
Digoxin (Lanoxin)	Safe during lactation, provided maternal serum levels are monitored and kept within the therapeutic range during the first 2 months of lactation
Quinidine (Quinora), guanethidine (Ismelin), propranolol (Inderal)	May cause arrhythmias in the infant
	Safe in therapeutic doses
Reserpine (Serpasil), hydralazine hydrochloride (Apresoline)	Powerful antihypertensives that may cause adverse effects in adults and infants; therefore, not recommended (see Table 3–3)
Diuretics	
Thiazide diuretics (chlorothiazide [Diuril], hydrochlorothiazide [Esidrix])	Decrease milk production in a poorly hydrated woman. Fluid and electrolyte imbalances may develop in the infant

(continued)

Table 10–10 447

Table 10–10
Adverse Effects Induced in Infants When Common Medications Are Transmitted in Breast Milk (continued)

Medication Category	Adverse Effects in Infants
Thyroid Hormones Liotrix	Safe during lactation but can mask symptoms of congenital hypothyroidism An infant's thyroid function should be checked before maternal replacement therapy begins
Antithyroids	All antithyroid medications are goitrogenic; therefore when treatment for hyperthyroidism is necessary, the infant's circulating thyroid hormones should be measured frequently; propylthiouracil is the medication usually preferred Iodides are contraindicated If exposure to radioactive iodine is necessary, breast feeding should be discontinued
Antacids (Amphojel, Maalox)	Safe unless taken in excessive doses, then the mother may develop electrolyte imbalance
Laxatives	Safe during lactation, the exception being danthron (Modane), which may cause colic or diarrhea in the infant
Miscellaneous Drugs Pyridoxine (Vitamin B_6)	Pyridoxine may inhibit lactation, especially in high doses; therefore, mothers having difficulty establishing a milk supply should be advised to take multivitamins that do not contain pyridoxine

(continued)

Table 10–10
**Adverse Effects Induced in Infants When Common
Medications Are Transmitted in Breast Milk** (continued)

Medication Category	Adverse Effects in Infants
Miscellaneous Drugs (continued)	
Alcohol	Doses greater than 1 g/kg of mother's weight may inhibit the milk ejection reflex
Caffeine	Doses higher than 2 g/kg may completely block the sucking-induced oxytocin release Infants are more sensitive to the effects of caffeine than adults because they do not eliminate this stimulant efficiently; consequently, the infant may become restless or irritable or have a reduced appetite
Nicotine	Cigarette smoke is highly irritating to the infant's respiratory tract; additionally, large amounts of nicotine (over a pack of cigarettes/day) may induce restlessness, diarrhea, vomiting, and tachycardia in the infant
Hormones Oral contraceptives (Envoid, others)	Diminish milk production May alter maternal blood levels of many nutrients; consequently, infant nutrient inadequacies may develop Nutrients that may be decreased in blood are albumin, high-density lipoproteins, calcium, phosphorus, magnesium, zinc, pyridoxine, thiamine, riboflavin, folacin, cobalamin, and ascorbic acid Nutrients that may be increased in blood are retinol (vitamin A), triglycerides, alpha and beta globulins, iron, copper, and glucose Glucose tolerance curves shift upward but the shape of the curve is unchanged

(Adapted from Wicklund S: Special report: Drugs for two in lactation. Am J Nurs 82:1428, 1982; and Worthington
BS: Pregnancy, lactation and oral contraception. Nurs Clin North Am 14:281, 1979)

Table 10–11 449

Table 10–11
Factors That Enhance and Inhibit Lactation

Category	Factors That Enhance Lactation	Factors That Inhibit Lactation
Sedatives	Minimal sedation during delivery	Drugs during labor and delivery may sedate the infant; consequently, the sucking reflex will be reduced
Breast Feeding	Breast feeding as soon as possible after delivery Develops the baby's sucking reflex Provides the benefits of colostrum (see Chap. 11) Stimulates peristalsis and segmentation in the infant's GI tract Stimulates the flow of mature milk	Delayed feeding can reduce colostrum benefits and inhibit the flow of mature milk Other benefits of early feeding will be impaired
Emotions	Rooming-in Emotional support from the husband, nursing staff, obstetrician, pediatrician, and family members enhances milk let-down (breast feeding alone initially may be more relaxing for the mother, creating less apprehension, and less distraction for the infant)	Anxiety about the ability to breast feed or apprehension about an adequate milk supply can inhibit the production of oxytocin, which stimulates milk let-down
Nourishment	Adequate intake of nutrient-dense foods and fluids	Inadequate intake of calories and fluids can reduce milk volume
Rest	Rest	Fatigue impairs the let-down reflex
Feeding	Avoid use of supplementary bottles If glucose and water solutions are necessary, owing to a traumatic birth, give with an eye dropper or spoon	Giving glucose and water with a bottle that has a nipple that does not simulate the breast nipple will confuse the infant

(continued)

Table 10–11
Factors That Enhance and Inhibit Lactation (continued)

Category	Factors That Enhance Lactation	Factors That Inhibit Lactation
	Feeding frequently (as often as 10–12 times a day in the beginning) and emptying breast completely after feeding lead to maximum milk production	Scheduled feeding may decrease milk supply. Additionally, the infant becomes "starved," which increases his sucking reflex and may cause nipple irritations
	Expression of the breast may be by hand or electric or hand pump	Incomplete drainage of the breast can decrease milk yield by impeding blood flow to the mammary tissue
		Breast may become engorged, without complete drainage, which impairs the infant's ability to suck properly and may induce mastitis
Holding infant	Holding the infant close to the breast and teasing the infant's mouth and cheek with the nipple stimulate feeding.	Holding the infant far away from the breast inhibits the sucking action and may cause nipple irritation
	When sucking begins, place the nipple plus the entire areola in the infant's mouth to prevent nipple irritation	
Nipple care	Good nipple care improves infant feeding	Improper nipple care can cause infant contamination or maternal discomfort, complications that can interrupt infant feeding
	Proper nipple care includes	Severe bacterial contamination induces vomiting and diarrhea, with resultant dehydration and electrolyte losses
	Keeping the nipple clean	
	Stimulating the nipples prior to lactation	
	Keeping nipples dry; however, drying agents such as soaps or alcohol should be avoided since these agents may enhance cracking (also, avoid using plastic liners in bras, which hinder air circulation)	

(continued)

Table 10–11 451

Table 10–11
Factors That Enhance and Inhibit Lactation (continued)

Category	Factors That Enhance Lactation	Factors That Inhibit Lactation
Positioning	Keep nipples soft by applying pure lanolin or vitamin A and D ointment Proper positioning during feeding prevents maternal and infant fatigue Proper positioning suggestions for the mother are Lie on your side supported by pillows Sit in a chair that has arm rests and a supportive back, with a footstool	Improper positioning of the mother fatigues mother and infant; consequently, feeding time will be shortened
Solid foods	Avoid supplementary solid foods in the infant's feeding plan until weaning is desired	Feeding solid foods decreases the infant's hunger, which leads to less frequent and vigorous sucking; consequently, milk production is reduced Solid foods inhibit iron and calcium absorption from breast milk
Medications	If medications are essential to maintain mother's health, breast feed before taking medications Discontinue breast feeding if adverse symptoms in the infant will be severe	Many medications are transmitted in human milk that can have adverse effects in the infant (see Table 10-10)
Smoking	Abstain or limit cigarette smoking	Cigarette smoking reduces the volume of milk produced; see Table 10–10 for other adverse effects

Bibliography

American Nursing Association: Hypertension in pregnancy. Am J Nurs 82:791, 1982

Anderson L, Dibble MV, Turkki PR et al: Nutrition in Health and Disease, 17th ed. Philadelphia, JB Lippincott, 1982

Avery GB (ed): Neonatology: Pathophysiology and Management of the Newborn, 2nd ed. Philadelphia, JB Lippincott, 1981

Billups NF (ed): American Drug Index, 27th ed. Philadelphia, JB Lippincott, 1983

Brunner LS, Suddarth DS: The Lippincott Manual of Nursing Practice, 3rd ed. Philadelphia, JB Lippincott, 1982

Christensen DJ: Diagnosis of anemia. Postgrad Med 73:293, 1983

Committee on Nutrition of the Mother and Preschool Child: Food and Nutrition Board, Assembly of Life Sciences, National Research Council, Nutrition Services in Perinatal Care. Washington, DC, National Academy Press, 1981

Grant NF, Worley RJ: Hypertension in Pregnancy: Concepts and Management. New York, Appleton–Century–Crofts, 1980

Haltstead JA: Geophagia in man: Its nature and nutritional effects. Am J Clin Nutr 21:1384, 1968

Hinton SM, Kerwin DR: Maternal Infant and Child Nutrition: A Resource Book for Health Professionals. Chapel Hill, Health Sciences Consortium, 1981

Howard RB, Herbold NH: Nutrition in Clinical Care, 2nd ed. New York, McGraw–Hill, 1982

La Leche League International: The Womanly Art of Breast Feeding, 3rd ed. Franklin Park, IL, La Leche League International, 1982

Lull CB, Kimbrough RA (eds): Clinical Obstetrics. Philadelphia, JB Lippincott, 1953

National Diabetes Data Group: Classification and diagnosis of diabetes mellitus and other categories of glucose intolerance. Diabetes 28:1039, 1979

Pike RL, Gursky DS: Further evidence of deleterious effects produced by sodium restriction during pregnancy. Am J Clin Nutr 28:883, 1970

Robinson CH, Lawler MR: Normal and Therapeutic Nutrition, 16th ed. New York, Macmillan, 1982

Schulman PK: Hyperemesis gravidarum: An approach to the nutritional aspects of care. Perspective in Practice 80:537, 1982

Stephenson PE: Physiologic and psychotropic effects of caffeine on man. J Am Diet Assoc 71:240, 1977

Wicklund S: Special report: Drugs for two in lactation. Am J Nurs 82:1428, 1982

Workshop on Nutrition of the Child: Maternal Nutritional Status and Fetal Outcome. Am J Clin Nutr (Suppl) 34:655, 1981

Worthington BS: Pregnancy, lactation and oral contraception. Nurs Clin North Am 14:281, 1979

Worthington–Roberts BS, Vermeersch J, Williams SR: Nutrition in Pregnancy and Lactation, 2nd ed. St Louis, CV Mosby, 1981

chapter 11

Life Cycle

Description

Infancy is the period from birth to age 1 year.
- Neonatal Period. First 28 days after birth
- Postnatal Period. From 29 days after birth to 1 year

Characteristics of a Healthy Infant

An infant who is born at the appropriate gestational age (AGA, 37–42 wk), weighs more than 2500 g, is fully developed for age, and is free of disease is considered healthy.

Nutritional Care Plans for Infants

Goals

Provide sufficient calories, high biologic protein, vitamins, minerals, and fluids to meet the nutritional needs of the infant for steady weight and height gain and optimal structural and mental development

Introduce the infant to a variety of natural flavors, early in life, so that the desire for unfavorable substances (*e.g.*, sugar and salt) will not be enhanced

Provide nutritional care plans that will alleviate or reduce common adverse symptoms (*e.g.*, diarrhea)

Provide nutritional care plans for the high-risk infant that will restore and enhance continuous support of metabolic functions as well as supply the caloric and nutrient requirements for optimal structural and mental development

Long-term goal, to motivate good eating behavior that will maintain optimal structural and mental development throughout the life cycle; that is, establish food as a pleasurable means of nourishing the body as well as the spirit, as an alternative to using food as an emotional pacifier

General Factors

Interview Chart (Components With Special Significance, Revealed by Parent or Guardian)

- Gestational Age. Determines caloric and nutrient needs; estimates infant's developmental readiness to ingest, digest, absorb, store, and utilize food and its breakdown products
- Ethnic and Religious Background. Background factors may reveal maternal and infant nutrient stores or nutrient inadequacies that may develop during lactation (*e.g.*, vitamin B_{12} deficiencies in infants and mothers who habitually eat a vegan diet). Additionally, they may determine when and what types of solid foods will be introduced to the infant
- Socioeconomic Factors. Socioeconomics influence the type of feeding (breast *vs.* bottle) offered; presently, the more educated and affluent the mother, the more inclined she is to breast feed.
- Obstetrical History. Complications upon delivery may have interrupted infant's feeding program; frequent pregnancies may have depleted maternal stores.
- Medical History of Infant and Immediate Family. Parental illnesses or genetic background may induce congenital illnesses (*e.g.*, inborn errors of metabolism); in such cases, modified nutritional care plans must be instituted (see High-Risk Infant).
- Allergies. A history of allergies in family members may indicate that modified milk formulas (*e.g.*, soy protein formulas [Prosobee]) must be instituted.
- Appetite. Increased appetite may mean that the formula concentration or breast milk volume is inadequate. A new type of formula or feeding method may be indicated. In contrast, a decreased appetite may indicate that the infant has impaired sucking development or appetite control.
- Elimination Habits. Infants with firm or loose stools (not similar to the stools of breast-fed infants) may need a formula or feeding method adjustment. Calories, fluids, and other nutrients will have to be increased to replace losses in infants with diarrhea. Frequent urination will increase fluid needs.

- Sleeping Patterns. Patterns of sleep determine caloric activity needs. Wakeful infants need higher caloric, nutrient, and fluid intake. Sleepy babies may also need higher caloric, nutrient, and fluid intakes at any one feeding if they sleep through other feedings. Additional medical and nutritional assessment data should be obtained if the infant cries or sleeps too frequently.

- Medications. Sedatives or tranquilizers taken by breast-feeding mothers may impair infant sucking, which ultimately reduces weight gain. Dietary supplements (*e.g.*, iron supplements) taken by the infant may cause gastrointestinal (GI) distress. Medications should be eliminated, changed, or reduced whenever possible. Breast feeding may have to be discontinued if weight loss is excessive.

Nutritional Assessment Data

Nutritional assessment data are used to determine if the infant is developing in a manner that will enable him to reach his optimal structural and mental capacity. Each individual infant develops at a different rate, however, so comparing him to standards may not always be an effective measure of his progress. The criteria that more accurately measure an infant's progress may be expressed as answers to these questions: Does he have a steady weight and height gain, moderate increases in subcutaneous fat, firm muscle development, good elimination habits, good eating and sleeping patterns, a good emotional outlook on life, and a normal curiosity toward his surroundings? If he is progressing in this fashion, he is probably developing properly.

- Diet History. When obtaining a diet history for a small infant, special emphasis should be placed on methodology of feeding (breast *vs.* bottle), feeding frequency, quantity of food (appetite) consumed daily and at each meal (compare findings to Table 11–1), quantity and type of dietary supplements being administered, family allergy history, adverse symptoms following a feeding (*e.g.*, excessive crying or diarrhea), sleeping patterns (influence caloric needs), and defecation habits (influence nutrient needs).

  In later infancy, emphasis should be placed on milk intake (excessive intake can curtail solid food intake), infant's solid food likes (*e.g.*, sweets) and dislikes, types of foods refused consistently (may indicate nutrient inadequacies), dexterity and desire to feed himself, and activity patterns (influence energy requirements per unit of body weight).

- Anthropometric Measurements
  1. Weight. Obtain infant's birth weight, gestational age, present weight, and weight progress over a period of time. Obtain present weight of a nude infant by placing him on a scale that measures to the nearest gram (see advanced nutritional texts for weighing procedures). Then compare the infant's weight prog-

Table 11–1
**Approximate Quantities of Milk Consumed by an
Average Infant During the First 6 Months of Life**

	g	oz
1st day	10	1/3
2nd day	90	3
3rd day	190	6 1/3
4th day	300	10
5th day	350	11 1/2
6th day	390	13
7th day	470	15 2/3
3rd week	500	16
4th week	600	20
8th week	800	26 1/2
12th week	900	30
24th week	1000	33

(Anderson L, Dibble MV, Turkki PR, et al: Nutrition in Health and Disease, 17th ed. Philadelphia, JB Lippincott, 1982)

ress to the norm by simply ascertaining that he has doubled his birth weight in 6 months, not 4 or 7 months, and tripled his birth weight in 1 year, when applicable. The more complex comparison, to establish his progress against the norm, is to compare his progress to physical growth charts. If the infant's progress is estimated to fall above the 90th percentile of these standards, he should be monitored for obesity; if he falls below the 10th to 5th percentiles, he should be monitored for malnutrition and growth failure. Advanced nutritional assessment data (*e.g.*, triceps skinfold measurements) should be obtained if the infant falls within the latter two categories (see Chap. 1).

2. Length or Height. Obtain infant's birth length, gestational age, present length, and length over a period of time. Recumbent length (*i.e.*, length that is measured on a table with a movable head piece and movable foot piece; see advanced nutritional texts for measuring procedures) is the measure used to assess present length in infants. Failure to measure in this manner may underestimate the infant's progress by 2 cm. To estimate the individual infant's progress against the norm, compare his findings to physical growth charts. If the findings confirm that the infant is small of stature (*i.e.*, below the 3rd percentile) he may be malnourished (however, genetic and environmental factors also influence stature).

3. Brain Growth. Head circumference measurements are used to measure how rapidly brain-cell growth is developing in the infant. It is theorized, but not proven, that a small head may indi-

cate malnutrition, which could subsequently affect central nervous system functions such as perception, attention, learning, and language development. However, the clinician should always remember that head circumference must be compared to overall size before any conclusions may be drawn. Additionally, she must remember that a head circumference that is grossly inappropriate to body size may also be a severe complication.

- Physiological and Biochemical Data
  1. Vital Signs
     a. Respiration. Low-birth-weight infants have a higher incidence of respiratory complications. Consequently, initial feedings may be delayed; the methodology, nutrient composition, and quantity of food may also need adjustment.
     b. Fever. Basal metabolic rates are escalated during fever to meet heat loss and stress alterations. Caloric and fluid intake needs to be increased.
  2. Laboratory Data
     a. Blood Analysis
        (1) Hemoglobin. Normal is 10 to 12 g/dl, but this may vary with age and hematocrit (normal, 31%–34%). Nutritional anemia is prevalent in infants who have low iron stores or low intake of iron. In addition, megaloblastic anemia may develop in infants whose mothers had low intake of folic acid and vitamin B_{12} during pregnancy.
        (2) Fasting Blood Sugar (FBS). Low levels (hypoglycemia) in an infant at birth may indicate that the mother has diabetes mellitus, had gestational diabetes, or was in poor nutritional status (*i.e.*, the flow of nutrients to the infant through the placenta was impaired) during pregnancy.
        (3) Albumin. Low levels, below 3.5 g/dl, may indicate malnutrition.
     b. Urine. An infant is unable to concentrate urine as well as an adult; therefore, excessive urination may rapidly precipitate dehydration.
     c. Stools. Excessively loose or firm stools may indicate that the methodology of feeding, nutrient composition, or quantity of the feeding needs adjustment. Abnormal stools (*e.g.*, greasy or frothy) may be indicative of celiac disease or cystic fibrosis. In these cases, major dietary adaptations are needed (see Chaps. 7 and 8 for the dietary adaptations required in these disorders).
- Clinical Evaluations. Clinical signs that an infant is probably progressing properly are steady weight gain, healthy smooth skin, firm muscles, moderate amounts of subcutaneous fat, normal tooth eruption at about 5 to 6 months with 6 to 12 teeth by 1 year, and a vig-

orous and happy outlook toward his surroundings. Clinical signs with nutritional implications that may denote poor development are given in Table 1–9.

Specific Factors
Nutritional Care Plans for Healthy Infants
Methodology of Feeding

The methodology of infant feeding is first and foremost the mother's choice. She should be encouraged to breast feed since human milk has many infant and maternal benefits, but she should not be made to feel guilty if she prefers another method of feeding. After she has made her choice, the health team and family members should offer ongoing support, encouragement, and therapeutic intervention should she encounter difficulties with her chosen feeding method.

- Feeding the Newborn
  1. Breast Feeding, Colostrum
     a. Description. A clear yellowish secretion from the breasts during the first 10 days after delivery
     b. Characteristics. In comparison to mature milk, colostrum has higher concentrations of protein, sodium, potassium, chloride, sulfur, copper, zinc, iodine, and vitamin A and lower concentrations of carbohydrate, fats, and water-soluble vitamins.
     c. Benefits of Colostrum Feeding for the Infant
        (1) Colostrum contains secretions of immunologic properties, that is, antibodies. These antibodies provide passive protection for the neonatal GI surface against microorganisms and intestinal antigens during the period before the active development of secretory immunity.
        (2) Colostrum aids in the development of digestive enzymes.
        (3) Colostrum stimulates GI peristalsis and segmentation.
        (4) Colostrum stimulates the flow of mature milk.
     d. Benefits of Colostrum Feeding for the Mother
        (1) Enhances placenta release
        (2) Helps uterus contract
        (3) Enhances mature milk flow
  2. Bottle Feeding
     a. Description. A semiclear liquid feeding of glucose and water
     b. Characteristics. A 5% glucose (D_5W) and water solution that is lower in protein and electrolytes than is colostrum is administered for 24 to 72 hours, depending upon the infant's size, followed by a formula feeding prescribed by the physician

    c. Benefits of Bottle Feeding for the Infant*

      (1) Sustains life

      (2) Provides glucose for the brain and prevents dehydration

    d. Benefits of Bottle Feeding for the Mother. Allows the infant to be nourished if the mother cannot or prefers not to breast feed

• Feeding the Older Neonate and Infant

  1. Breast Feeding, Mature Milk

    a. Description. A yellowish white opaque fluid

    b. Characteristics. Human milk is a solution composed of protein, sugar, water, and salts in which a variety of fatty compounds are suspended (see Tables 11–2 and 11–3);† its composition varies from human to human, from one period of lactation to another, from one time of day to another; also, the concentrations of some nutrients are influenced by the maternal diet and other environmental factors (*e.g.*, medications)

    c. How to Breast Feed the Infant

      (1) Hold the baby close to avoid his pulling on the nipple

      (2) Talk to and cuddle the baby while feeding

      (3) Burp the baby during and after feeding

      (4) Do not rush

      (5) See Factors that Enhance or Inhibit Lactation, Table 10–11

    d. Benefits of Human Milk for Normal Infants

      (1) Nutrient Benefits

        (a) Caloric Content. Although human milk, cow's milk, and commercial formulas may have a similar caloric content, human milk may be most beneficial to the infant because the caloric content of fore-milk and hind-milk differ, the latter having more protein and fat. It is theorized that this change in composition, during a feeding, may serve as a signal in aiding appetite control; the infant may be gradually motivated to withdraw from the breast and cease eating when satiated. Consequently, he does not overfeed, which may ultimately curtail early obesity development. Additionally, the breast-fed infant must suck harder and feed more often to obtain adequate intake; thus, he is more active and uses more energy to obtain energy, reducing his chances of obesity.

---

* If the infant has a sucking disorder, he may need nourishment by eyedropper or parenterally.

† See tables at the end of this chapter.

(b) Protein. The protein content of human milk is lower than that of cow's milk; however, the bioavailability of the protein present and the composition of the protein and amino acids differ markedly from those of cow's milk. Commercial formulas simulate the protein content and composition found in human milk as accurately as possible. Some of the protein compositional changes in human milk *versus* cow's milk that may benefit the infant are as follows:

i. The biologic value of mature human milk is higher than that of cow's milk.

ii. The reduced protein content of human milk reduces the renal solute load in the infant, reducing his chances of dehydration.

iii. The low aromatic amino acid content of human milk may reduce the amount of protein that must be metabolized by an immature liver.

iv. Human milk has a casein/albumin–globulin whey ratio of casein to lactalbumin, 40:60, *versus* casein to lactalbumin, 76:24 in cow's milk. The high lactalbumin value in human milk facilitates infant digestion because it forms a softer, smaller, more flocculent curd than does casein, which forms a tougher, larger, cheesier curd.

v. The major whey proteins in human milk, α-lactalbumin and lactoferrin with B-lactoglobulin present in insignificant amounts, may impair bacterial growth. Alpha-lactalbumin is a specific protein component of the enzyme lactose synthetase. Lactoferrin is an iron-binding protein that inhibits bacterial, especially *Escherichia coli*, multiplication.

vi. Taurine and cystine amino acids are found in higher concentrations in human milk. Taurine is important in the development and function of the brain and retina. It is also important in the conjugation of bile acids. Cystine is essential for growth and development. Conversion of methionine to cystine by cystathionase is late to develop; thus, increased amounts of cystine in breast milk facilitates growth and development. Hypermethioninemia, however, may damage the central nervous system.

vii. The amino acids that are in lower concentrations in human milk are phenylalanine and tyrosine, which, when in high concentrations, may adversely affect development of the central nervous system, especially in the premature infant.

viii. Human milk contains more nucleotides, which supply more nonprotein nitrogen (25%) *versus* cow's milk (6%). This increased concentration of nonprotein nitrogen may enhance growth and anabolism.

(c) Carbohydrates. Mature human milk contains more lactose (7%) than cow's milk (4.8%). Lactose stimulates the growth of microorganisms, which subsequently produce organic acids and synthesis of many B vitamins. Lactose also enhances the growth of fermentative rather than putrefactive bacteria in the intestinal tract. A small amount of undigested lactose in the colon is also fermented to lactic acid by Lactobacillus bifidus, a nitrogen-containing oligosaccharide in human milk that enhances the growth of lactobacillus (Table 11–4) and augments the low (acidic) *p*H of the intestines. An acidic *p*H augments lysozome stability and enhances calcium, phosphorus, magnesium, and other trace metal absorption. In addition, the osmotic effect of nondigested lactose in the colon may be the factor responsible for the loose stool characteristic of the breast-fed infant.

(d) Lipids (Including Cholesterol). The total fat content of human and whole cow's milk is similar, but the fatty acid compositon, positional distribution of the fatty acids on the triglyceride molecule, and the cholesterol content differ markedly.

i. The major fatty acids in human milk are oleic, palmitic, and linoleic acids. Linoleic acid, an essential fatty acid, constitutes approximately 10% of the fatty acids, or 5% of total calories, in human milk while the linoleate in cow's milk provides only 1% to 2% of the total calories. Linoleic acid must make up at least 2% to 3% of the dietary intake, or an essential fatty acid deficiency may develop, which is believed to be manifested in the infant as thickening and drying of the skin, eruption in the diaper area, and eczema. Additionally, linoleic and linolenic acids are converted to long-chain polyunsaturated fatty acids (PUFAs). These PUFAs are important for cell membrane and prostaglandin synthesis.

Note, however, that the fat content of human milk, with the exception of cholesterol, can be influenced by the maternal diet. Commercial formulas provide adequate linoleic acid by substituting vegetable oils for butterfat.

ii. The position of fatty, especially palmitic, acids on the glycerol molecule to form a triglyceride is different in human milk. This positional difference seems to enhance fat absorption and digestion. Additionally, human milk contains several fat-digesting enzymes (lipases), which may facilitate hydrolysis of milk triglycerides, further enhancing fat digestion.

iii. The length of the fatty acid chains on the triglyceride molecule in human milk is longer than that in cow's milk. This appears to perturb bacteria and virus membranes.

iv. The cholesterol content of human milk is two to three times higher than that of cow's milk and seven times higher than that of commercial formulas. It is not known whether or not the infant benefits from high cholesterol levels, but it is hypothesized that the high levels of cholesterol in human milk may enhance myelination of the central nervous system, enhance synthesis of steroid hormones and bile salts, or enhance regulation of the feedback mechanism that controls the buildup and breakdown of cholesterol in the cell. It is suspected, but not proven, that this enhanced regulation may lead to lower plasma cholesterol levels throughout the life cycle.

(e) Minerals. The mineral content of human milk is approximately three times lower than that of cow's milk, and the relative amounts of various elements differ (*e.g.,* the copper concentration is higher and the calcium concentration is lower in human milk), as does the bioavailability of some minerals (*e.g.,* iron). The following details the differences of the minerals of greatest concern.

i. Iron. The concentration of iron in human milk is approximately 0.3 mg/liter of mature human milk until 5 to 6 months of age. This concentration is lower than the iron concentration of cow's milk (0.5 mg/liter), and commercial formulas (1.4 mg to 12.5 mg/liter if fortified). However, 49% of the iron in human milk is absorbed while only 10% of cow's milk iron is absorbed. Supplementation of iron before 4 to 6 months of age is recommended by some clinicians (*e.g.*, Fomon recommends 7 mg ferrous sulfate/day), but not by others, to prevent nutritional anemia in the infant.

ii. Zinc. Human milk contains less zinc, 1.8 mg, than does cow's milk, 3.9 mg; however, its bioavailability is higher than in cow's milk. Zinc enhances growth and development.

iii. Calcium and Phosphorus. Human milk contains the more desirable calcium-to-phosphorus ratio, which is 2:1. This ratio appears to augment the infant's growth, bone and tooth development, normal cellular functions, and enzymatic reactions. Formulas have a calcium-to-phosphorus ratio of close to 1:1 or 1:1.5, which may induce neonatal hypocalcemia and convulsions and possibly postnatal rickets and tetany.

iv. Fluoride. The concentration of fluoride in human milk is not believed to be high enough to protect against caries later in life. Consequently, supplementation is recommended.

v.   Sodium, Potassium, and Chloride. Human milk concentrations of these electrolytes are approximately three times lower than the concentrations in cow's milk. The beneficial effect of these lower levels is a reduced renal solute load in the infant.

(f) Vitamins. Human milk from a healthy, well-nourished mother supplies sufficient levels of vitamins for the infant, with the possible exception of vitamin D.

i.   Water-Soluble Vitamin Concentrations. The concentration of vitamins, especially water-soluble vitamins, in human milk may be influenced by maternal diet or maternal nutritional status (*i.e.*, the extent of maternal stores). The vitamin of most concern in maternal diet and stores is vitamin B_{12}, because concentrations can be minimal or lacking in vegan mothers. This inadequacy can induce pernicious anemia in the infant and mother if supplements are not administered. Other supplements, especially folic acid and vitamin C, may also be needed if maternal intake is low. However, it is more beneficial to enhance the mother's dietary intake of nutrient-dense foods than to give supplements to the infant, whenever possible.

ii. Fat-Soluble Vitamin Concentrations. Concentrations of fat-soluble vitamins are influenced less by maternal diet, but low concentrations, especially of vitamin A, have been observed when the maternal diet has a low fat content. Infant vitamin E requirements are generally met by human milk unless maternal intake of polyunsaturated fats is excessively high. Infants fed commercial formulas that are not fortified with vitamin E will need vitamin E supplements, since the fat content of these formulas is predominantly polyunsaturated vegetable oils. The nonaqueous content of vitamin D in human milk is lower than that in cow's milk. Supplementation to prevent rickets, therefore, has been recommended. Recently, however, it has been found that human milk contains substantial amounts, 0.9 mg/dl, of vitamin D in the aqueous phase as a sulfate conjugate. This amount is equivalent to the concentration of vitamin D in cow's milk and formulas. Most clinicians still recommend supplementation, however.

(g) Fluids. Human milk appears to contain enough fluid to meet the infant's requirements. Cow's milk, however, is a more concentrated milk that must have water added in order to simulate human milk.

(2) Immunologic Benefits. The major anti-infective properties of human milk are found in the whey protein fraction. Some of the anti-infectious factors and their functions are presented in Table 11–4. Additionally, allergies are rare in infants fed breast milk because human milk does not contain emulsifiers or thickening agents, as do evaporated milk and commercial formulas. These may precipitate allergic reactions in hypersensitive infants. The overall benefits of the anti-infective factors found in colostrum and mature milk are lower incidences of diarrhea; respiratory diseases, including colds; generalized infections; childhood diseases; ear infections; necrotizing enterocolitis; and hospitalization.

(3) Anatomical Benefits

(a) The infant, not the mother, controls the flow of milk, which may prevent swallowing difficulties and subsequent speech and dental problems that develop later in life.

    (b) Milk cannot enter the eustachian canals when the infant is held, as it can when the infant is fed on its back with the bottle propped. Consequently, the incidence of otitis media (inflammation of the middle ear) is reduced.

    (c) Breast-fed infants usually have lower weight gain during the first year of life than formula-fed infants. This may decrease fat cell hyperplasia and resultant obesity.

e. Contraindications for Breast Feeding

   (1) The mother has poor nutritional status. Nutrient deficiencies may develop in the infant if the quantity and quality of the mother's diet or nutrient stores are inadequate.

   (2) The infant shows signs of a malnutrition that has been induced by inadequate quantities of breast milk, primary sucking disorder, or an appetite control deficiency. If the malnutrition is not corrected by adequate caloric and nutrient intake, marked cachexia and hypernatremia dehydration may develop, which could lead to a central nervous system insult.

   (3) The mother is exposed to excessive quantities of environmental chemicals such as chlorinated hydrocarbon insecticides (DDT), polychlorinated biphenyls (PCBs), and polybrominated biphenyls (PBBs).

   (4) The mother consumes excessive quantities of alcohol, nicotine, caffeine, psychoactive drugs (*e.g.,* lithium), and other medications (*e.g.,* oral contraceptives), which are transmitted in breast milk (see Table 10–10 and Chap. 10, List of Drugs Excreted in Human Milk, for the adverse effects that specific medications may have on the infant).

   (5) The infant has hyperbilirubinemia. It is theorized that some human milk shows high levels of lipoprotein lipase activity, which may increase free fatty acid concentration, which, in turn, is proposed to have an inhibitory effect on bilirubin conjugation.

   (6) The infant has a primary disease (*e.g.,* galactosemia), or gestational abnormalities are present in the infant. In these situations, the quantity and quality of the nutrients in breast milk may aggravate the disorder. In most conditions, however, especially gestational abnormalities, breast milk may be given along with other supplementary feedings, if desired.

   (7) The mother has several other small children or is pregnant.

   (8) The mother is overanxious, does not have the desire to breast feed, or cannot breast feed conveniently because she is employed outside the home. In these situations, the

mother may transmit feelings of hostility and anxiety to the infant, not feelings of love. Bottle feeding and having other people help with feedings may be more beneficial to the infant.

    f. Benefits of Breast Feeding for the Mother

        (1) *Uterine contraction* is hastened by the release of oxytocin, a hormone that facilitates milk ejection and also enhances uterine contractions.

        (2) *Return to pre-pregnancy weight,* if desired, is accelerated since maternal fat stores are used for milk production.

        (3) *Nutrient quantity and quality* seem to be adjusted to infant needs (*e.g.,* easier to digest, absorb, and excrete); thus, infant may be more content.

        (4) It is *more economical* than commercial formula feeding, even though the mother must consume more food to enhance milk production.

        (5) It is *convenient.* Milk is always available, no preparation time is necessary, and temperature is controlled.

2. Bottle Feeding, Full-Strength Formula

    a. Description. Milk-based formulas or substitute-milk-based formulas are fed through a bottle. Generally, the amount and type of formula to be used for feeding the newborn is prescribed by the physician. Various factors are considered in this selection: the infant's gestational age and intrauterine growth, the infant's sex, infant and maternal complications, caloric and nutrient needs to reach and maintain optimal growth and development, fluid needs, cost, ease of preparation, and availability.

    b. Classifications. There are three basic formulas:

        (1) Modified cow's milk, that is, evaporated whole cow's milk that has added water and sugar

        (2) Prepared commercial formulas, which are available in a variety of forms: powdered, concentrated-liquid, and ready-to-feed

        (3) Milk-substitute commercially prepared formulas that are made to meet the needs of infants with complications who require elimination of cow's milk

    c. Characteristics

        (1) Evaporated whole cow's milk formulas contain sterilized evaporated milk (see Sample Evaporated Milk Formula). This heat treatment produces a finer curd and a more digestible fat. Water must be added in proportions of 1.5 ml:1 kcal in order to produce a reduced renal solute load. Sugar is added in the form of dextrose or corn syrup in

order to simulate the high sugar content of human milk. Evaporated milk is usually fortified with vitamin D, but supplements of some B-complex vitamins such as folic acid and pyridoxine may be needed. These vitamins are readily destroyed by heat.

Sample Evaporated Milk Formula

A 7-lb (3.2-kg) infant requires 100–130 kcal/kg/day or 320–384 kcal

Ingredient	Amount
Evaporated milk ———————	1 oz/lb or 7 oz
Sugar (corn syrup or lactose) ——	1 tbsp for every 5 oz milk; Total, 1½ tbsps
Water —————————————	Added in quantities that allow the infant to obtain 2¼ oz total formula/lb/day
	7-lb baby × 2¼ oz = 16 oz total
	9 oz water added +
	7 oz milk = 16 oz
	divided by 6 feedings = 2⅔ oz per feeding

(2) Prepared commercial formulas are made to simulate human milk as nearly as possible. The nutrient and caloric levels of these formulas are regulated by the American Academy of Pediatrics and the Food and Drug Administration. During commercial preparation, these formulas have been modified in the following ways: milk protein has been denatured and diluted to produce a softer, more flocculent curd, which is more easily digested by the infant, and to reduce the renal solute load. Dilution also reduces the calcium concentration. Butterfat may be removed and vegetable oils used as a substitute. This adjustment increases the amount of unsaturated fatty acid, particularly the essential fatty acid, linoleic acid. Fat in this form appears to be better digested and absorbed than is butterfat. Dialysis may also be used to reduce the sodium content of cow's milk. Milk dilution, however, may reduce the caloric level of the milk; consequently, additional lactose is added in order to simulate the caloric content, 20 kcal/oz, of human milk. Vitamins and minerals are added in quantities that simulate human milk or eliminate the need for additional supplementation (see Tables 11–5 and 11–6 for specific formula ingredients and nutrient content).

(3) Milk Substitutes. Commercially prepared formulas are used when infants are born with a sensitivity to the prote-

ins in cow's milk. This sensitivity may cause irritability or violent illness. Several commercial preparations have been devised that contain no cow's milk at all. The proteins substituted are soybeans (*e.g.,* Prosobee) and meat proteins (*e.g.,* MBF). They may also be used when one or more amino acids must be removed (*e.g.,* Lofenalac). Additionally, milk substitute formulas may be used when an infant has a lactose intolerance or galactosemia. In these conditions, cow's milk is removed from the formula. Soy isolates replace the milk protein, and corn syrup or sucrose replaces the lactose (*e.g.,* Prosobee and Isomil, see Table 11–5). All substitute milk formulas are properly supplemented with adequate quantities of substitute nutrients, to replace those that are removed; therefore, they simulate human milk as accurately as possible (see Table 11–5 for specific formulas).

d. Preparation of the Formula. Formula is sterilized to minimize bacterial growth and to provide a finer curd. Overheating, however, will denature the protein and destroy water-soluble vitamins, especially vitamin B_6. If formulas require added water, only the amount recommended should be added because too much water may cause overhydration and too little, dehydration in the infant. Sterilization is accomplished by the following methods:

(1) Terminal Sterilization. Clean bottles are filled with formula and then sterilized (placed in boiling water for 25 min). This is the most popular method; it is easiest and reduces the chances of formula contamination and water loss during preparation.

(2) Aseptic Method. The bottles, nipples, and all equipment used in preparation are sterilized by being boiled in water for a specified length of time. Tap water, if used in the formula, is boiled for 5 minutes. Formula is added after the equipment is clean. The chances of contaminating the formula are higher than with terminal sterilization. Water often boils away, breaking bottles or destroying nipples. The likelihood of touching and contaminating nipples is increased.

(3) Clean Method. Formula is poured into clean, not sterilized, bottles so that the chances of contamination are increased.

(4) Newer methods of placing sterilized formula into disposable bottles may be used. Caution should be exercised, however, to minimize chances of contamination when the formula is poured into the bottle.

    e. Preparation of Formula Prior to Feeding

       (1) If formula has been stored in the refrigerator, it may be heated to room temperature. The mother should test the temperature by shaking a few drops on her wrist. (If the mother's wrist is toughened to heat, the formula may burn the infant's tongue.)

       (2) Place refrigerated bottles in pan of hot water before feeding.

       (3) Older infants may tolerate cold formula without heating.

    f. Feeding the Formula

       (1) Hold, cuddle, and talk to the infant. Do not prop the bottle, which impairs emotional contact and increases the chances of aspiration.

       (2) Check nipple, but do not touch it, before feeding to make sure that the milk flow is not too slow or too fast.

       (3) Hold the bottle up so that air does not accumulate in the nipple.

       (4) Always burp the infant during and after a feeding.

       (5) Do not rush.

       (6) Throw away leftover formula.

       (7) Do not force infant to finish the bottle. This encourages overfeeding, which may lead to obesity.

       (8) Do not allow bottles filled with formula or juice to remain in the crib overnight. This induces caries. Substitute water.

       (9) Do not habitually give an infant a bottle to pacify him. This encourages using food as an emotional pacifier throughout life. Substitute love or use other means (*e.g.,* activity) as a diversion.

    g. Benefits of Bottle Feeding Over Breast Feeding for the Infant*

       (1) Nutrient compositions of commercial formulas can be adjusted to individual needs when complications exist.

       (2) Most commercial formulas are similar to breast milk, so they can be used if the mother becomes ill or is unavailable.

    h. Disadvantages of Bottle Feeding (Instead of Breast Feeding) for the Infant

       (1) The major anti-infective properties found in human milk are not found in formulas.

---

* A bottle feeding offered with love, warmth, and responsiveness to the infant's needs does not impair an infant's chances for normal psychological development.

(2) If cow's milk formulas are used, the high protein content may induce hyperammonemia, vomiting, and coma. The high protein content of cow's milk may also induce GI bleeding in the infant, with subsequent iron loss and anemia.

(3) Sucking mechanisms to procure food through the artificial nipple may differ; consequently, swallowing difficulties that impair tooth placement may develop.

(4) If sucrose is added instead of lactose, the infant may develop a "sweet tooth," because sucrose tastes sweeter than lactose in equal quantities. Additionally, the sweet taste may increase consumption and precipitate obesity.

(5) If a low-volume concentrated formula is consumed, resulting in a high renal solute load, adverse symptoms such as oliguria, weight loss, fever, and hypernatremia may develop.

(6) If the formula is overheated, some nutrients may be destroyed or the water content may not be adequate.

(7) The amount of feeding consumed can be controlled by the mother, not the infant, which can precipitate obesity.

i. Benefits of Bottle Feeding for the Mother. The mother does not have to be available for every feeding, and the father can participate in feeding.

j. Disadvantages of Bottle Feeding (Instead of Breast Feeding) for the Mother

(1) Uterine contraction is delayed.

(2) Postpartum weight loss may be impaired.

(3) Formula may not be as easily digested or absorbed; thus the infant may be colicky, constipated, or irritable or spit up frequently.

(4) Time must be set aside to procure and prepare the formula. Improper preparation may cause contamination and adverse symptoms in the infant such as vomiting, diarrhea, fever, and dehydration.

Caloric and Nutrient Increases During Normal Infancy

• Calories. Caloric requirements are greater during infancy than at any other time during the life cycle. Consequently, the caloric requirements per unit of body weight are much higher than in the adult. Generally an AGA infant thrives when he consumes 150 to 200 ml/kg/day of milk for the first 6 months. The energy procured by the infant who consumes this amount of human milk, or its equivalent, is approximately 100 to 130 kcal/kg/day. This estimate is based on the premise that the average caloric density of human milk is 67 kcal/ml, or 20 kcal/oz, for pooled human milk. The macronutrient distribution in infant feedings to provide these caloric needs is given in Tables 11–2 and 11–3.

The approximate difference between the caloric needs of an infant, 100 to 130 kcal/kg/day, and an adult, 30 to 35 kcal/kg/day, is 70 to 100 kcal/kg/day. The infant's caloric requirements are increased to meet his escalated caloric expenditures (Table 11–7). But as an infant matures, his caloric requirements decrease; therefore, his caloric intake from 6 months to 1 year should be 90 to 100 kcal/kg/day.

- Protein. Protein requirements are increased during infancy to provide the nitrogen needed for synthesis of new tissue, maturation of tissue, and maintenance of already existing tissue. In order to meet these needs, the recommended intake for an infant under 6 months of age is 2.2 g/kg/day of protein. From 6 months to 1 year, this intake should be reduced to 2.0 g/kg/day and, after 1 year, to 1 to 1.5 g/kg/day. Human milk contains approximately 1.2 g of protein/100 ml of milk. Therefore, if a 7-lb (3.2-kg) baby consumes his recommended fluid intake of 150 to 200 ml/kg/day (150 ml × 3.2 = 480 ml, 200 ml × 3.2 = 640 ml), he will obtain his protein requirement of 5.76 to 7.68 g/day (2.2 g × 3.2 = 7.04 g/day).

This amount of protein is adequate to meet the infant's needs but not excessive enough to overload his immature kidneys. Cow's milk, however, supplies 3.3 g of protein/100 ml of milk, which leads to an excessive renal solute load, which can precipitate dehydration without dilution. In addition, the high protein content of cow's milk can induce enteric bleeding, which can subsequently lead to anemia if the milk is not diluted properly. Sterilization of cow's milk does not alleviate this complication. The content of protein in commercially prepared formulas is similar to that concentration in human milk.

Table 11–7
**Estimated Caloric Expenditures
of an Infant Until 6 Months of Age**

Caloric Expenditure Category	Caloric Expenditure per Kilogram of Body Weight
Resting caloric expenditure	50–50
Activity	10–25
Growth	20–35
Others (calories wasted in stools, increased heat losses due to an increased surface area/lb, the thermogenic effect of food utilization formerly called the *specific dynamic action* [SDA])	20–20
Total daily caloric expenditure	100–130

- Carbohydrates and Fats. Carbohydrates and fats are required by the infant to meet his caloric needs, but there are no recommended daily allowances for these two nutrients for the infant or the adult. It is recommended, however, that lactose, not sucrose, be the chief source of carbohydrate energy, because it has beneficial effects in the infant's intestines. It is also recommended that polyunsaturated fats, which contain linoleic acid, not saturated fats, be the chief source of fat energy. It must also be remembered that fats are needed to transport fat-soluble vitamins (A, D, E, and K).

- Vitamins and Minerals. All vitamins and minerals are increased during infancy in proportion to body weight in order to promote growth and development and act as coenzymes and cofactors in enzymatic reactions that enhance body functions and energy production. Most clinicians agree that these increased infant needs can be met if a mother who is breast feeding eats a varied, nutrient-dense, calorically adequate diet or if an infant is fed an evaporated milk formula that is fortified or a commercially prepared formula that simulates the composition of human milk or is fortified, when the simulation is not possible. Meeting these requirements without supplementation, however, is difficult because the composition of human milk reflects maternal dietary intake, especially the concentration of water-soluble vitamins, fat-soluble vitamin A, sodium, and fatty acids which also alters vitamin E requirements. The nutrient concentrations affected the least by maternal diet are calcium, iron, and cholesterol. Consequently, if the mother does not eat a properly balanced diet consistently, her milk may have an inadequate supply of some nutrients.

  Since human milk differs from mother to mother, the optimal formula and fortification standards for each individual infant become difficult to determine. Therefore, most clinicians, but not all, recommend that the following factors be considered before nutrient supplements are given to the infant:

1. The nutritional status of the infant and mother
2. The anticipated dietary intake of the mother (*e.g.*, is she a vegetarian?)
3. What solid foods will be introduced to the infant when he is weaned
4. The projected nutrient composition of these foods

   After assimilating this information, clinicians can then decide when and what types of vitamins and minerals should supplement the infant's diet. The general pattern of supplementation agreed upon by most clinicians at present is listed below:

1. Iron. Newborn infants who are breast fed should be given 7 mg of ferrous sulfate, or its equivalent, each day as a dietary supplement in order to assure a daily iron absorption of 0.5 mg (10% absorption rate). Other clinicians do not recommend this supple-

mentation until 4 to 6 months of age because they claim that additional iron may saturate the bacteriostatic protein in human milk, lactoferrin, which could ultimately reduce its effectiveness. Iron also may induce adverse symptoms such as constipation, vomiting, diarrhea, tooth discoloration, and zinc deficiency syndromes, since iron impairs zinc absorption. When the infant reaches 4 to 6 months of age, however, clinicians generally agree that the infant should receive iron supplements because his iron stores may be low or depleted by then. Iron-fortified cereals, meats with heme iron, or artificial supplements can be used to supply iron requirements. Cow's milk should not be introduced until later because it may cause enteric bleeding with subsequent iron loss. Infants fed commercially prepared formulas will not usually need supplementation, because most of these formulas are already fortified.

2. Fluoride. Most clinicians agree that infants fed breast milk, cow's milk, and commercially prepared formulas should be given 0.25 ml/day of fluoride as a dietary supplement, even though tap water may be fluorinated.

3. Vitamin K. Most clinicians recommend parenteral administration of vitamin K in newborns in order to prevent hemorrhagic disease. This practice is advocated because microbial production of vitamin K in the colon may be impaired, in the sterile gut of the infant, for several days.

4. Vitamin D. Most clinicians recommend that an infant who is breast fed or one who is fed an unfortified formula be given 400 IU (10 μg)/day of vitamin D as a dietary supplement, especially if the infant has very little exposure to the sun. This supplementation is still practiced at present, despite the recent finding of a water-soluble form of vitamin D in breast milk. Vitamin D supplementation is recommended in order to limit the occurrence of infantile rickets. Levels higher than those recommended may induce calcification of the soft tissues and renal complications.

   Multivitamin supplementation is usually recommended for the premature infant since his milk or formula consumption, or both, may be only one third that of the full-term infant.

• Fluid. Fluid needs in normal healthy infants are increased by 50% over adult needs. The fluid-to-calorie ratio, then, in infants is 1.5 ml/kcal instead of the 1 ml/kcal ratio recommended for adults. To meet these additional needs, the infant must consume approximately 150 ml/100 kcal (5 oz)/kg/day. This amount of fluid and the appropriate fluid-to-calorie ratio are provided by breast milk (67 kcal/100 ml), if the mother consumes adequate fluids and calories daily (see Chap. 10 for calorie, nutrient, and fluid requirements during lactation). Fluid intake can also be met by cow's milk and commercially prepared formulas if they are diluted according to directions. Increased intake of fluids is needed in the infant to maintain growth; to replace losses from the GI tract in the form of metabolized wastes (stools), from the urinary tract (inability to concentrate urine), and from the skin (greater surface area in relation to body weight than in adults); and to dilute and excrete the renal solute load, which is, collectively, the end product of protein metabolism (urea) and the electrolytes sodium, chloride, and potassium.

Nutrients Decreased During Normal Infancy

There are no recommended nutrient decreases for infants. However, most clinicians recommend that excessive intake of refined sugars and of carbohydrates in the form of complex carbohydrates (young infants do not have a sufficient supply of pancreatic amylase to hydrolyze large quantities of complex carbohydrates, *e.g.*, cereals) be curtailed. They also recommend that sodium and fat intake be limited.

Dietary Adaptations for a Full-Term Healthy Infant

- Early infancy (4–6 months)
  1. Feed the infant breast milk, evaporated milk formula, or commercially prepared formulas. Skim milk formulas are not recommended (see Table 11–2; see Table 11–1 for the approximate quantities of milk a growing infant should consume during the first 6 months of life).
  2. Avoid introducing solid foods during this time because they reduce the infant's desire to breast feed, thus reducing the volume of milk produced, and because the infant's neuromuscular ability to cope with solid foods is not properly developed (see List of Developmental Signs that relate to infant feeding).

Developmental Signs With Feeding Implications

Birth–3 months

Rooting reflex (turns mouth toward any object that brushes the cheek, including the nipple)

Sucks and swallows

Tongue thrusts when fed by spoon

Random motion of hands

Unable to sit, even with support

4–6 months

Sucking becomes voluntary

Extrusion reflex diminishes; back-and-forth tongue movements begin

Lip closure develops, allowing infant to take some fluid from a cup

Reaches for and grasps an object
Learns to close hands over the bottle
Hand-to-mouth movements begin
Sits supported

6–12 months

Chewing ability develops
Voluntarily brings hands to mouth
Feeds with fingers
Can handle cup and some utensils without assistance
Sits alone, creeps, crawls, or walks

(After Hinton SM, Kerwin DR: Maternal, Infant, and Child Nutrition: A Resource Book for Health Professionals. Chapel Hill, NC, Health Services Consortium, 1981)

3. A breast-fed infant should receive supplements of vitamin D, fluoride, and iron if prescribed by the physician.

4. Wean the baby gradually to minimize infant and maternal discomfort. Eliminate the least favorite feeding first, then wait a few days before eliminating another feeding. Substitute milk in a cup if the child is developmentally ready. If not, give a bottle.

- Later Infancy (6 months–1 year). If the child is developmentally ready at 4 to 6 months of age, introduce solid foods (Table 11–8). Complementary feeding is likely to be required sooner by a boy than by a girl, mainly because of differing size and growth rates.

- Guidelines for Introducing New Foods

1. Introduce a single-ingredient food first (*e.g.*, iron-fortified rice cereal), either homemade or commercially prepared. Thereafter, only one new food a week should be offered. This facilitates detecting a food intolerance.

2. Hold the child while introducing solid foods so that the experience is similar to breast or bottle feeding.

3. Initially dilute solid food to make it fairly liquid—the consistency of smooth cream soup. Gradually change the consistency to a more solid one as the infant learns to propel food to the back of his mouth with his tongue.

4. Increase the infant's fluid intake because solid foods have more protein and electrolytes than does breast milk or formula; thus, they increase the renal solute load.

   a. If juices are added, as a means of increasing the fluid intake, offer them only in a cup. Offering fruit juices in a bottle increases the likelihood of developing caries, owing to the increased time that bacteria and sucrose may remain on the teeth.

b. If water is given in a bottle, avoid using honey on the nipple, because this enhances caries production, and because honey has been known to induce botulism in infants.

5. Introduce new foods before offering the breast or bottle.

6. Introduce new foods in small portions (*e.g.*, teaspoons) at the meal the child enjoys most, and only when he is rested.

7. If the infant rejects a new food (*i.e.*, he appears to dislike the texture [*e.g.*, Jell-O]), offer it again in a few days. If he continually rejects a new food, respect his wishes and offer another food of equivalent nutrient density. Keep in mind that an infant has more taste buds than does an adult; thus, foods may taste differently to him than they do to the mother.

8. To enhance the infant's consumption and swallowing reflex, place food well back on the tongue, using a small blunt-ended spoon.

9. Establish good eating habits. Do not add salt, fat, or sugar (unless caloric needs are increased for activity) to home-prepared or commercial foods. Natural flavors, enjoyed early, enhance life-long good eating habits.

10. Give a variety of foods, after tolerance is established, in order to ensure that nutrient balances and intake are adequate.

11. Offer the child small amounts of foods frequently, rather than large amounts of foods at one sitting. Keep in mind that a newborn infant's stomach capacity for food is only 2 tablespoons and that of an infant aged 1 year is only 1 cup (an adult's capacity is 2 quarts). Consequently, if you offer too much food, the child becomes frustrated and irritable. These emotions precipitate maternal distress, and the meal hour becomes a time for "battle."

12. As a child's development increases from 6 months to a year, offer him foods that he can chew, feel with his hands (this is no time for table manners), and consume without maternal assistance (*e.g.*, zwieback or dry toast). The latter also enhances dexterity.

13. Do not offer foods that are difficult to consume (*e.g.*, peas) until the child is developmentally ready in order to limit frustration.

• Usual Sequence of Introducing New Solid Foods. Strained enriched iron-fortified cereals → mild-flavored strained fruits and juices (except orange juice, which may cause allergic reactions) → strained mild-flavored vegetables → strained meats and egg yolks (avoid egg whites, which may cause allergic reactions) → finger foods (*e.g.*, dry breads) → puddings → mixed dishes, either junior foods or appropriate ones from the table → solid foods from the table that are bland, easy to chew (cut in small pieces), and free of nuts, seeds, raisins, and bones.

- Preparing Foods at Home. If a mother wants to prepare her own baby foods at home in a blender, food mill, or food processor, she should follow these guidelines:

1. Start with a single food

2. Properly cook all foods to ensure tenderness and enhance digestibility

3. Limit nutrient destruction by
   a. Using as little water as possible when cooking vegetables or fruits; use leftover fluid to enhance consistency
   b. Not overcooking
   c. Cutting up foods just before blenderizing, not storing them cut-up
   d. Refrigerating all foods that are to be used for future feedings
   e. Preparing servings in small portions to avoid having to use leftovers

4. Limit bacterial contamination of home-prepared foods by
   a. Using only fresh unspoiled or undamaged foods
   b. Thoroughly cleaning, washing, and trimming all foods and thoroughly cleaning all equipment
   c. Properly cooking foods before blenderizing to inactivate undesirable enzymes or bacteria
   d. Preparing foods in small portions and refrigerating immediately (ice-cube trays are good guides to serving sizes and allow proper storage of frozen foods)
   e. Refrigerating all foods that are not eaten by the baby immediately; better still, avoid leftovers by making small portions that can be eaten in one meal and freeze the rest (keep in mind that babies dehydrate rapidly if vomiting or diarrhea is induced by food contamination)

5. Choose different foods from the Basic Four Food Groups, after tolerance is tested, to introduce variety and ensure nutrient density

6. Avoid adding salt, sugar, honey, or fat, which add extra calories and introduce inappropriate taste desires

7. Avoid beets, spinach, carrots, and collard greens, for some clinicians believe that these induce methemoglobinemia (iron becomes oxidized and is unable to transport oxygen or carbon dioxide), and infant may become cyanotic

8. Add fluids to foods to accomplish desired consistency; offer additional fluids at meals and between meals to be sure that fluid requirements are being met

Meal Plan Modifications

- Rigidity of feedings, every 3 to 4 hours, for breast-fed and bottle-fed infants is no longer considered desirable. Rigidity frustrates the infant, creating stress that enhances caloric needs, and ultimately weight gain may be impaired. Presently, it is thought that the time to feed an infant is when he is hungry, whether there are 2-, 3-, 4-, or even 5- hour intervals between feedings. Care should be taken not to confuse hunger with other emotions, however, for overfeeding may induce poor habits that ensure lifelong obesity.
- Do not introduce semisolid foods until the infant is developmentally ready (see List of Developmental Signs with Feeding Implications).
- Offer small portions of foods frequently. Remember that an infant's GI tract can assimilate only 2 tablespoons to 1 cup of food at a time.
- As the infant grows older, limit whole milk consumption to one fourth to one third of the calories, so that he will desire a sufficient quantity of various foods.
- Avoid forced feeding of a child who is no longer hungry. For instance, if an older infant appears to be eating less food as he grows older, remember that he now can participate in other activities (*e.g.*, crawling and exploring) so that his interest in food may waver.

Behavioral Modifications

1. Establish good, desirable eating patterns early
   a. Allow the child to eat only in one room, preferably the kitchen or dining room
   b. Have him rest before meals
   c. Encourage him to sit while eating in a well-balanced chair with his feet on the ground
   d. Obtain utensils that fit his body size and that he can easily manipulate without spilling or breaking; this alleviates infant and maternal frustration
   e. Adapt dish size to child's consumption capacity so that he can eat all his food without having to overeat
   f. Use hot water in some custom-made children's dishes so that food remains warm and palatable
   g. Allow child to eat leisurely but not slowly enough that he loses interest
   h. Allow child to eat with the family whenever possible, to introduce him to acceptable mealtime behavior; but do not insist on perfect manners at this time, because he needs to explore the textures, feel, color, and smell of food

2. Set a good example; remember, children mimic their parents' behavior (if Daddy refuses a food, the child will also)

3. Avoid distractions during meal hours (do not allow him to sit in front of the TV set)

4. Read labels on all commercially prepared food; remember, the first ingredient on the label signifies the food in the highest concentration (*e.g.*, buy beef and gravy junior foods, not gravy and beef junior foods, which may be mostly water); additionally, look for added ingredients that may not be necessary or beneficial (*e.g.*, monosodium glutamate)

5. Last, enjoy the infant's growing period and teach him that pleasurable eating nourishes the spirit as well as the body

Dietary Adaptations for Common Disorders During Infancy

See Table 11–9.

Nutritional Care Plans for High-Risk Infants

Low-Birth-Weight Infant (LBWI)

- Description. LBWI is a general term for all infants who weigh 2500 g or less, irrespective of the cause (*e.g.*, impaired intrauterine growth) or age of gestation (*e.g.*, fewer than 37 wk). This new term was devised when it became apparent that not all neonates of 2500 g or lower were premature or preterm (*i.e.*, fewer than 37 wk gestational age).

- Classifications and Characteristics. Widely used terms for classifying these infants further are listed below. In order to determine in which classification an infant falls, he is assessed by the pediatrician according to the Dubowitz scale, based upon both external physical and neurologic characteristics. After assessment, the pediatrician then prescribes the appropriate treatment, including feedings, that will alleviate the life-threatening disorders, sustain life, and allow the infant to "catch up" to a normal infant's growth and development pattern.

  1. Average-for-gestational-age infant (AGAI), who is also LBW. An AGAI (37–42 wk) who is fully developed for his gestational age but low in birth weight (fewer than 2500 g)

  2. Small-for-gestational-age infant (SGAI), also referred to as small for dates. A full-term or near full-term infant (37–42 wk) who is small for gestational age (*e.g.*, has an inappropriate weight gain or neurologic, structural, physiological, and biochemical development)

3. Preterm infant (PTI), formerly called a premature infant. An AGAI who is immature; that is, born before term (fewer than 37 wk), which means that the infant's weight and development is appropriate for his age but he is immature

4. Very-low-birth-weight infant (VLBI). An infant who weighs under 1500 g at birth

- Symptoms. Hypoglycemia, hypoalbuminemia, hypothermia, hypocalcemia, hyperbilirubinemia, and many respiratory disorders including hyaline membrane disease may occur; these infants also have a poorly developed GI and excretory system, tire easily, and often have sucking and swallowing disorders.

- Nutritional Care Plan. No protocol has been set for the nutritional care plans for the LBWI. Each infant has different assessment values and abilities to procure nourishment. Some infants will need to be fed parenterally if, after testing with sterile water, their respiratory and GI tracts appear too immature to handle enteral feedings. Others will need to be fed continuously with a pump or every 2 hours by nasogastric gavage if their gag reflex or ability to suck or swallow is impaired. However, the quantity of food tolerated by the infant by this feeding method may be very small; consequently, parenteral feedings may also be needed. Other infants who show no signs of respiratory distress, a normal gag and swallowing reflex, absence of abdominal distress, and acceptance of the feeding with only minimal residual volume on prefeeding aspiration may be fed small oral feedings (*e.g.*, Similac/Special Care) by an oral gastric tube feeding or a soft "preemie" nipple. In other cases, the infant may be fed human milk by bottle, breast, or gavage, or he may be fed by a combination of methods (Table 11–10). The methodology of feeding and the composition of the feeding for an LBWI constitute a complicated decision that requires constant adjustment and monitoring by specially trained members of the health team. Consequently, only a general discussion of the possible progression, types, benefits and disadvantages, and caloric and nutrient composition of these oral feedings can be discussed in this book.

1. Methodology of Feeding. Parenteral, gavage, or oral feedings (see Table 11–10), depending upon the infant's development and freedom from complications; usual feeding progression: 12 times/24 hr (every 2 hr) gavage feedings; 8 times/24 hr (every 3 hr) nipple-fed; 6 times/24 hr (every 4 hr) nipple-fed

2. Nutrients Increased. In general, all nutrients need to be increased for LBWIs, because their storage levels are low, and they need increased amounts of calories and nutrients to promote tissue synthesis and enhance the organ maturity and weight gain that did not occur during the third trimester of intrauterine growth. Additionally, the metabolic rate and body composition of infants with similar weights but dissimilar gestational ages differ;

consequently, nutrient requirements differ. Very generally, then, the recommended caloric intake of a LBWI is 110 to 150 kcal/kg/day (normal, 100–130 kcal/kg/day). The recommended macronutrient distribution to provide these calories should resemble that of a normal-term infant, which is 7% to 16% protein, 30% to 65% carbohydrate, and 40% to 55% fat. The lower protein and higher fat concentrations are recommended when the infant is unable to metabolize and excrete a high renal solute load. See Dietary Adaptations for feedings that meet these caloric requirements and special formulas (Table 11–5). Multivitamin and mineral supplements may be necessary and balances adjusted in order to enhance tissue synthesis and caloric utilization and to provide stores. See advanced nutrition texts for more detailed information on the quantity and quality of nutrients needed for a LBWI.

3. Nutrients Decreased. No nutrient decreases are recommended for the LBWI unless high intake of one nutrient impairs absorption or utilization of another (*e.g.*, vitamin E and iron imbalances). In addition, nutrient intake may have to be adjusted if a high GI osmotic load leads to other complications such as necrotizing enterocolitis (NEC).

4. Dietary Adaptations

   a. Breast feeding frequently if the infant can suck properly and gains weight steadily

   b. Bottle feeding specialized commercially prepared formulas such as Similac/Special Care and Enfamil Premature in the hospital (see Table 11–5)

   c. Combinations of bottle, breast, or gavage feedings. The infant must be monitored closely for signs of impending complications such as aspiration.

5. Meal Plan Modifications

   a. Rigid feedings are not recommended; breast-fed infants should feed on demand and bottle-fed infants should be fed as frequently as 10 times/day

   b. Feedings must be small because the infant's stomach capacity is not fully developed

   c. Excessive feeding may increase resting metabolism at the expense of growth as well as sometimes causing intestinal milk bolus obstruction

Large-for-Gestational-Age Infant (LGAI) and Postmature Infant

• Descriptions
  LGAI. An infant who weighs more than 3300 g at 40 weeks' gestation

Postmature or post-term infant. An infant born after 42 weeks' gestation

- Characteristics. The infant usually weighs more than 3300 g at birth. He may have signs of hypoglycemia or other adverse symptoms if the mother had gestational or traditional diabetes mellitus (see gestational diabetes in Chap. 10 and diabetes mellitus in Chap. 5).
- Nutritional Care Plan. See nutritional care plan for healthy infants. Maintain caloric intake at lowest possible level advised to ensure normal growth and development. See rationales and dietary adaptations for obesity (Table 11–9) and nutritional care plans for obesity (Chap. 6). See nutritional care plans for gestational diabetes (Chap. 10) and diabetes mellitus (Chap. 5).

Dietary Adaptations for Acute Diarrhea

The essential elements of nutritional care for acute diarrhea in infants are the following:

1. Replacement of electrolytes (*e.g.*, sodium, chloride, potassium) and base (bicarbonate or lactate)
2. Replacement of fluid and other nutrient losses
3. Maintenance and prevention of further tissue catabolism, including the intestinal mucosa
4. A progression of feeding that prevents further nutrient losses or dehydration such as
   a. Intravenous feedings of glucose, water, and electrolytes if the infant is not vomiting
   b. Hyperalimentation if infant is losing additional nutrients and fluids through vomitus as well as stools (see Chap. 2 for the caloric, nutrient, and fluid content of parenteral feedings)
   c. Oral feedings
      (1) Give an oral rehydration solution. The solution recommended by the World Health Organization is similar to an intravenous infusion but it may be administered by the enteral route. The formula packet (see reference) should be mixed with 1 liter of the cleanest available water. Give other liquids and solids as tolerated.
      (2) See mild diarrhea feeding progression, Table 11–9
   d. If infant shows signs of lactose intolerance such as abdominal cramping, give soy-based, lactose-free formulas such as Isomil and Prosobee (see Table 11–5)

Anemia

Folic Acid Deficiency Megaloblastic Anemia

See Chapter 10. Folic acid deficiency may be induced in breast-fed infants if the mother consumes excessive quantities of alcohol. It may also be induced in formula-fed infants, especially those who are fed evaporated milk formulas that have been overheated. Dietary adaptations are to

- Give folic acid supplements during pregnancy to prevent depleted stores in infants
- Limit intake of alcoholic beverages by the mother
- Supplement the infant's diet with 4 μg of folacin/100 kcal/day if the infant is fed unfortified milk formulas
- Give folacin-fortified cereals to the older infant

Pernicious Anemia

A form of megaloblastic anemia induced by a vitamin B_{12} deficiency (see Chap. 10). The mother may have had inadequate intake of vitamin B_{12} during pregnancy; thus infant stores are low. Additionally, if a mother with low levels of vitamin B_{12} breast feeds, the infant's intake of vitamin B_{12} may be insufficient. Dietary adaptations are to

- Advise mother to take 1 to 1.5 μg of vitamin B_{12} daily throughout pregnancy and lactation; supplements may be taken orally or parenterally
- Give parenteral injections or oral supplements of vitamin B_{12} to infants if stores and intake are low

Hemolytic Anemia

Enhanced Breakdown of Red Blood Cells. Vitamin E stores in the infant are low or depleted at birth; this is especially prevalent in the LBWI. Dietary adaptations are

- A supplement of 0.5 mg/kg/day of alpha-tocopherol, especially for premature infants
- Limited iron supplementation if high intake impairs vitamin E absorption

Nutritional Anemia

See Table 11–9 and Chapter 10

Malabsorption Syndromes*

Celiac Disease

Nutritional care plans used for the dietary treatment of celiac disease are discussed in Chapter 7.

Cystic Fibrosis

Nutritional care plans used for the dietary treatment of cystic fibrosis are discussed in Chapter 8.

---

*Other malabsorption syndromes are beyond the scope of this book.

Inborn Errors of Metabolism

Phenylketonuria (PKU)

- Description. An inborn error in the metabolism of the essential amino acid phenylalanine
- Characteristics. High blood levels of phenylalinine (Phe) in excess of 20 mg/dl (normal, 1–3 mg/dl) and phenylpyruvic acid in the urine (normal, 0–trace) are evident as soon as the infant ingests milk. The common defect responsible for these raised blood levels is a lack of the hepatic enzyme phenylalanine hydroxylase which converts Phe, in excess of the quantity required from structural proteins, to tyrosine. Consequently, when blood levels are excessive, Phe is metabolized by its alternate pathway to phenylpyruvic acid, which is spilled into the urine; thus the name *phenylketonuria.*
- Symptoms. Light-colored skin and hair, irritability, and hyperactivity that leads to convulsive seizures or mental retardation if left untreated
- Nutritional Care Plan
    1. Goal. To provide the infant's daily requirements of calories, protein (including enough Phe for tissue synthesis), and all other nutrients to promote optimal structural, physiological, and mental development
    2. Methodology. Oral feedings
    3. Nutrients Increased. Carbohydrates and fats to enhance caloric intake and spare proteins for tissue synthesis
    4. Nutrients Decreased. The content of phenylalanine in the diet is limited to a prescribed level the infant can tolerate. Tolerance means that the plasma levels of Phe are maintained at approximately 4 to 8 mg/dl for the first year, 6 to 14 mg/dl from 1 to 4 years, and 10 to 20 mg/dl above 4 years of age. The usual tolerance level ranges from 250 to 500 mg/Phe/day. However, if serum Phe levels decrease below 2 mg/dl, as the result of excessively stringent dietary restrictions, growth retardation and generalized malnutrition may develop. Consequently, the dietary intake of Phe must be continuously revised as the infant grows in order to maintain optimal, but not excessive, blood levels of Phe.
    5. Dietary Adaptations
        a. Infants are given a commercially prepared formula (Lofenalac), from which 95% of the phenylalanine has been removed. Lofenalac contains unsaturated fat, carbohydrate, and all the vitamins, minerals, and amino acids (including tyrosine, but only a small amount of Phe) that are required by the infant (see Table 11–5).
        b. Small amounts of milk or other formula may be mixed with the Lofenalac in order to provide the essential quantity of Phe needed for tissue synthesis.

    c. As the infant grows older, Phenyl-Free may be substituted for Lofenalac to meet energy needs (see Table 11–5). In addition, solid foods that contain low amounts of Phe such as tapioca and fruit ices are added to the diet to meet increased caloric and nutrient growth needs. However, other foods with high levels of Phe will have to be eliminated completely (*e.g.*, milk).

  6. Meal Plan Modifications. Daily meals are planned by the use of food exchange lists that relate to the phenylalanine, protein, and kilocalorie content of common foods. See advanced nutritional texts and diet manuals for the use of these exchange lists.

- Behavioral Modifications
  1. Blood plasma must be analyzed frequently.
  2. All foods taken by the infant must be recorded to ensure that calories and nutrients, including Phe, are adequate to meet growth and development needs.
  3. Most foods must be prepared and consumed at home to assure that the daily Phe intake is being met but not exceeded.
  4. All food labels must be read; for example, the new artificial sweetener aspartame is composed of two amino acids, phenylalanine and aspartame. High intake of this substance could unbalance the recommended Phe blood level.

Galactosemia

- Description. An inherited disorder caused by a deficiency of four enzymes essential to the normal conversion of galactose into glucose in the body
- Characteristics. Inadequate breakdown of galactose to glucose and intermittent galactosuria, commonly caused by the lack of the enzyme galactose 1-phosphate uridyl transferase; without this enzyme or other galactose-metabolizing enzymes, galactose metabolites such as galactose 1-phosphate accumulate abnormally in the body, causing tissue damage that precipitates chronic nutritional failure plus severe liver and brain damage (which can result in mental retardation)
- Early Symptoms. Vomiting, diarrhea, growth failure, and possibly infantile cataracts
- Nutritional Care Plan
  1. Goal. Maintenance of the erythrocyte level of galactose 1-phosphate at lower than 3 mg/dl and the reduction of urinary galactose to below 10 mg/dl
  2. Methodology. Oral feedings
  3. Nutrients Increased. All those that promote "catch up" growth (*e.g.*, protein) if the infant has deteriorated after birth because of

the disorder; supplements of calcium, vitamin D, and riboflavin may also be needed by the older infant if milk substitutes are not consumed

4. Nutrients Decreased. Carbohydrates that contain lactose that can be hydrolyzed to galactose (*e.g.,* milk sugar), plus all other carbohydrates that contain galactose directly, such as organ meats (*e.g.,* liver, pancreas, and brain)

5. Dietary Adaptations
   a. Soybean milk (*e.g.,* Prosobee) substituted for breast milk, cow's milk, or milk-based formulas
   b. As infant grows, all solid, commercially prepared infant foods that contain milk or milk solids plus all other products that contain milk such as ice cream, milk sherbets, cheese, breads, casseroles, and luncheon meats must be eliminated
   c. In severe cases, all food that contains traces of galactose such as peaches, lentils, and many others must be limited or eliminated (see advanced nutritional texts and hospital diet manuals for a complete listing of foods that contain lactose and galactose and the quantity contained in each food)

6. Meal Plan Modifications. Daily meals must be planned without the addition of milk or milk products. For accuracy, galactose-free diet lists may be used; consult advanced texts for galactose contents in foods

- Behavioral Modifications
  1. Blood and urine must be analyzed frequently.
  2. Most foods must be prepared and consumed in the home in order to ensure that daily galactose intake is not exceeded.
  3. All food labels must be read because some foods have hidden sources of galactose (*e.g.,* luncheon meats)

Other Inborn Errors of Metabolism

Nutritional care plans for other inborn errors of metabolism such as maple syrup urine disease are beyond the scope of this book. Readers desiring information on these diseases should consult advanced nutritional texts or hospital diet manuals.

Chronic Illnesses*

Diabetes Mellitus

Nutritional care plans for the dietary treatment of juvenile, insulin-dependent diabetes mellitus are discussed in Chapter 5.

---

* Other chronic illnesses such as congenital heart disease are beyond the scope of this book. Readers desiring information on these diseases should consult advanced nutritional texts or hospital diet manuals.

Epilepsy

Nutritional care plans for the dietary treatment of epilepsy are discussed in Chapter 9.

Nurses' Responsibilities in the Nutritional Care of the Infant

Initiate Good Care

The motivational level of the mother to feed her newborn infant the nutrients he requires to reach his optimal mental and physical development is extremely high. However, she is not always certain what these nutritional requirements are, nor does she know what, how much, or how often she must feed her infant in order to meet his nutritional needs. Therefore, providing her with this knowledge is the responsibility of the health team. It must also be remembered that introducing sound eating habits during infancy (*i.e.,* limited caloric intake plus limited salt, refined sugar, and fat intake) may be beneficial in the prevention of disorders that could otherwise decrease the infant's life span.

The nurse's responsibility for the initiation of sound eating habits in the infant is to provide professional information to the mother, while she is hospitalized, so that she will not be apprehensive about the infant's nutritional care when she goes home. This information should be related by the dietitian; however, if she is not available, the nurse may have to assume this role. She should only assume this responsibility, however, if she has kept abreast of scientific advances (*e.g.,* benefits of breast feeding vs. bottle feeding) in nutrition. Whether the nurse does the instructing or whether that is the province of another member of the health team, the nurse should use her position as health-team member closest to the mother to *offer encouragement* and *reinforce information* on what type of formula should be fed, if applicable; how feedings should be prepared or what factors enhance lactation (Table 10–11); how much food should be fed; and how often the infant should be fed. This enhanced knowledge should relieve the mother's anxieties and thus ensure continuation of sound infant eating habits in the home environment.

Participate in Care

In the Hospital

- Assist the mother while she is feeding her infant by providing emotional support and technical assistance so that she can continue acceptable techniques at home. This is especially important when the mother is breast feeding; however, the mother who is bottle feeding a first-born infant will also need assistance.

- Observe and assess the effectiveness of the feeding (*e.g.,* are mother's breasts still full? Is the infant contented after feeding?).
- Motivate and encourage the mother to continue to breast feed, if she desires, by using your position of trust to assure her that her baby is doing well. Also, assure her that she is learning the art of breast feeding well and will be able to continue feeding her baby at home without assistance.
- Remove feelings of guilt if the mother cannot or does not care to breast feed her baby. Assure her that formula feedings simulate breast milk; therefore, the baby will be receiving his nutritional requirements. Also assure her that his emotional needs can be met if she holds, cuddles, and talks to the baby during feeding as she would if she were breast feeding.

In the Physician's Office or Clinic

- Monitor and assess feeding effectiveness by weighing and measuring the infant at each visit. Record weights and lengths and compare them to standards. However, it should be remembered that genetics as well as geography influence an infant's measurements; consequently, even if the infant's recordings are below standard, he may still be developing well if his records show an adequate, steady upward trend. Additionally, breast feeding mothers should be told that breast-fed infants usually gain weight more slowly than do formula-fed infants. To relieve her apprehension about this slow weight gain, assure her that this may be a beneficial (less likelihood of obesity), not a detrimental progression.
- Provide information early in the infant's care about the addition of solid foods to the diet: when foods should be introduced, what types of food should be introduced, how they should be introduced (*e.g.,* one at a time), how much should be introduced, and how home-prepared baby foods should be made and stored to decrease the chances of contamination.

Coordinate Care

Coordinate health-team meetings in the hospital, clinic, and physician's office, if possible. These coordinated meetings should include several members of the health team (*i.e.,* nurse, physician, dietitian, and social worker). During these meetings, the following should be established

- A feeding protocol within the hospital or community
- A system for summarizing pertinent nutritional data (flow sheets)
- A means of providing organized professional nutritional education throughout the infants' first years of life for members of the health team as well as for the mothers

Between meetings, obtain, observe, assimilate, and then report subjective as well as objective information that will be beneficial to other members of the health team during follow-up sessions.

- Subjective information to be reported includes any evidence of maternal apprehension about her ability to feed her infant; information about the mother's lifestyle, such as drinking and smoking habits, especially if she is breast feeding (see Tables 10–1, 10–10, and 10–11); and information the mother reveals about her ability to procure or prepare food for her baby when she returns home.
- Objective information to be monitored and reported
  1. Structural Data. Present weight of the breast-feeding mother and infant and excessive deviations from past weights
  2. Vital Signs. Raised body temperature in the mother or infant; respiration changes in the infant
  3. Laboratory Data. Changes in blood sugar levels in the infant (*e.g.*, hypoglycemia), deviations in stool or urine specimens in the infant
  4. Clinical Signs. Color changes in the infant that may indicate jaundice, signs of irritability in the infant, appetite changes in the mother or infant

Reinforce and Follow Up Care*

The nurse's role in the follow-up care of an infant is of great magnitude, for she may be the only member of the health team who is consistently available to *monitor the progress* of the infant throughout his lifetime, within the community. If the nurse is to monitor this progress effectively and offer assistance when necessary, however, she must obtain the following knowledge:

1. A good background in infant nutrition, which will teach her the nutrient needs of normal infants during each stage of development
2. A good background in normal nutrition so that she can assess what nutrient increases or decreases are necessary during infancy
3. Up-to-date information on the types of infant formulas and feedings presently available (*e.g.*, their names and nutrient composition and how much must be fed daily in order to provide the infant's caloric, nutrient, and fluid needs)
4. A good ability to portray her knowledge to the mother (*i.e.*, good counseling skills)

---

* If the nurse acquires the knowledge to perform Nos. 2, 4, 5, 6, and 7 efficiently she will also be able to help most clients obtain good nutritional knowledge throughout their life cycle.

5. A good ability to recognize abnormal growth and development patterns in order to adjust the feeding program appropriately or make referrals if needed

6. A good ability to utilize and coordinate available community services and agencies that provide reliable food and nutritional resources

7. A good ability to teach her clients what federally funded food-assistance programs are available, what the eligibility requirements are, and how they may apply for this assistance.

Nutritional Care Plans for the Child, Adolescent, Young Adult, and Older Adult

The scope of this book does not permit a detailed discussion of the nutritional assessment values, nutrient recommendations, and detailed nutritional care plans for individuals throughout the remainder of the life cycle. Therefore, only the most common disorders having nutritional implications, plus the dietary adaptations that may alleviate adverse symptoms or nutrient inadequacies, are discussed here. See Tables 11–11 to 11–14.

Table 11-2
Distribution of Energy in Infant Milk Feedings (Percent)

Nutrient	Milk Feeding Source			
	Human	Commercial Formula	Whole Cow's Milk	Skim Cow's Milk*
Protein	8	9	21	40
Carbohydrate	37	42	34	57
Fat	55	49	45	3

* Skim milk is not recommended for infant feeding because it does not meet the caloric requirements and does not contain linoleic acid, an essential fatty acid required by infants.
(Reprinted with permission of Hinton SM, Kerwin DR: Maternal, Infant, and Child Nutrition: A Resource Book for Health Professionals. Chapel Hill, NC, Health Sciences Consortium, 1981)

Table 11–3
Comparison of Recommended Dietary Allowances for Normal Infants With Composition of Human Milk, Cow's Milk, and Milk-Based Formula

Nutrient	Dietary Allowances		Human Milk, (per 1000 ml*)	Cow's Milk, Whole Milk (per 1000 ml)	Milk-Based Formula (per 1000 ml)
	0–6 Months	6–12 Months			
Weight, kg	6	9			
lb	13	20			
Height, cm	60	71			
in	24	28			
Water, ml			897	894	875
Energy, kcal	kg × 115	kg × 105	718	620	670
Protein, g	kg × 2.2	kg × 2.0	10.6	33.4	15–16
Fat, g			44.9	33.9	36–37
Carbohydrate, g			70.6	47.3	70–72
Vitamin A, RE	420	400	656	315	340–500
IU	1400	2000	2470	1279	1700–2500
Vitamin D, μg	10	10		10†	10
Vitamin E, mg TE	3	4	1.3–3.3	5.7	5.7–8.5
Ascorbic acid, mg	35	35	51	10	55
Thiamine, mg	0.3	0.5	0.14	0.39	0.4–0.7
Riboflavin, mg	0.4	0.6	0.37	1.65	0.6–1.0
Niacin, mg NE	6	8	2.0	0.85	7–9
Vitamin B_6, mg	0.3	0.6	0.11	0.43	0.3–0.4
Vitamin B_{12}, μg	0.5	1.5	0.46	3.63	1.5–2.0
Folacin, μg	30	45	51	51	50–100
Calcium, mg	360	540	328	1208	550–600
Phosphorus, mg	240	360	144	945	440–460

(continued)

494 *Life Cycle*

Table 11–3
Comparison of Recommended Dietary Allowances for Normal Infants With Composition of Human Milk, Cow's Milk, and Milk-Based Formula (continued)

Nutrient	Dietary Allowances		Human Milk, (per 1000 ml*)	Cow's Milk, Whole Milk (per 1000 ml)	Milk-Based Formula (per 1000 ml)
	0–6 Months	6–12 Months			
Sodium, mg	115–350‡	250–750‡	141	498	250–390
Potassium, mg	350–925‡	425–1275‡	523	1544	620–1000
Magnesium, mg	50	70	31	132	40–50
Iodine, µg	40	50	30–100		40–70
Iron, mg	10	15	0.3	0.5	1.4–12.5§
Zinc, mg	3	5	1.8	3.9	2.0–4.0

* One liter of human milk = 1.025 g; 1 liter of cow's milk = 1.017 g
† Assumes fortification of cow's milk with 10 µg vitamin D
‡ Allowances for sodium and potassium are ranges considered to be safe and adequate
§ Values for formula not fortified and fortified with iron

(Food and Nutrition Board: Recommended Dietary Allowances, 9th ed. Washington, DC, National Research Council—National Academy of Sciences, 1980)

Table 11-4 495

Table 11-4
Anti-infectious Factors in Human Milk

Factor	Function
Bifidus factor	Converts lactose to lactic acid, which lowers the intestinal *p*H and interferes with the growth of many enteropathogenic bacteria
Secretory IgA (sIgA), IgM, and IgG	Act against bacterial invasion, especially *E. coli* of the mucosa or colonization of the gut (slow bacterial- or viral-neutralizing capacity [*e.g.*, enterovirus], activate alternative complement pathway)
Antistaphylococcus factor	Inhibits systemic staphylococcus infection
Lactoferrin	Binds iron and inhibits bacterial multiplication, especially of *E. coli*
Lactoperoxidase	Kills streptococci and enteric bacteria
Complement (C_3, C_4)	Promotes opsonization (the rendering of bacteria and other cells susceptible to phagocytosis)
Interferon	Inhibits intracellular viral replication
Lysozyme	Lyses bacteria through destruction of their cell wall
B_{12} binding protein	Renders vitamin B_{12} unavailable for bacterial growth
Lymphocytes	Synthesize secretory IgA; may have other roles such as producing the antiviral substance interferon
Macrophages	Synthesize complement, lactoferrin, lysozyme, and other factors; carry out phagocytosis and probably other functions
Lipid factors, fatty acids, and monoglycerides	Perturbation of bacteria and virus membranes

(Adapted from Worthington–Roberts BS: Lactation and human milk: Nutritional considerations. In Worthington–Roberts BS, Vermeersch J, Williams SR: Nutrition in Pregnancy and Lactation, 2nd ed. St Louis, CV Mosby, 1981)

Table 11–5
Special Formulas With Vitamins and Minerals Added

Product and Producer	Protein	Carbohydrate	Fat	Special Comments	Osmolality (kg H_2O)	Uses
Soy-Based, Lactose-Free						
Isomil (Ross Laboratories, Columbus, OH 43216)	Soy isolate	Corn syrup, sucrose	Coconut and soy oils	Concentrate or ready to feed. Iron-fortified only	250 mOsm	Diarrhea, cow's milk allergy, lactase deficiency
Prosobee (Mead-Johnson Laboratories, Evansville, IN 47721)	Soy isolate	Corn syrup, solids	Soy and coconut oils	Concentrate, ready to feed. Iron-fortified only; now lactose- and sucrose-free	180 mOsm	Cow's milk sensitivity, lactose or sucrose intolerance, galactosemia, diarrhea
Soyalac (Loma Linda Foods, Riverside, CA 92515)	Soybean solids and methionine	Corn syrup, solids, sucrose	Soybean oil	Concentrate	273 mOsm	Cow's milk allergy
I-Soyalac (Loma Linda Foods)	Soy isolate	Sucrose, modified tapioca starch	Soy oil	Concentrate; corn- and lactose-free	206 mOsm	Cow's milk allergy, galactosemia
Nursoy (Wyeth Laboratories, Philadelphia, PA 19101)	Soy isolate, methionine added	Sucrose	Oleo, coconut, safflower, and soy oils	Concentrate, ready to feed	296 mOsm	Cow's milk allergy
RCF (Ross)	Soy isolate	To be added	Soy and coconut oil	Carbohydrate must be added Concentrate		Diarrhea, disaccharide intolerance

(continued)

Table 11–5 497

Table 11–5
Special Formulas With Vitamins and Minerals Added (continued)

Product and Producer	Protein	Carbohydrate	Fat	Special Comments	Osmolality (kg H₂O)	Uses
Non-soy, Lactose-Free *(continued)*						
Nutramigen (Mead–Johnson)	Enzymatically hydrolyzed and charcoal treated casein	Sucrose, tapioca starch	Corn oil	Powder (9.5 g/2 oz $H_2O = 20$ kcal/oz) 15% calories from protein	479 mOsm	Diarrhea, cow's milk allergy, intact protein sensitivity
MBF, meat-base formula (Gerber Products Co., Fremont, MI 49412)	Beef heart	Sucrose, tapioca starch	Sesame oil	Concentrate	207.8 mOsm	Cow's milk allergies
Pregestimil (Mead–Johnson)	Casein hydrolysate, amino acids	Corn syrup solids, modified tapioca starch	Corn oil, medium-chain triglycerides	Powder (9.7 g/2 oz $H_2O = 20$ kcal/oz) 14% calories from protein	348 mOsm	Diarrhea, disaccharidase deficiency, steatorrhea
Lofenalac (Mead–Johnson)	Casein hydrolysate processed to remove most of phenylalanine, amino acids added	Corn syrup solids, tapioca starch	Corn oil	Powder (9.4 g/2 oz $H_2O = 20$ kcal/oz) 15% calories from protein Phenylalanine content, approximately 0.08%	454 mOsm	Infants with phenylketonuria

(continued)

Table 11–5
Special Formulas With Vitamins and Minerals Added (continued)

Product and Producer	Protein	Carbohydrate	Fat	Special Comments	Osmolality (kg H₂O)	Uses
Non-Soy, Lactose-Free *(continued)*						
Phenyl-Free (Mead–Johnson)	Phenylalanine-free food amino acids	Sucrose, corn syrup solids, modified	Corn oil	Powder (98.5 g/13.5 oz H₂O = 25 kcal/oz) 16 oz formula = 1 day intake 20% calories from protein	420 mOsm	Children over 2 years with PKU
MSUD Diet Powder (Mead–Johnson)	Amino acids free of branched-chain amino acids isoleucine, leucine, and valine	Corn syrup solids and modified tapioca starch	Corn oil	Powder (9 g/2 oz H₂O = 20 kcal/oz)	358 mOsm	Maple syrup urine disease
Other Special Formulas						
Portagen (Mead–Johnson)	Sodium caseinate	Sucrose, corn syrup solids	Medium-chain triglyceride oil, corn oil	Powder (9.5 g/2 oz H₂O = 20 kcal/oz) 14% calories from protein; 43% from fat	158 mOsm	Fat malabsorption

(continued)

Table 11-5 499

Table 11-5
Special Formulas With Vitamins and Minerals Added (continued)

Product and Producer	Protein	Carbohydrate	Fat	Special Comments	Osmolality (kg H_2O)	Uses
Other Special Formulas (continued)						
Probana (Mead–Johnson)	Whole and nonfat cow's milk, banana powder, casein hydrolysate	Dextrose, lactose, banana powder	Corn oil, butterfat	Powder (9.8 g/2 oz H_2O = 20 kcal/oz) 24% calories from protein; 29% from fat	592 mOsm	Diarrhea, steatorrhea
Similac PM60/40 (Ross Laboratories)	Partially demineralized whey, sodium caseinate	Lactose	Corn and coconut oils	Powder (8.56 g/2 oz H_2O = 20 kcal/oz) 60:40 lactalbumin: casein Electrolyte composition similar to human milk	260 mOsm	Renal and cardiac disease
SMA, S-29 (Wyeth Laboratories)	Electrodialyzed whey	Lactose	Oleo, coconut, safflower, and soy oils	Powder (8.4 g/2 oz H_2O = 20 kcal/oz) Very low in electrolytes	310 mOsm	Acute congestive heart failure, acute renal disease
SMA, S-14 (Wyeth Laboratories)	Nonfat milk	Lactose	Oleo, coconut, safflower, and soy oils	Powder (7.4 g/2 oz H_2O = 20 kcal/oz) 9% calo-	280 mOsm	Leucine-induced hypoglycemia

(continued)

Table 11-5
Special Formulas With Vitamins and Minerals Added (continued)

Product and Producer	Protein	Carbohydrate	Fat	Special Comments	Osmolality (kg H₂O)	Uses
Other Special Formulas (continued)						
				...ries from protein; low in leucine (33 mg/oz)		
Special Formulas for Preterm Infants						
Enfamil Premature (Mead–Johnson)	Demineralized whey, nonfat milk solids	Corn syrup solids	Medium-chain triglyceride oils, corn and coconut oils	Available for hospital use only, ready to feed 12% calories from protein; 48% calories from fat; 24 kcal/oz	300 mOsm	Growing low-birth-weight infants
Similac/Special Care Infant Formula	Whey and casein, 60:40	Lactose, corn syrup solids	Medium-chain triglycerides, corn and coconut oils	Available in 4-oz bottles ready to feed, hospital use only 11% total calories from protein; 46% total calories from fat; 42% total calories from carbohydrate 24 kcal/oz	300 mOsm	Growing low-birth-weight infants

(continued)

Table 11-5 501

Table 11-5
Special Formulas With Vitamins and Minerals Added (continued)

Product and Producer	Protein	Carbohydrate	Fat	Special Comments	Osmolality (kg H_2O)	Uses
Other Products						
Casec (Mead–Johnson)	Dried, soluble calcium caseinate derived from skim milk curd	Trace	Butterfat	Powder (4.7 g contains 4 g protein, 75 mg calcium, 2.7 mg sodium, and 17 kcal)		Protein supplement or for designing individualized formulas
MCT Oil (Mead–Johnson)	None	None	Triglycerides of medium-chain fatty acids	Liquid (68% C_8 fatty acids, 24% C_{10} fatty acids)		Substitution for energy from long-chain fatty acids
Polycose (Ross Laboratories)	None	Glucose polymers derived from controlled hydrolysis of corn starch	None	Powder (8 g = 30 calories; 9.2 mg sodium) Liquid (1 oz = 60 calories; 17.4 mg sodium)	850 mOsm	Carbohydrate supplement for formulas

(Anderson L, Dibble MV, Turkki PR et al: Nutrition in Health and Disease, 17th ed, pp 596–597. Philadelphia, JB Lippincott, 1982)

Table 11–6
Average Nutrient Content of Commercially Prepared Milk-Based Formulas (Per 100 ml)

	Enfamil[†]	Similac[‡]	SMA[§]
Energy, kcal	67	68	67
Protein, g	1.5	1.55	1.5
Type of protein	Nonfat cow milk	Nonfat cow milk	Demineralized whey and nonfat cow milk
Fat, total, g	3.7	3.6	3.6
Saturated, g	1.2	1.4	1.6
Unsaturated, g	2.5	2.2	2.0
Type of fat	Soy, coconut	Coconut, soy	Oleo, coconut, soy, safflower
Cholesterol, mg	1.4	1.6	3.3
Carbohydrate, g	7.0	7.2	7.2
Type of carbohydrate	Lactose	Lactose	Lactose
Ash, g	0.4	0.4	0.3
Calcium, mg	55	51	44
Phosphorus, mg	46	39	33
Iron, mg	0.15 (1.27)*	0.15 (1.2)*	(1.3)*
Iodine, mcg	46	10	7
Copper, mcg	63	60	48
Magnesium, mg	4.7	4.1	5.3
Zinc, mg	0.42	0.50	0.37
Sodium, mg	28	22	15
Potassium, mg	70	78	56
Vitamin A, IU	251	250	264
Vitamin D, IU	42	40	42

(continued)

Table 11–6 503

Table 11–6
**Average Nutrient Content of Commercially Prepared
Milk-Based Formulas (Per 100 ml)** (continued)

	Enfamil[†]	Similac[‡]	SMA[§]
Vitamin E, mg	1.3	1.5	1.0
Vitamin K, mcg	7	9	6
Ascorbic acid, mg	5.5	5.5	5.5
Thiamine, mcg	53	65	71
Riboflavin, mcg	63	100	106
Niacin equiv, mg	0.8	0.7	1.0
Pyridoxine, mcg	42	40	42
Pantothenic acid, mg	0.32	0.30	0.21
Vitamin B_{12}, mcg	0.21	0.15	0.11
Folacin, mcg	10.6	10.0	5.3

* Sold as "Iron-Fortified."
† Producer, Mead–Johnson Laboratories, Evansville, IN 47721
‡ Producer, Ross Laboratories, Columbus, OH 43216
§ Producer, Wyeth Laboratories, Philadelphia, PA 19101
(Anderson L, Dibble MV, Turkki PR et al: Nutrition in Health and Disease, 17th ed. Philadelphia, JB Lippincott, 1982)

Table 11-8
Introducing New Foods Into an Infant's Diet

When to Introduce	Approximate Total Daily Intake of Solids	Description of Foods and Hints About Giving Them
4–5 months (6–7 months if infant is breast fed)	Dry cereal, start with ½ tsp (dry measurement), gradually increase to 2–3 tbsp Vegetables, start with 1 tsp, gradually increase to 2 tbsp Fruit, start with 1 tsp, gradually increase to 2 tbsp Divide food among 4 feedings/day (if possible)	Cereal, offer iron-enriched baby cereal or plain Cream of Rice first. Begin with single grains (rice, barley, corn). Mix cereal with an equal amount of breast milk, formula, or water. Vegetables, try a mild-tasting vegetable first (carrots, squash, peas, green beans). Stronger-flavored vegetables (spinach, sweet potatoes) may be tried after the infant accepts some mild-tasting ones. Fruits, mashed ripe banana and unsweetened, cooked, bland fruits (apples, peaches, pears) are usually well liked. Apple juice and grape juice (unsweetened) may be introduced. Initially, dilute juice with an equal amount of water. Introduce one new food at a time, and offer it several times before trying another new food. Give a new food once a day for a day or two; increase to twice a day as the infant begins to enjoy the food. Watch for signs of intolerance. Include some foods that are good sources of vitamin C (other than orange juice).
5–6 months (6–7 months if infant is breast fed)	Dry cereal, gradually increase up to 4 tbsp Fruits and vegetables, gradually increase up to 3 tbsp of each	Meat, offer pureed or milled poultry (chicken or turkey) followed by lean meat (veal, beef); lamb has a stronger flavor and may not be as well liked initially. *(continued)*

Table 11–8 505

Table 11–8
Introducing New Foods Into an Infant's Diet (continued)

When to Introduce	Approximate Total Daily Intake of Solids	Description of Foods and Hints About Giving Them
	Meat, start with 1 tsp and gradually increase to 2 tbsp Divide food among 4 feedings/day (if possible)	Liver is a good source of iron; it may be accepted at the beginning of a meal with a familiar vegetable. Continue introducing new cereals, fruits, and vegetables as the infant indicates he is ready to accept them, but always one at a time.
6–8 months (7–9 months if infant is breast fed)	Dry cereal, up to ½ c Fruits and vegetables, up to ¼ to ½ c of each Meats, up to 3 tbsp Divide food among 4 feedings/day (if possible)	Soft table foods may be introduced (*e.g.*, mashed potatoes and squash and small pieces of soft, peeled fruits). Toasted whole-grain or enriched bread may be added when the infant begins chewing. If introduction of solids is delayed until now, it is not necessary to use strained fruits and vegetables. Continue using iron-fortified baby cereals.
8–12 months	Dry cereal, up to ½ c Bread, about 1 slice Fruits and vegetables, up to ½ c of each Meat, up to ¼ c Divide food among 4 feedings/day (if possible)	Table foods may be added gradually. Cut table foods into small pieces. Start with ones that do not require too much chewing (cooked, cut green beans and carrots, noodles, ground meats, tuna fish, soft cheese, plain yogurt). If fish is offered, check closely to be sure there are no bones in the serving. Mashed, cooked egg yolk and orange juice may be added at about 9 months of age. Sometimes offer smooth peanut butter or thoroughly cooked dried peas and beans in place of meat.

(Suitor CW, Hunter MF: Nutrition: Principles and Application in Health Promotion, p 86. Philadelphia, JB Lippincott, 1980)

Table 11–9
**Nutritional Care Plans, Dietary Adaptations, and
Rationales for Disorders Common During Infancy**

Disorder	Rationales	Dietary Adaptations
Colic		
Abdominal cramping and profuse crying after eating	Feeding milk-based formulas instead of breast feeding (the more concentrated the formula [*e.g.*, cereal added], the more intense the distress)	Breast feed Do not add solids to formula
	Distention due to swallowed air	Burp the infant frequently during feedings
	Gas formed by bacterial fermentation of undigested food	Lactose is the most desirable sugar in infant formulas Avoid feeding complex carbohydrates to small infants; the infant's enzymatic (amylase) ability to digest them is inadequate
	Overfeeding, underfeeding, feeding too fast	Adjust nipple size if feeding seems to be flowing too fast or too slow; stop feeding when infant appears satisfied
	Formula feedings that are too hot or too cold	Experiment with various temperatures (some infants tolerate cold formulas better than hot)
	Low body temperatures or distraction in the infant	Swaddle the infant; body temperatures rise, extremities are restricted
	Maternal or infant anxiety or fatigue	Mother and infant should rest before feedings; assure mother that this symptom lessens with age, and that the infant is being sufficiently nourished and developing adequately

(continued)

Table 11-9 507

Table 11-9
**Nutritional Care Plans, Dietary Adaptations, and
Rationales for Disorders Common During Infancy** (continued)

Disorder	Rationales	Dietary Adaptations
Vomiting		
Large amounts of food regurgitated after feeding	Viral infections Bacterial multiplication caused by unclean breasts Bacterial multiplication caused by formula contamination, due to unclean equipment, improper sterilization techniques, or improper storage Obstruction or other serious illnesses such as pyloric stenosis	Consult physician Improve nipple care (see Table 10-11) Check preparation of formula techniques (see preparation of formula in this chapter) Avoid reusing formula from previous feedings Consult physician
Regurgitation		
Small amounts of foods regurgitated after feeding; known as "spitting up"	Fatigue Swallowing air Force feeding more than the small infant's stomach can store and assimilate Formulas that have a high fat concentration, especially butterfat; fat enhances satiety, food remains in the stomach for longer periods	Allow infant to rest before feedings Be sure bottle is held high enough to prevent air formation in the nipple Adjust feeding position if breast feeding The young infant's stomach capacity is only 2 tbsp or 1 oz (see Table 11-1 for the recommended amounts of feedings to give small infants) Breast feed if possible Adjusting concentration of formula to infant's needs will lessen incidence of spitting up

(continued)

Table 11-9
**Nutritional Care Plans, Dietary Adaptations, and
Rationales for Disorders Common During Infancy** (continued)

Disorder	Rationales	Dietary Adaptations
Regurgitation *(continued)*		
		Feed formulas that have fat in the form of vegetable oils, not butterfat (*e.g.*, Similac or Enfamil)
Mild Diarrhea		
Diarrhea of 1–4 days' duration	Viral infection	General dietary adaptations and feeding progression to alleviate the symptom in infants and the young child:
		NPO for 12–24 hours
		Progress to clear fluids such as tea, Coke, and Popsicles (not ice cold)
		If symptom has not subsided in 24 hours, give electrolyte solutions with minimal glucose (*e.g.*, Lytren or Pedialyte), if prescribed by the physician
		Progress to a dilute formula as diarrhea subsides (*i.e.*, a dilution of 1:3 on the first day; 1:2 on the second day, 1:1 on the third day, and full formula on the fourth day)

(continued)

Table 11–9 509

Table 11-9
**Nutritional Care Plans, Dietary Adaptations, and
Rationales for Disorders Common During Infancy** (continued)

Disorder	Rationales	Dietary Adaptations
Mild Diarrhea (continued)		If solid foods are tolerated, use foods contained in the Brat Diet, which increase electrolytes, caloric intake, and pectin intake, the last of which thickens stools (*e.g.,* bananas, rice without butter, apple [the less ripe and more solid the better], tea, and sometimes toast without butter)
		If milk is allowed, as diarrhea subsides, use skim milk instead of whole milk; do not boil the milk because water will evaporate, increasing the renal solute load
	Excessive bacterial multiplication caused by contaminated formula or equipment	Check sterilization techniques
		See recommended techniques in this chapter; throw away unused formula after feeding
	Formulas that contain cow's milk (*e.g.,* evaporated milk formulas)	Breast feed or feed the infant commercially prepared formulas such as Enfamil instead of evaporated milk formulas
		If lactose intolerance suspected, substitute Isomil or other lactose-free formula for commercial formulas with lactose
		(continued)

Table 11–9
**Nutritional Care Plans, Dietary Adaptations, and
Rationales for Disorders Common During Infancy** (continued)

Disorder	Rationales	Dietary Adaptations
Mild Diarrhea (continued)		
	Feeding solid foods too soon	Young infants cannot digest complex carbohydrates efficiently; carbohydrate ferments, causing diarrhea
	Formulas that contain high fat concentrations or high concentrations of butterfat	Substitute formulas with lower fat concentrations for a few days, such as Probana Use formulas that contain vegetable oils, not butterfat, such as Similac and Enfamil
	Allergies	See Allergy in this table Severe or prolonged diarrhea in the infant or child may neccessitate hospitalization of the child to prevent dehydration; consult pediatrician whenever diarrhea continues more than 24 hours
Constipation		
Firmness of the stool and the difficulty of evacuation are the criteria used to diagnose constipation (breast-fed infants normally have several loose [not watery] stools each day)	Feeding too concentrated a formula (*e.g.*, evaporated milk formulas that have not been diluted properly).	Breast feed or use commercially prepared formulas that have already been diluted (expensive) Give additional water between formula feedings
	Feeding a formula with insufficient carbohydrate	Add additional sugar to evaporated milk formulas but only on the advice of the physician Do not increase sugar intake by spreading honey on the nipple or pacifier; honey

(continued)

Table 11–9 511

Table 11–9
**Nutritional Care Plans, Dietary Adaptations, and
Rationales for Disorders Common During Infancy** (continued)

Disorder	Rationales	Dietary Adaptations
Constipation (continued)		
	Excessive milk intake in older infants	has been known to cause botulism in infants
		Decrease milk intake in older infants; substitute solid foods such as fruits and vegetables if tolerated
		Increase intake of water and fruit juices
Nutritional Anemia		
Hemoglobin levels of < 11 g/dl usually indicate nutritional anemia (iron-deficiency anemia) in infancy	Inadequate iron stores at birth, especially prevalent in LBW infants	Breast feed or feed commercially prepared formulas that have been fortified with iron
	Inadequate intake of iron and other nutrients (e.g., protein and vitamin B_6) necessary for hemoglobin production in mother and infant	Give iron supplements to the mother during pregnancy and lactation (see Chapter 10 for recommended intake)
		Give iron supplements to infants (see this chapter for recommended intake)
	Cow's milk formulas that cause enteric bleeding	Do not give small infants whole milk; substitute commercially prepared formulas
Allergy		
An immunologic reaction or hypersensitivity to a substance, which produces such symptoms as irritability, mucous and bloody diarrhea, eczema, respiratory distress, and poor weight gain in the infant	In young infants, usually caused by protein foods, especially cow's milk	Breast feed, which is associated with a lower incidence of allergic reactions
	Highly allergenic foods that should be used with caution in the older infant are cow's milk, egg whites, wheat (contains	Substitute soy-based formulas such as Prosobee for milk-based formulas
		Introduce new foods one at a time; test in-

(continued)

Table 11-9
Nutritional Care Plans, Dietary Adaptations, and
Rationales for Disorders Common During Infancy (continued)

Disorder	Rationales	Dietary Adaptations
Allergy (continued)	gluten), seafood, nuts, citrus fruits (especially orange juice and tomatoes), chocolate, and cocoa	fant's reaction to this food for several days before adding a new food to the diet
Obesity May place the infant in the high-risk category; see large-for-gestational-age infant in this chapter	Mother had gestational or traditional diabetes mellitus Force feeding the infant, which means giving the infant more food than he takes willingly at each feeding Feeding too frequently Feeding too concentrated a formula	See high-risk pregnancies in Chapters 5 and 10 Breast feed; the breast-fed infant regulates the amount of food desired, not the mother If bottle feeding, allow the infant to stop feeding when he is no longer interested Feed on demand, not on a rigid schedule Do not add solid foods to the infant's feeding until he is 4–6 months of age

Table 11-10 513

Table 11-10
Feeding Progression, Benefits, and Disadvantages of Recommended Oral Feedings for Low-Birth-Weight Infants

	Bottle Feeding	Breast Feeding
Feeding Progression	NPO until development is assessed Distilled water, followed (as individually tolerated) by Half-strength specially prepared LBW and preterm formulas (see dietary adaptations and Table 11-5) Full-strength formula fed as frequently as possible (as many as 10–12 times/day) Feeding an infant every 2–3 hr may tire the infant—he may be using the calories he is acquiring merely to obtain nourishment rather than to enhance his growth. Consequently, many pediatricians recommend alternating bottle and gavage feeding (feeding a bottle every 8 hrs with gavage feedings in between)	NPO until development is assessed Distilled water or colostrum Full-strength colostrum Full-strength human mature milk fed as frequently as infant desires If the infant is unable to obtain milk from the breast, which is usual in infants weighing less than 2000 g, the mother may express her milk and have it fed by bottle or gavage if the infant is hospitalized. If mother's milk is not available, milk may be obtained from milk banks. However, the latter may have some nutrient changes (see Benefits, below).
Benefits	Premature formulas have a high caloric content (80–100 kcal/ml) and protein content (2.8 g/ml), rapidly which enables the infant to "catch up" The type and distribution of nutrients (*e.g.*, calcium) can be adjusted when the infant's structural development is impaired. They can also be adjusted when other complications such as hypoglycemia are present	Milk from mothers who give birth prematurely may have a higher protein content, as well as other nutrient composition alterations, including a more digestible fat (see Disadvantages, p. 514). In addition, the mother is able to participate in the care of her infant, which is beneficial to them both (see Benefits of Human Milk for Normal Infants)

(continued)

Table 11–10
**Feeding Progression, Benefits, and Disadvantages of
Recommended Oral Feedings for Low-Birth-Weight Infants** (continued)

	Bottle Feeding	Breast Feeding
Disadvantages	See Benefits of Human Milk for Normal Infants	The protein and mineral content of breast milk may be inadequate to meet the nutrient needs of the VLBWI or severely immature infant. However, it has been found that the milk of a mother who has a preterm infant has a higher concentration of protein, calcium, iron, and magnesium and a lower concentration of lactose and sometimes sodium. On the basis of these findings, it is now theorized that the milk of a LBW infant's own mother may meet his qualitative and quantitative nutrient requirements better than mature human milk. Forman still recommends supplementing 1–2 bottles of concentrated formula daily, however, to assure adequate weight gain (human milk contains only 67 kcal/100 ml), skeletal mineralization, and increased length

Table 11–11 515

Table 11–11
**Dietary Adaptations for Common Conditions
With Nutritional Implications in the Child**

Disorders	Nutritional Implications	Dietary Adaptations
Physiological		
Weight gain with resultant obesity	Caloric and other nutrient requirements are not as high as in infancy (see RDAs, Appendix IV). Mother force feeds and uses food as an emotional pacifier. Usually sweet foods are offered: "Are you hurt? Have a cookie." Weight gain is enhanced if caloric intake remains the same as during infancy and activity is not escalated. Furthermore, when child is overweight activity is decreased.	Foods included in daily meals to meet total energy needs should have nutrient density, not empty calories. See recommendations for preventing or alleviating obesity Chapter 6. Encourage increased energy expenditure especially if energy intake remains the same as in infancy.
Growth rate declines with resultant decreased food consumption	Protein requirements decrease when growth (tissue synthesis) declines. Reduced from 2 g for the first year to 0.8 g throughout the remainder of the life cycle	
Dental caries	Sweet intake increases owing to environmental influences (*e.g.*, peers and advertising).	Milk intake should be reduced to 3-4 glasses/day so that other foods (*i.e.*, meats) can be introduced to provide other nutrients (*e.g.*, iron). See Chapter 7 for a more detailed discussion of the development and prevention of dental caries.
Nutritional anemia	Iron stores and intake may be low.	See Dietary Adaptations for anemia in Chapter 10 and during infancy in this chapter.
Poor digestion	Eating rushed meals and skipping meals, especially breakfast, when child attends school.	Introduce child to sound eating habits; have him rise in time to eat a good breakfast.

(continued)

Table 11–11
**Dietary Adaptations for Common Conditions
With Nutritional Implications in the Child** (continued)

Disorders	Nutritional Implications	Dietary Adaptations
		Intellectual levels decline with hunger. Encourage local schools to obtain federally supported breakfast and lunch programs. These programs are of no use if food is not consumed, however, so palatable meal plans should be advocated.
Appetite declines due to decreased growth rate and environmental distractions	Food consumption is less. Meats and vegetables are most frequently refused. Mother attempts to increase food consumption; meal time becomes a battle.	Avoid highly seasoned meats and vegetables or meats that are difficult to manage. Vitamin and mineral supplements may be needed until food consumption increases. Keep eating time pleasurable; allow child to eat with the family. Introduce manners gradually. Family members should practice all food habits and manners recommended to the child.
Psychological		
Outside environment influences eating habits — peers and advertising	Consumption of refined sugars, salt, and fat increases. Peers introduce fast-food establishments. Advertising, especially on TV, introduces child to junk foods. Food consumption is curtailed if food is eaten in front of the TV set (distraction).	Obtain games that introduce child to good sound eating habits. Invite peers to play along also. Monitor TV programs for undesirable eating habits. Set good eating behavioral patterns by allowing the child to eat only in one room, preferably the kitchen.

(continued)

Table 11–11 517

Table 11–11
**Dietary Adaptations for Common Conditions
With Nutritional Implications in the Child** (continued)

Disorders	Nutritional Implications	Dietary Adaptations
Psychological (continued)		
Snacking—peer influence, rushed meals enhance hunger between meals	Snacking impairs appetite for nutrient-dense foods; nutritional inadequacies or imbalances may develop.	Avoid snacks before meals. Do not limit snacking completely; as part of the lifestyle, offer nutrient-dense snacks instead (*e.g.*, cheese cubes, carrot sticks, popcorn).
Fad dieting (often begins in girls during puberty; boys also fad diet to improve athletic abilities)	Nutrient inadequacies or imbalances may develop. Excessive dieting may lead to anorexia nervosa. Carbohydrate loading to increase glycogen stores and endurance may lead to nutrient imbalances and inadequacies.	Nutrition-education programs that explain the hazards involved in fad dieting should be taught to parents as well as to children. Offer an alternative such as school-weight programs so that undesirable plans will not be continued. See Chapter 6 for the hazards of fad dieting and professionally recommended alternatives.

Table 11–12
Dietary Adaptations for Common Conditions
With Nutritional Implications in the Adolescent

Disorders	Nutritional Implications	Dietary Adaptations
Physiological		
Growth is escalated	Caloric and other nutrient requirements are increased (see RDAs, Appendix IV).	Increase intake of nutrient-dense foods at mealtimes and as snacks. Milk intake should be increased to 4 cups/day. Vitamin and mineral supplements may be needed, especially iron supplements if meat intake is low. Girls may need supplements more than boys; their caloric intake is often lower.
Alcohol, drugs (*e.g.*, OCAs and addictive drugs) and cigarette smoking	Drug and nutrient interactions may impair nutrient ingestion, digestion, absorption, and utilization.	Programs that explain the hazards of alcohol, drugs, and smoking should be part of the public-school educational curriculum. See nutrient and drug interactions in Chapter 8 (alcohol), Chapter 10 (OCAs and nicotine), and Table 10–10.
Pregnancy	Caloric and nutrient requirements increase above those required for a young adult. Adolescent's body is also growing (see RDAs, Appendix IV).	See rationales for caloric and nutrient increases and Dietary Adaptations, Chapter 10.
Anemia	See Table 11–11 and Chapter 10.	See Table 11–11 and Chapter 10.

(continued)

Table 11–12 519

Table 11–12
**Dietary Adaptations for Common Conditions
With Nutritional Implications in the Adolescent** (continued)

Disorders	Nutritional Implications	Dietary Adaptations
Psychological		
Loneliness, frustration, anxiety, lack of identity and control over one's life, which lead to rebellion against parental control	Binge eating. Food is used as an emotional tranquilizer. Junk foods are consumed more than nutrient-dense foods. This is a means of rebellion against parents. Habit forming; may lead to obesity or anorexia nervosa.	Alleviate emotional stress, if possible; settle for a grade of B instead of pushing for an A. See Chapter 6 for professional methods to alleviate obesity or anorexia nervosa.

Table 11–13
Dietary Adaptations for Common Conditions With Nutritional Implications in the Young Adult

Disorders	Nutritional Implications	Dietary Adaptations
Physiological		
Growth, development, and BMR decline	Caloric and nutrient requirements are less than those of the adolescent (see RDAs, Appendix IV). Consequently, maintenance of adolescent caloric intake may lead to obesity.	Reduced intake of high caloric foods is recommended. Increase intake of nutrient-dense foods that provide needed nutrients as well as calories.
Activity levels decline; individual becomes an armchair "watcher" rather than participant	If caloric intake remains the same as during adolescence, especially in men, obesity may be induced.	Increase moderate activity. See Chapter 6 for professional methods used to prevent and alleviate obesity.
Constipation	Increased intake of highly refined foods that are inexpensive and easy to prepare and store impairs defecation. A rushed lifestyle prevents allowing time for defecation.	Increase fluids and complex carbohydrates. See Chapter 7 for dietary habits that prevent or alleviate constipation. Allow time for defecation, preferably after breakfast.
Chronic illness (*e.g.*, hypertension); symptoms often ignored	Continuation of undesirable eating habits may aggravate the condition. Eating patterns and behavioral patterns may need alterations.	Dietary adaptations for chronic diseases usually must be practiced for a lifetime. Consequently, the client must be motivated and instructed by well-trained professionals. See Dietary Adaptations for chronic diseases throughout this book.
Psychological		
Stress	Stress increases nutrient requirements (*e.g.*, vitamin C). Meals are often rushed or skipped to meet deadlines.	Allow time for breakfast. Take a nutrient-dense lunch to work in order to increase protein, vitamin, and mineral intake.

(continued)

Table 11–13 521

Table 11–13
**Dietary Adaptations for Common Conditions
With Nutritional Implications in the Young Adult** (continued)

Disorders	Nutritional Implications	Dietary Adaptations
Psychological *(continued)*		
Drugs, alcohol, and cigarette smoking to relieve stress	See Table 11–12.	See Table 11–12.
Other		
Economics—purchasing material articles (*e.g.,* furniture) rather than food	Intake of inexpensive carbohydrates that are easy to prepare and store is often substituted for nutrient-dense, high biologic protein foods such as meat. In contrast, individuals with high incomes may consume too much meat and too little complex carbohydrate.	Encourage consumption of mixed dishes (*i.e.,* dishes that combine many foods, thus contributing a variety of nutrients to the diet). This advice may apply to the affluent as well as to the economically embarrassed because high intake of one nutrient (*e.g.,* meat fat) as well as low intake may cause adverse side affects (*e.g.,* atherosclerosis).

Table 11–14
**Dietary Adaptations for Common Conditions
With Nutritional Implications in the Older Adult***

Disorders	Nutritional Implications	Dietary Adaptations
Physiological		
BMR ↓ and body composition changes: ↑ fat, ↓ lean tissue, ↓ bone density	Continuous high intake of fat without increased activity will lead to enhanced deposition of body fat, commonly called *obesity*. Inactivity may also enhance bone reabsorption.	Since body composition normally changes with age, in order to prevent excessive deposition of fat or reabsorption of bone in the older adult, the general dietary recommendations are to eat a variety of foods from the Basic Four Food Groups daily. The minimum quantities recommended will provide approximately 1200 kcal, the minimal amount of calories recommended for a woman. See Tables 1–5 to 1–8.
Sense of smell and taste changes	Changes in the sense of smell, taste, and sight of food decrease production of saliva, which ultimately reduces liquidation of food. Impaired liquidation of food inhibits swallowing.	Foods served to the older adult should not only be nutritionally adequate, they must also be palatable: if they stimulate the desire for consumption, with resultant salivary production, they will nourish the spirit as well as the body, which ultimately enhances digestion and absorption. Eat a varied diet to assure adequate nutrient intake.
GI tract—decreased HCl and gastrin secretion with possible resultant anemia	Nutrient inadequacies of vitamin A, B-complex, and zinc may impair taste. This causes symptoms of indigestion. It impairs absorption of iron, calcium, and vitamin B_{12}.	Eat small, frequent, nutrient-dense meals; chew foods well; and decrease intake of fats, which retard gastrin secretion.

(continued)

Table 11-14 523

Table 11–14
**Dietary Adaptations for Common Conditions
With Nutritional Implications in the Older Adult*** (continued)

Disorders	Nutritional Implications	Dietary Adaptations
Physiological (continued)		
		Reduce intake of foods that provide calories but few other essential nutrients such as foods with concentrated amounts of alcohol, sugar, fat, and oil.
		Increase moderate exercise; it enhances digestion.
		Vitamin and mineral supplements may be needed.
Surface and villus height of small intestines reduced	Absorption of essential nutrients is impaired, especially vitamin A, thiamine, folic acid, calcium, and iron.	A varied diet is essential to supply nutrient requirements.
		Vitamin and mineral supplements may be needed if caloric and food intake is inadequate.
		Limit intake of fat, which inhibits calcium absorption.
		See Table 11–13.
Decreased motility in the large intestines causes constipation	Overconcern about bowel changes precipitates high consumption and use of laxatives. High intake of some laxatives (*e.g.*, mineral oil) may impair the absorption of vitamins A, D, E, and K. See Table 7–1.	
Structural differences—loose and missing teeth, ill-fitting dentures, and periodontal disease	Alterations in chewing decrease intakes of many nutrient-dense foods (*e.g.*, meat and raw fruits). Client restricts food intake to soft-textured foods that are easy to chew (*e.g.*, cake and pasta).	Fruits and vegetables that are easy to chew should be recommended (*e.g.*, applesauce and mashed carrots).
		Mixed dishes that contain all three major macronutrients plus vitamins and minerals

(continued)

Table 11–14
**Dietary Adaptations for Common Conditions
With Nutritional Implications in the Older Adult*** (continued)

Disorders	Nutritional Implications	Dietary Adaptations
Physiological *(continued)*		
		should be encouraged (*e.g.*, tuna and cheese casseroles).
		Moderate amounts of bran can be added to cereals or mixed dishes to minimize constipation.
Bone density and mineralization decreases, leading to osteoporosis	Inactivity leads to bone reabsorption.	Increase moderate activity.
	Other possible causes of osteoporosis are high phosphorus-to-calcium intake, high protein-to-calcium intake, and low intake of vitamin D, which leads to decreased absorption of calcium.	Increase calcium intake to 1200 mg/day. Fortified vitamin D milk is the best source of calcium, but excessive intake may induce lactose intolerance symptoms. If these symptoms occur, cheese, which is low in lactose, should be added to casseroles and cream sauces. Food intake may not be sufficient to meet the requirements, however, so supplements of vitamin D (400 IU/day, 10 μg) and calcium may be indicated.
	Combined use of alcohol, antacids, and other drugs reduces calcium and phosphorus absorption from the intestines, which ultimately increases its reabsorption from the bone.	
Arthritis	Pain and malformation may inhibit the ability to procure, prepare, and ingest food.	Individual should be introduced to home nursing services or Meals on Wheels if disability is severe enough to cause impaired nutritional status.
		See Chapter 9 for Dietary Adaptations for individuals with arthritis.

(continued)

Table 11–14 525

Table 11–14
Dietary Adaptations for Common Conditions
With Nutritional Implications in the Older Adult* (continued)

Disorders	Nutritional Implications	Dietary Adaptations
Physiological *(continued)*		
Mental changes. Presenility or Alzheimer's disease	Individual may forget to eat or be incapable of procuring or preparing food.	Visiting nursing service plus Meals on Wheels should become a part of the individual's care.
	Recent dietary research has indicated that high intakes of aluminum or low intake of lecithin and choline may precipitate the disease.	At present, not enough evidence is available to warrant eliminating or increasing intake of these substances to prevent or alleviate this disease.
Impaired eyesight and hearing	Ability to procure, prepare, and ingest food may be impaired.	Individual should be introduced to home nursing services or Meals on Wheels if disability is severe enough to cause impaired nutritional status.
		See Chapter 1 for the recommended methodology of feeding the blind.
		See Table 11–11 and Chapter 10.
Anemia	See Table 11–11 and Chapter 10.	
Chronic illness (*e.g.,* diabetes mellitus and coronary heart disease)	Individuals with these conditions have often, but not always, consumed excessive quantities of fat, alcohol, refined sugar, and salt throughout the life cycle. These dietary habits may have enhanced the progression of the disease.	Dietary alterations may be necessary. The severity of the adjustment, however, should depend on the individual's age. For instance, a newly diagnosed diabetic who is 85 needs only refined sugar removed from his diet, not a detailed dietary regimen.
		See related chapters in this book for the dietary adaptations recommended in chronic diseases.

(continued)

Table 11–14
**Dietary Adaptations for Common Conditions
With Nutritional Implications
in the Older Adult*** (continued)

Disorders	Nutritional Implications	Dietary Adaptations
Psychological		
Physical appearance changes	Individual is vulnerable to claims that food supplements provide eternal youth.	Nutrient-dense or fortified foods that provide needed calories, protein, vitamins, and minerals should be emphasized. Individual should be taught that in the long run food is less expensive than supplements. Food for the most part also contains more than one nutrient. For instance, an orange contains vitamin C, vitamin A, potassium, and fluid, while a supplement may contain only vitamin C.
Loneliness, "nobody needs me, nobody cares," fear, changing roles, feelings of rejection, loss of independence	Food is a symbol of friendship, prestige, creativity, and reward. Consequently, when individuals eat alone, they lack these feelings and food becomes just something to do to relieve hunger; what is in it does not matter. Nutritional status declines.	Encourage individuals who are mobile to have "pot luck" or "bring your own" dinners and attend Title III C, formerly Title VII, lunches in their community. These lunches are federally subsidized; therefore, they are inexpensive. Immobile shut-ins should be introduced to and helped to obtain Meals on Wheels because these meals also provide some social contact with the deliverer of the meals.
		These community meals are based on the Basic Four Food Groups and provide ⅓ of the daily RDAs.

(continued)

Table 11–14 527

Table 11–14
**Dietary Adaptations for Common Conditions
With Nutritional Implications in the Older Adult*** (continued)

Disorders	Nutritional Implications	Dietary Adaptations
Psychological *(continued)*		
Economic reverses cause embarrassment and depression	An excess of refined carbohydrates is often consumed for they are inexpensive, easy to carry (even up stairs), easy to prepare, and easy to chew. Deficiencies and nutrient imbalances (*e.g.,* more thiamine is needed with high carbohydrate intake but less is supplied in highly refined carbohydrate foods) occur.	Foods available in the market for the older adult should be adjusted to provide individual foods in small containers (less waste and contamination) and easy-to-open packages. Additionally, essential nutrients should be added by means of fortification, if necessary, in order to improve or maintain the nutritional status of the older adult.

* Classifications: mature adult (68 yr and below), aging adult (69–76 yr), elderly adult (77–85 yr), aged adult (86 yr and older)

Bibliography

Anderson L, Dibble MV, Turkki PR et al: Nutrition in Health and Disease, 17th ed. Philadelphia, JB Lippincott, 1982

Brady MS, Rickard KA, Ernest JA et al: Formulas and human milk for premature infants: A review and update. J Am Diet Assoc 81:547, 1982

Brooke OG: Nutrition in the preterm infant. Lancet 1:514, 1983

Foman SJ, Strauss RG: Nutrient deficiencies in breast-fed infants. N Engl J Med 299:355, 1978

Harzer G, Haug M, Dieterich I et al: Changing patterns of human milk lipids in the course of the lactation and during the day. Am J Clin Nutr 37:612, 1983

Hinton SM, Kerwin DR: Maternal Infant and Child Nutrition. Chapel Hill, NC, Health Sciences Consortium, 1981

Hirschhorn N: Oral rehydration therapy for diarrhea in children—a basic primer. Nutr Rev 40:97, 1982

Howard RB, Herbold NH: Nutrition in Clinical Care. New York, McGraw–Hill, 1982

Kabara JJ: Lipids as host-resistance factors of human milk. Nutr Rev 38:65, 1980

Kaye R, Oski FA, Barness LA: Core Textbook of Pediatrics, 2nd ed. Philadelphia, JB Lippincott, 1982

Kohrs MB, Kamath SK (eds): Symposium on nutrition and aging. Am J Clin Nutr (Suppl) 36:735, 1982

La Leche League International: The Womanly Art of Breast Feeding, 3rd ed. Franklin Park, IL, La Leche League International, 1982

Lebenthal E (ed): Textbook of Gastroenterology and Nutrition in Infancy. New York, Raven Press, 1981

Miranda R, Saravia NG, Ackerman R et al: Effect of maternal nutritional status on immunological substances in human colostrum and milk. Am J Clin Nutr 37:632, 1983

Pemberton CM, Gastineau CF (eds): Mayo Clinic Diet Manual. Philadelphia, WB Saunders, 1981

Pipes PL: Nutrition in Infancy and Childhood. St Louis, CV Mosby, 1977

Psiaki D, Olson C, Kaplowitz D: Breast Feeding: Division of Nutritional Sciences. Ithaca, NY, Cornell University Press, 1980

Rivlin RS, Young EA (eds): Symposium on evidence relating selected vitamins to health and disease in the elderly population in the U.S. Am J Clin Nutr (Suppl) 36:977, 1982

Robinson CH, Lawler MR: Normal and Therapeutic Nutrition, 16th ed. New York, Macmillan, 1982

Rowland TW, Zori RT, Lafleur WR et al: Malnutrition and hypernatremic dehydration in breast-fed infants. JAMA 247:1016, 1982

Roy S: Perspectives on adverse effects of milks and infant formulas used in infant feeding. J Am Diet Assoc 82:373, 1983

Suitor CW, Hunter MF: Nutrition: Principles and Application in Health Promotion. Philadelphia, JB Lippincott, 1980

Suskind RM (ed): Textbook of Pediatric Nutrition. New York, Raven Press, 1981

Whitehead RF: Nutritional aspects of human lactation. Lancet 1:167, 1983

Williams SR: Nutrition and Diet Therapy. St Louis, CV Mosby, 1981

Worthington–Roberts BS, Vermeersch J, Williams SR: Nutrition in Pregnancy and Lactation, 2nd ed. St Louis, CV Mosby, 1981

Appendix I

Height and Weight Tables

Table I–1 531

Table 1–1
Average Weights of Men by Height and Age Group: 1959 and 1979 Build and Blood Pressure Studies* (Graduated Weight in Shoes and Indoor Clothing in Pounds)

| | Men By Age Group, 1959 and 1979 Studies | | | | | | | | | | | |
| | 15–16 years | | | 17–19 years | | | 20–24 years | | | 25–29 years | | |
Height	1959 Study	1979 Study	Weight Change	1959 Study	1979 Study	Weight Change	1959 Study	1979 Study	Weight Change	1959 Study	1979 Study	Weight Change
5′ 2″	107	112	+5	119	128	+9	128	137	+9	134	140	+6
3″	112	116	+5	123	129	+6	132	136	+4	138	141	+3
4″	117	121	+4	127	132	+5	136	139	+3	141	143	+2
5″	122	127	+5	131	137	+6	139	143	+4	144	147	+3
6″	127	133	+6	135	141	+6	142	148	+6	148	152	+4
7″	132	137	+5	139	145	+6	145	153	+8	151	156	+5
8″	137	143	+6	143	150	+7	149	157	+8	155	161	+6
9″	142	148	+6	147	155	+8	153	163	+10	159	166	+7
10″	146	153	+7	151	159	+8	157	167	+10	163	171	+8
11″	150	159	+9	155	164	+9	161	171	+10	167	175	+8
6′0″	154	162	+8	160	168	+8	166	176	+10	172	181	+9
1″	159	168	+9	164	174	+10	170	182	+12	177	186	+9
2″	164	173	+9	168	179	+9	174	187	+13	182	191	+9
3″	169	178	+9	172	185	+13	178	193	+15	186	197	+11
4″	175	184	+9	176	190	+14	181	198	+17	190	202	+12

(continued)

Table 1-1
Average Weights of Men by Height and Age Group: 1959 and 1979 Build and Blood Pressure Studies* (Graduated Weight in Shoes and Indoor Clothing in Pounds)(continued)

| Height | Men By Age Group, 1959 and 1979 Studies | | | | | | | | | | | |
| | 30-39 years | | | 40-49 years | | | 50-59 years | | | 60-69 years | | |
	1959 Study	1979 Study	Weight Change	1959 Study	1979 Study	Weight Change	1959 Study	1979 Study	Weight Change	1959 Study	1979 Study	Weight Change
5' 2"	137	142	+5	140	142	+2	142	141	−1	139	140	+1
3"	141	143	+2	144	144	0	145	145	0	142	144	+2
4"	145	147	+2	148	149	+1	149	150	+1	146	149	+3
5"	149	151	+5	152	154	+2	153	155	+2	150	153	+3
6"	153	156	+3	156	158	+2	157	159	+2	154	158	+4
7"	157	160	+4	161	163	+2	162	164	+2	159	163	+4
8"	161	165	+5	165	167	+2	166	168	+2	163	167	+4
9"	165	170	+4	169	172	+3	170	173	+3	168	172	+4
10"	170	174	+5	174	176	+2	175	177	+2	173	176	+3
11"	174	179	+5	178	181	+3	180	182	+2	178	181	+3
6'0"	179	184	+5	183	186	+3	185	187	+2	183	186	+3
1"	183	190	+7	187	192	+5	189	193	+4	188	191	+3
2"	188	195	+7	192	197	+5	194	198	+4	193	196	+3
3"	193	201	+8	197	203	+6	199	204	+5	198	200	+2
4"	199	206	+7	203	208	+5	205	209	+4	204	207	+3

*The 1959 Build and Blood Pressure Study reflects data collected during the years 1935 through 1954. The 1979 Build and Blood Pressure Study reflects data collected during the years 1954 through 1972. (Ad Hoc Committee of the New Build and Blood Pressure Study. Association of Life Insurance Medical Directors of America and Society of Actuaries)

Table I-1 533

Table 1-2
Average Weights of Women by Height and Age Group: 1959 and 1979 Build and Blood Pressure Studies* (Graduated Weight in Shoes and Indoor Clothing in Pounds)

| Height | Women By Age Group, 1959 and 1979 Studies | | | | | | | | | | | |
| | 15-16 years | | | 17-19 years | | | 20-24 years | | | 25-29 years | | |
	1959 Study	1979 Study	Weight Change	1959 Study	1979 Study	Weight Change	1959 Study	1979 Study	Weight Change	1959 Study	1979 Study	Weight Change
4'10"	97	101	+4	99	103	+4	102	105	+3	107	110	+3
11"	100	105	+5	102	108	+6	105	110	+5	110	112	+2
5'10"	103	109	+6	105	111	+6	108	112	+4	113	114	+1
1"	107	112	+5	109	115	+6	112	116	+4	116	119	+3
2"	111	117	+6	113	119	+6	115	120	+5	119	121	+2
3"	114	121	+7	116	123	+7	118	124	+6	122	125	+3
4"	117	123	+6	120	126	+6	121	127	+6	125	128	+3
5"	121	128	+7	124	129	+5	125	130	+5	129	132	+3
6"	125	131	+6	127	132	+5	129	133	+4	133	134	+1
7"	128	135	+7	130	136	+6	132	137	+5	136	138	+2
8"	132	138	+6	134	140	+6	136	141	+5	140	142	+2
9"	136	142	+6	138	145	+7	140	146	+6	144	148	+4
10"	†	146		142	148	+6	144	149	+5	148	150	+2
11"	†	149		147	150	+3	149	155	+6	153	156	+3
6'10"	†	152		152	154	+2	154	157	+3	158	159	+1

(continued)

Table 1-2
Average Weights of Women by Height and Age Group: 1959 and 1979 Build and Blood Pressure Studies* (Graduated Weight in Shoes and Indoor Clothing in Pounds) (continued)

Women By Age Group, 1959 and 1979 Studies

Height	30–39 years			40–49 years			50–59 years			60–69 years		
	1959 Study	1979 Study	Weight Change	1959 Study	1979 Study	Weight Change	1959 Study	1979 Study	Weight Change	1959 Study	1979 Study	Weight Change
4'10"	115	113	−2	122	118	−4	125	121	−4	127	123	−4
11"	117	115	−2	124	121	−3	127	125	−2	129	127	−2
5'0"	120	118	−2	127	123	−4	130	127	−3	131	130	−1
1"	123	121	−2	130	127	−3	133	131	−2	134	133	−1
2"	126	124	−2	133	129	−4	136	133	−3	137	136	−1
3"	129	128	−1	136	133	−3	140	137	−3	141	140	−1
4"	132	131	−1	140	136	−4	144	141	−3	145	143	−2
5"	135	134	−1	143	139	−4	148	144	−4	149	147	−2
6"	139	137	−2	147	143	−4	152	147	−5	153	150	−3
7"	142	141	−1	151	147	−4	156	152	−4	157	155	−2
8"	146	145	−1	155	150	−5	160	156	−4	161	158	−3
9"	150	150	0	159	155	−4	164	159	−5	165	161	−4
10"	154	153	−1	164	158	−6	169	162	−7	†	163	
11"	159	159	0	169	162	−7	174	166	−8	†	167	
6'0"	164	164	0	174	168	−6	180	171	−9	†	172	

* The 1959 Build and Blood Pressure Study reflects data collected during the years 1935 through 1954. The 1979 Build and Blood Pressure Study reflects data collected during the years 1954 through 1972.

† Average weights omitted in classes with too few cases for analysis.

(Ad Hoc Committee of the New Build and Blood Pressure Study. Association of Life Insurance Medical Directors of America and Society of Actuaries)

Table I-3
Metropolitan Life Insurance Company Height and Weight Charts*†

To make an approximation of frame size, extend the arm and bend the forearm upward at a 90° angle. Keep fingers straight and turn the inside of the wrist toward the body. If you have a caliper, use it to measure the space between the two prominent bones on *either side* of the elbow. Without a caliper, place thumb and index finger of your other hand on these two bones. Measure the space between your fingers against a ruler or tape measure. Compare it with the table below that lists elbow measurements for *medium-framed* men and women. Measurements lower than those listed indicate a small frame. Higher measurements indicate a large frame.

Men

Height	Elbow Breadth
5'2"–5'3"	2½"–2⅞"
5'4"–5'7"	2⅝"–2⅞"
5'8"–5'11"	2¾"–3"
6'0"–6'3"	2¾"–3⅛"
6'4"	2⅞"–3¼"

Women

Height	Elbow Breadth
4'10"–4'11"	2¼"–2½"
5'0"–5'3"	2¼"–2½"
5'4"–5'7"	2⅜"–2⅝"
5'8"–5'11"	2⅜"–2⅝"
6'0"	2½"–2¾"

Men

Height	Small Frame	Medium Frame	Large Frame
5' 2"	128–134	131–141	138–150
5' 3"	130–136	133–143	140–153
5' 4"	132–138	135–145	142–156
5' 5"	134–140	137–148	144–160
5' 6"	136–142	139–151	146–164

Women

Height	Small Frame	Medium Frame	Large Frame
4'10"	102–111	109–121	118–131
4'11"	103–113	111–123	120–134
5' 0"	104–115	113–126	122–137
5' 1"	106–118	115–129	125–140
5' 2"	108–121	118–132	128–143

(continued)

Table I-3 535

Table I-3
Metropolitan Life Insurance Company Height and Weight Charts*† (continued)

Men				Women			
Height	Small Frame	Medium Frame	Large Frame	Height	Small Frame	Medium Frame	Large Frame
5' 7"	138–145	142–154	149–168	5' 3"	111–124	121–135	131–147
5' 8"	140–148	145–157	152–172	5' 4"	114–127	124–138	134–151
5' 9"	142–151	148–160	155–176	5' 5"	117–130	127–141	137–155
5'10"	144–154	151–163	158–180	5' 6"	120–133	130–144	140–159
5'11"	146–157	154–166	161–184	5' 7"	123–136	133–147	143–163
6' 0"	149–160	157–170	164–188	5' 8"	126–139	136–150	146–167
6' 1"	152–164	160–174	168–192	5' 9"	129–142	139–153	149–170
6' 2"	155–168	164–178	172–197	5'10"	132–145	142–156	152–173
6' 3"	158–172	167–182	176–202	5'11"	135–148	145–159	155–176
6' 4"	162–176	171–187	181–207	6' 0"	138–151	148–162	158–179

* 1983 Metropolitan Life Insurance Company weight tables by height and size of frame, for people aged 25 to 59, in shoes with 1" heels and wearing five pounds of indoor clothing for men, three pounds for women. Adjustments should be made when weighing hospitalized clients without shoes and for those wearing lighter clothing.

† Desirable weight is defined as the weight associated with lowest mortality or greatest longevity. It is not the weight that minimizes morbidity or incidence of disease. Similarly, desirable weight is not necessarily the weight that optimizes job performance nor is it the weight at which appearance is best. Because the terms *ideal* and *desirable* mean different things to different people (and since there is a difference between average mean weight and desirable weight for longevity), these terms are no longer being used in the Metropolitan Life Insurance Company Chart titles.

Example: The average weight of a 40- to 49-yr-old 5'9" man is 172 lb +3 while the desirable weight for longevity is 148 to 160 lb for a medium-framed man (see other tables in Appendix I).

Appendix II

Nutrient Composition of Selected Enteral Formulas

Table II–1
Composition of Selected Formulas

			Composition per 100 ml		
Product and Manufacturer	Caloric Density (kcal/ml)	How Supplied	kcal	Protein	Fat
Intact Protein and Protein Isolates: Low-Lactose, Low-Residue					
Ensure Ross	1.06	240-ml bottles and cans	106	3.7 g; 14% of kcal Sodium and calcium caseinates Soy protein isolate	3.7 g; 31.5% of kcal Corn oil
Ensure Osmolite Ross	1.06	240-ml bottles and cans; 960-ml cans	106	3.6 g; 13.6% of kcal Sodium and calcium caseinates Soy protein isolate	3.8 g; 32.3% of kcal MCT oil† Corn oil Soy oil
Ensure Plus Ross	1.50	240-ml cans	150	5.5 g; 14.7% of kcal Sodium and calcium caseinates Soy protein isolate	5.3 g; 32% of kcal Corn oil
Isocal Mead–Johnson	1.04	240-ml bottles and cans; 360-ml and 960-ml cans	104	3.4 g; 12.9% of kcal Sodium and calcium caseinates Soy protein isolate	4.4 g; 38.5% of kcal Soy oil MCT oil†
Precision High Nitrogen Diet Doyle	1.05	82-g packet; mix with 240 ml of water to yield 285 ml	105	4.4 g; 17% of kcal Egg albumin	0.05 g; 0.4% of kcal Soybean oil
Precision Isotonic Diet Doyle	0.96	58-g packet; mix with 240 ml of water to yield 260 ml	96	2.9 g; 11.8% of kcal Egg albumin	3 g; 28.2% of kcal Vegetable oil
Precision LR Diet Doyle	1.11	84-g packet; mix with 240 ml of water to yield 285 ml	111	2.6 g; 9.5% of kcal Egg albumin	0.08 g; 0.6% of kcal Soy bean oil
Precision Moderate Nitrogen Diet Doyle	1.21	77-g packet; mix with 240 ml of water to yield 275 ml	121	3.9 g; 13% of kcal Egg albumin	3.8 g; 28% of kcal Soybean oil
Hydrolyzed Protein and Amino Acids: Low-Lactose, Low-Residue, Chemically Defined Formula					
Flexical Mead–Johnson	1	56-g packet; mix with 207 ml of water to yield 250 ml	100	2.2 g; 9% of kcal Hydrolyzed casein Crystalline amino acids	3.4 g; 30% of kcal Soy oil MCT oil†
Vital Ross	1	78-g packet; mix with 255 ml of water to yield 300 ml	100	4.2 g; 16.7% of kcal Hydrolyzed whey, soy, and meat proteins Free essential amino acids	1 g; 9.3% of kcal Sunflower oil
Vivonex Eaton	1	80-g packet; dilute to 300 ml	100	2.1 g; 8.5% of kcal Crystalline amino acids	0.1 g; 1.3% of kcal Safflower oil
Vivonex HN Eaton	1	80-g packet; dilute to 300 ml	100	4.2 g; 18.26% of kcal Crystalline amino acids	0.1 g; 0.78% of kcal Safflower oil
Intact Protein Containing Milk: Moderate- and Low-Residue					
Compleat-B Doyle	1	250-ml bottles and 400 ml cans	100	4 g; 16% of kcal Intact meat, beef, and wheat protein	4 g; 36% of kcal Corn oil Beef fat
Carnation Instant Breakfast§** Carnation	1.22	34-35 g packets; mix with 240 ml of whole milk to yield 260 ml	122	5.8 g; 22.1% of kcal Whole Nonfat milk Sodium caseinate Soy protein isolate	3.1 g; 28% of kcal Milk fat

Table II–1 539

Composition per 100 ml

Carbohydrate	Lactose (g)	Sodium (mEq)	Potassium (mEq)	Chloride (mEq)	Calcium (mg)	Phosphorus (mg)	Osmolality* mOsm/kg of Water	Moisture (% wt/vol)
14.5 g; 54.5% kcal Corn syrup solids Sucrose	0	3.2	3.25	2.9	52.8	52.8	450	84
14.3 g; 54% of kcal Corn syrup solids Glucose polymers (Polycose)	0	2.3	2.3	2.3	54.2	54.2	300	83
19.7 g; 53.3% of kcal Corn syrup solids Sucrose	0	4.6	4.9	4.5	63	63	600	‡
13 g; 49.6% of kcal Corn syrup solids	0	2.3	3.3	2.9	62.5	52.1	350	78
21.8 g; 83% of kcal Maltodextrin Sucrose	0	4.3	2.3	3.4	35.1	35.1	557	‡
14.4 g; 60% of kcal Glucose oligosac- charides Sucrose	0	3.3	2.5	2.9	65.4	65.4	300	‡
24.9 g; 89.9% of kcal Maltodextrin Sucrose	0	3.0	2.2	3.1	58.4	58.4	500–545	‡
18.2 g; 59% of kcal Maltodextrin Sucrose	0	4.5	2.3	3.1	60.6	60.6	395	‡
15.4 g; 61% of kcal Sucrose Dextrin Citrate	0	1.5	3.2	3.5	60.0	50.0	723	‡
18.5 g; 74% of kcal Glucose, oligosac- charides and polysaccharides Sucrose Cornstarch	0	1.7	3.0	1.9	66.6	66.6	450	86
22.6 g; 90.2% of kcal Glucose oligosac- charides	0	3.7	3.0	5.1	44.3	44.3	500–1180	85
21.0 g; 80.96% of kcal Glucose, oligosac- charides	0	3.3	1.8	5.2	26.7	26.7	810–1150	85
12 g; 48% of kcal Maltodextrin Lactose	2.4	6.8	3.4	2.3	62.5	168.7	490	80
13.5 g; 49.9% of kcal Sucrose Corn syrup solids Lactose	9.5	4.2	7.2	‡	137.1	110.5	‡	‡

(continued)

Table II–1
Composition of Selected Formulas (continued)

				Composition per 100 ml	
Product and Manufacturer	Caloric Density (kcal/ml)	How Supplied	kcal	Protein	Fat

Intact Protein Containing Milk: Moderate- and Low-Residue (continued)

Product and Manufacturer	Caloric Density (kcal/ml)	How Supplied	kcal	Protein	Fat
Meritene liquid§ Doyle	1	240-ml and 300-ml cans	100	6.1 g; 24% of kcal Concentrated skim milk Sodium caseinate	3.4 g; 30% of kcal Vegetable oil Monoglycerides and di- glycerides
Meritene powder‡ and milk** Doyle	1.06	Mix 32 g of pow- der with 240 ml of whole milk to yield 260 ml	106	6.9 g; 25.8% of kcal Whole milk Nonfat milk	3.5 g; 31.3% of kcal Milk fat
Sustacal liquid§ Mead–Johnson	1	240-ml, 360-ml, and 960-ml cans	100	6 g; 24.4% of kcal Concentrated skim milk Sodium and calcium caseinates Soy protein isolate	2.3 g; 20.1% of kcal Soy oil
Sustacal powder‡ and milk** Mead–Johnson	1.33	53-g packet; mix with 240 ml of whole milk to yield 270 ml	133	8 g; 24% of kcal Nonfat milk Whole milk	3.3 g; 22% of kcal Milk fat
Sustagen powder‡ and water Mead–Johnson	1.66	Mix 100 g of pow- der with 160 ml of water to yield 240 ml	166	10 g; 24% of kcal Nonfat milk Whole milk Calcium caseinate	1.4 g; 7.5% of kcal Milk fat

* Unflavored; the osmolality of the product varies with the flavor packet used. If the product is mixed with a soft drink or a juice rather than water, the osmolality of the mixing product should be included when the osmolality of a solution is determined.
† MCT = medium-chain triglycerides.
‡ Information not available
§ Values for vanilla flavor
** Whole milk added
(Pemberton CM, Gastineau CF [eds]: Mayo Clinic Diet Manual, 5th ed. Philadelphia, WB Saunders, 1981)

Table II–1 541

	Composition per 100 ml							
Carbohydrate	Lactose (g)	Sodium (mEq)	Potassium (mEq)	Chloride (mEq)	Calcium (mg)	Phosphorus (mg)	Osmolality* (mOsm/kg of Water)	Mositure (% wt/vol)
11.7g; 46% of kcal Sucrose Lactose Corn syrup solids	5.7	4.0	4.3	4.7	125.0	125.0	700–750	‡
11.9 g; 42.9% of kcal Lactose Corn syrup solids	9.8	4.0	7.1	6.5	217.9	181.6	690	‡
13.8 g; 55.2% of kcal Sucrose Lactose Corn syrup solids	1.7	4.0	5.3	4.4	100.0	91.7	625	‡
17.9 g; 54% of kcal Sucrose Lactose Corn syrup solids	11.4	5.3	8.6	5.0	214.8	177.8	756	‡
28.6 g; 68.5% of kcal Corn syrup solids Glucose	9.5	5.0	8.5	‡	304.8	228.6	1334	‡

Table II–2
Composition of Selected Supplements

Product and Manufacturer	Type	How Supplied	Amount to Give 100 kcal	Composition per 100 kcal				
				Protein (g)	Fat (g)	Carbohydrate (g)	Sodium (mEq)	Potassium (mEq)
Cal-Power General Mills	Carbohydrate source	Liquid: 1 carton = 8 fl oz (300 g)	55 g, liquid	0.06	0	27.2	0.24	0.07
Citrotein Doyle	Calorie supplement	Powder: ¼ cup = 33 g	26.3 g, dry wt	6.05	0.26	18.42	4.58	2.68
Controlyte Doyle	Calorie supplement: low-electrolyte, low-protein	Powder	19.8 g, dry wt	Trace	4.80	14.3	0.13	0.02
Hycal Beecham	Carbohydrate source	Liquid	40.7 ml, liquid	0.01	0.01	24.41	0.24	0.01
Lipomul-Oral Upjohn	Fat source	Liquid	16.7 ml, liquid	0.01	11.11	0.11	0.29	0.01
MCT Oil Mead-Johnson	Fat source: medium-chain triglycerides	Liquid: 1 tbsp = 14 g	12.05 g, liquid	0	12.05	0	0	0
Nonfat dry milk	Protein, calorie supplement	Powder: 1 tbsp = 7 g	28 g; 4 tbsp	10	0.2	14.6	6.5	12.6
Polycose Ross	Carbohydrate source: oligosaccharides	Powder: 1 tbsp = 8 g; Liquid: 1 bottle = 120 ml	25 g, dry wt; 50 ml, liquid	0	0	25	1.23	0.03

(continued)

(Pemberton CM, Gastineau CF [Eds]: Mayo Clinic Diet Manual, 5th ed. Philadelphia, WB Saunders, 1981)

Appendix III

Triceps Skinfold and Arm Circumference Measurements

Table III–1
Smoothed Percentile Values for Triceps Skinfolds for White Males From NHANES-I, 6–50 yr (Measurement in mm)

Age	Percentile						
	5th	10th	25th	50th	75th	90th	95th
yr							
6	5.0	6.1	7.2	8.8	10.6	13.1	16.5
7	5.1	6.1	7.3	9.4	11.7	15.0	18.1
8	5.2	6.1	7.5	9.8	12.7	16.8	19.7
9	5.3	6.0	7.5	10.1	13.4	18.3	21.1
10	5.3	5.9	7.5	10.2	13.8	19.4	22.3
11	5.3	5.7	7.4	10.2	13.9	20.1	23.2
12	5.2	5.5	7.3	9.9	13.8	20.4	23.8
13	5.1	5.4	7.1	9.6	13.6	20.3	24.1
14	5.0	5.2	6.9	9.3	13.2	19.9	24.1
15	4.9	5.1	6.7	9.0	12.9	19.4	23.9
16	4.7	5.1	6.6	8.7	12.7	18.9	23.6
17	4.6	5.1	6.5	8.7	12.6	18.6	23.2
18–20	4.4	5.2	6.5	9.2	13.4	18.7	22.2
21–23	4.4	5.3	6.6	9.9	14.3	19.6	22.1
24–26	4.8	5.4	7.2	10.9	15.6	21.1	23.3
27–29	5.0	5.7	7.7	11.3	15.8	21.0	23.9
30–32	5.3	6.4	8.9	12.1	16.0	20.4	23.9
33–35	5.2	6.6	9.3	12.5	16.1	20.3	23.4
36–38	5.0	6.2	9.0	12.3	16.0	20.2	22.6
39–41	5.0	5.9	8.7	11.9	15.8	19.9	22.7
42–44	5.1	6.1	8.4	11.3	15.5	19.6	23.6
45–47	5.3	6.5	8.5	11.4	15.5	19.9	24.1
48–50	5.7	6.8	8.3	11.5	15.3	20.7	24.5

Table III–2
**Smoothed Percentile Values for Triceps Skinfolds
for Black Males From NHANES-I 6–50 yr (Measurement
in mm)**

Age	Percentile						
---	5th	10th	25th	50th	75th	90th	95th
yr							
6	4.0	4.0	5.1	6.4	8.4	10.4	13.0
7	4.0	4.2	5.3	6.5	8.8	11.7	15.1
8	4.0	4.3	5.5	6.6	9.1	12.7	16.9
9	4.0	4.4	5.6	6.8	9.2	13.7	18.6
10	4.0	4.4	5.7	6.9	9.3	14.4	20.2
11	4.0	4.4	5.7	7.0	9.3	15.2	21.6
12	3.9	4.4	5.6	7.1	9.4	15.9	22.9
13	3.9	4.3	5.5	7.1	9.5	16.5	24.0
14	3.8	4.2	5.3	7.2	9.7	17.2	24.9
15	3.7	4.1	5.2	7.2	9.9	17.8	25.4
16	3.6	4.0	5.0	7.1	10.1	18.2	25.6
17	3.5	3.9	4.9	7.1	10.3	18.6	25.4
18–20	3.3	3.7	4.8	6.9	10.7	18.7	23.1
21–23	3.3	3.7	4.8	6.9	10.9	18.2	21.7
24–26	3.3	3.7	5.1	7.9	11.8	17.9	23.7
27–29	3.4	3.8	5.5	8.7	12.9	18.4	25.9
30–32	3.6	4.2	6.5	10.3	14.9	19.2	26.3
33–35	3.7	4.5	6.9	10.6	15.0	19.3	24.5
36–38	4.1	4.8	7.0	10.0	13.8	20.1	23.5
39–41	4.2	4.7	6.7	9.4	13.3	20.9	25.4
42–44	3.8	4.2	6.1	8.8	13.5	21.3	27.8
45–47	3.5	4.0	6.0	9.0	13.8	20.3	26.8
48–50	3.1	4.1	6.0	9.8	14.0	18.5	24.8

Table III–3 545

Table III–3
**Smoothed Percentile Values for Triceps Skinfolds
for White Females From NHANES-I 6–50 yr
(Measurement in mm)**

	Percentile						
Age	5th	10th	25th	50th	75th	90th	95th
yr							
6	5.8	6.1	7.7	9.6	11.6	13.4	15.6
7	6.1	6.5	8.3	10.5	13.0	15.5	18.6
8	6.4	7.0	8.9	11.4	14.5	17.6	21.4
9	6.8	7.5	9.6	12.3	15.9	19.6	24.0
10	7.1	8.0	10.2	13.2	17.2	21.5	26.2
11	7.5	8.6	10.9	14.1	18.4	23.1	28.0
12	7.9	9.1	11.5	14.9	19.4	24.5	29.4
13	8.2	9.6	12.0	15.6	20.2	25.7	30.5
14	8.5	10.1	12.5	16.2	21.0	26.5	31.3
15	8.8	10.5	12.9	16.8	21.6	27.2	31.9
16	9.1	10.9	13.3	17.3	22.1	27.7	32.5
17	9.2	11.1	13.6	17.8	22.5	28.0	32.9
18–20	9.6	11.4	14.1	18.6	23.4	28.9	34.0
21–23	9.6	11.4	14.3	18.9	23.9	29.7	34.6
24–26	9.9	11.4	14.9	19.7	25.5	32.0	35.8
27–29	10.0	11.7	15.3	20.3	26.5	33.2	36.7
30–32	10.7	12.7	16.5	21.8	28.1	34.5	38.3
33–35	11.2	13.2	17.0	22.3	28.5	34.6	38.4
36–38	12.0	13.6	17.9	22.6	28.7	34.7	37.6
39–41	12.0	13.6	18.2	22.9	29.0	34.9	37.7
42–44	11.7	13.9	18.8	24.3	30.2	35.8	39.7
45–47	11.7	14.3	19.2	24.9	30.6	36.1	40.7
48–50	12.7	15.4	19.9	25.0	30.2	36.2	40.6

Table III–4
Smoothed Percentile Values for Triceps Skinfolds
for Black Females From NHANES-I 6–50 yr
(Measurement in mm)

Age	Percentile						
	5th	10th	25th	50th	75th	90th	95th
yr							
6	3.7	4.8	6.1	7.4	9.7	11.3	19.4
7	3.9	5.0	6.6	8.1	10.9	14.2	21.1
8	4.1	5.4	7.2	9.0	12.2	17.1	23.0
9	4.5	5.8	7.8	10.1	13.6	19.8	24.9
10	4.9	6.2	8.3	11.1	14.9	22.3	26.9
11	5.4	6.7	8.9	12.0	16.3	24.3	28.7
12	5.8	7.1	9.4	12.9	17.6	25.9	30.3
13	6.3	7.4	9.9	13.7	18.8	27.2	31.7
14	6.6	7.7	10.4	14.4	19.9	28.1	32.8
15	6.9	7.8	10.8	14.9	20.8	28.8	33.6
16	7.0	7.9	11.1	15.4	21.6	29.4	34.1
17	7.1	7.9	11.4	15.8	22.3	29.9	34.5
18–20	7.2	8.4	12.2	16.9	23.8	31.5	34.7
21–23	7.5	9.1	12.7	17.7	24.6	32.5	34.8
24–26	8.4	10.6	13.8	19.8	26.8	33.5	36.5
27–29	8.7	10.6	14.5	21.0	28.5	34.0	38.1
30–32	8.6	9.9	16.3	23.8	31.9	36.5	41.9
33–35	8.7	10.2	17.3	25.0	33.1	38.1	43.4
36–38	9.6	12.3	18.9	26.1	33.3	39.8	44.7
39–41	9.7	13.2	19.2	26.0	32.8	39.9	44.6
42–44	8.6	12.3	18.9	25.8	32.0	40.2	43.6
45–47	8.0	11.3	18.5	26.0	32.5	40.7	43.4
48–50	8.8	11.1	18.4	26.8	34.8	41.4	44.7

Table III–5 547

Table III–5
Triceps Skinfold: Normal and Subnormal Standards for Adults' Triceps Skinfold Measurement (mm)

Sex	Normal Standard	90% of Standard	80% of Standard	70% of Standard	60% of Standard
Male	12.5	11.3	10.0	8.8	7.5
Female	16.5	14.9	13.2	11.6	9.0

Table III–6
Arm Circumference: Normal and Subnormal Standards for Adults' Arm Circumference Measurement* (cm)

Sex	Normal Standard	90% of Standard	80% of Standard	70% of Standard	60% of Standard
Male	29.3	26.3	23.4	20.5	17.6
Female	28.5	25.7	22.8	20.0	17.1

* To determine mid-upper arm muscle circumference, see formula in Chapter 1. (Reprinted with permission. Blackburn GL: Nutritional assessment: An overview. Clinical Consultations in Nutritional Support 1:10, 1981)

Table III-7
Percentiles of Upper Arm Circumference (mm) and Estimated Upper Arm Muscle Circumference (mm) for Whites of the United States Health and Nutrition Examination Survey I of 1971 to 1974

Percentile	Arm Circumference (mm)							Arm Muscle Circumference (mm)						
Age Group (yr)	5	10	25	50	75	90	95	5	10	25	50	75	90	95
Males														
1-1.9	142	146	150	159	170	176	183	110	113	119	127	135	144	147
2-2.9	141	145	153	162	170	178	185	111	114	122	130	140	146	150
3-3.9	150	153	160	167	175	184	190	117	123	131	137	143	148	153
4-4.9	149	154	162	171	180	186	192	123	126	133	141	148	156	159
5-5.9	153	160	167	175	185	195	204	128	133	140	147	154	162	169
6-6.9	155	159	167	179	188	209	228	131	135	142	151	161	170	177
7-7.9	162	167	177	187	201	223	230	137	139	151	160	168	177	190
8-8.9	162	170	177	190	202	220	245	140	145	154	162	170	182	187
9-9.9	175	178	187	200	217	249	257	151	154	161	170	183	196	202
10-10.9	181	184	196	210	231	262	274	156	160	166	180	191	209	221
11-11.9	186	190	202	223	244	261	280	159	165	173	183	195	205	230
12-12.9	193	200	214	232	254	282	303	167	171	182	195	210	223	241
13-13.9	194	211	228	247	263	286	301	172	179	196	211	226	238	245
14-14.9	220	226	237	253	283	303	322	189	199	212	223	240	260	264
15-15.9	222	229	244	264	284	311	320	199	204	218	237	254	266	272
16-16.9	244	248	262	278	303	324	343	213	225	234	249	269	287	296
17-17.9	246	253	267	285	308	336	347	224	231	245	258	273	294	312
18-18.9	245	260	276	297	321	353	379	226	237	252	264	283	298	324
19-24.9	262	272	288	308	331	355	372	238	245	257	273	289	309	321
25-34.9	271	282	300	319	342	362	375	243	250	264	279	298	314	326
35-44.9	278	287	305	326	345	363	374	247	255	269	286	302	318	327
45-54.9	267	281	301	322	342	362	376	239	249	265	281	300	315	326
55-64.9	258	273	296	317	336	355	369	236	245	260	278	295	310	320
65-74.9	248	263	285	307	325	344	355	223	235	251	268	284	298	306

(continued)

Table III–7
Percentiles of Upper Arm Circumference (mm) and Estimated Upper Arm Muscle Circumference (mm) for Whites of the United States Health and Nutrition Examination Survey I of 1971 to 1974 (continued)

Table III–7 549

Percentile	Arm Circumference (mm)							Arm Muscle Circumference (mm)						
Age Group (yr)	5	10	25	50	75	90	95	5	10	25	50	75	90	95
Females														
1–1.9	138	142	148	156	164	172	177	105	111	117	124	132	139	143
2–2.9	142	145	152	160	167	176	184	111	114	119	126	133	142	147
3–3.9	143	150	158	167	175	183	189	113	119	124	132	140	146	152
4–4.9	149	154	160	169	177	184	191	115	121	128	136	144	152	157
5–5.9	153	157	165	175	185	203	211	125	128	134	142	151	159	165
6–6.9	156	162	170	176	187	204	211	130	133	138	145	154	166	171
7–7.9	164	167	174	183	199	216	231	129	135	142	151	160	171	176
8–8.9	168	172	183	195	214	247	261	138	140	151	160	171	183	194
9–9.9	178	182	194	211	224	251	260	147	150	158	167	180	194	198
10–10.9	174	182	193	210	228	251	265	148	150	159	170	180	190	197
11–11.9	185	194	208	224	248	276	303	150	158	171	181	196	217	223
12–12.9	194	203	216	237	256	282	294	162	166	180	191	201	214	220
13–13.9	202	211	223	243	271	301	338	169	175	183	198	211	226	240
14–14.9	214	223	237	252	272	304	322	174	179	190	201	216	232	247
15–15.9	208	221	239	254	279	300	322	175	178	189	202	215	228	244
16–16.9	218	224	241	258	283	318	334	170	180	190	202	216	234	249
17–17.9	220	227	241	264	295	324	350	175	183	194	205	221	239	257
18–18.9	222	227	241	258	281	312	325	174	179	191	202	215	237	245
19–24.9	221	230	247	265	290	319	345	179	185	195	207	221	236	249
25–34.9	233	240	256	277	304	342	368	183	188	199	212	228	246	264
35–44.9	241	251	267	290	317	356	378	186	192	205	218	236	257	272
45–54.9	242	256	274	299	328	362	384	187	193	206	220	238	260	274
55–64.9	243	257	280	303	335	367	385	187	196	209	225	244	266	280
65–74.9	240	252	274	299	326	356	373	185	195	208	225	244	264	279

Appendix IV

Recommended Daily Dietary Allowances

Table IV–1 551

Table IV–1
Mean Heights and Weights and Recommended Energy Intake

Category	Age (Years)	Weight kg	Weight lb	Height cm	Height in	Energy Needs (With Range) kcal		Mj
Infants	0.0–0.5	6	13	60	24	kg × 115	(95–145)	kg × 0.48
	0.5–1.0	9	20	71	28	kg × 105	(80–135)	kg × 0.44
Children	1–3	13	29	90	35	1300	(900–1800)	5.5
	4–6	20	44	112	44	1700	(1300–2300)	7.1
	7–10	28	62	132	52	2400	(1650–3300)	10.1
Males	11–14	45	99	157	62	2700	(2000–3700)	11.3
	15–18	66	145	176	69	2800	(2100–3900)	11.8
	19–22	70	154	177	70	2900	(2500–3300)	12.2
	23–50	70	154	178	70	2700	(2300–3100)	11.3
	51–75	70	154	178	70	2400	(2000–2800)	10.1
	76+	70	154	178	70	2050	(1650–2450)	8.6
Females	11–14	46	101	157	62	2200	(1500–3000)	9.2
	15–18	55	120	163	64	2100	(1200–3000)	8.8
	19–22	55	120	163	64	2100	(1700–2500)	8.8
	23–50	55	120	163	64	2000	(1600–2400)	8.4
	51–75	55	120	163	64	1800	(1400–2200)	7.6
	76+	55	120	163	64	1600	(1200–2000)	6.7
Pregnancy						+300		
Lactation						+500		

The energy allowances for the young adults are for men and women doing light work. The allowances for the two older age groups represent mean energy needs over these age spans, allowing for a 2% decrease in basal (resting) metabolic rate per decade and a reduction in activity of 200 kcal/day for men and women over these age spans, allowing for a 2% decrease in basal (resting) metabolic rate per decade and a reduction in activity of 200 kcal/day for men and women over 75.... The customary range of daily energy output is shown for adults in parentheses, and is based on a variation in energy needs of ±400 kcal at any one age ... emphasizing the wide range of energy intake appropriate for any group of people.

Energy allowances for children through age 18 are based on median energy intake of children these ages followed in longitudinal growth studies. The values in parentheses are 10th and 90th percentiles of energy intake, to indicate the range of energy consumption among children of these ages....

(Recommended Dietary Allowances, Revised 1980. Food and Nutrition Board, National Academy of Sciences—National Research Council, Washington, D.C.)

Table IV-2
Vitamin, Protein, and Mineral Intakes Designed for the Maintenance of Good Nutrition of Practically All Healthy People in the United States*

	Age (years)	Weight		Height		Protein (g)	Fat-Soluble Vitamins				
		kg	lb	cm	in		Vitamin A (μg RE)[†]	Vitamin D (μg)[‡]	Vitamin E (mg α TE)[§]	Vitamin C (mg)	Thiamine (mg)
Infants	0.0–0.5	6	13	60	24	kg × 2.2	420	10	3	35	0.3
	0.5–1.0	9	20	71	28	kg × 2.0	400	10	4	35	0.5
Children	1–3	13	29	90	35	23	400	10	5	45	0.7
	4–6	20	44	112	44	30	500	10	6	45	0.9
	7–10	28	62	132	52	34	700	10	7	45	1.2
Males	11–14	45	99	157	62	45	1000	10	8	50	1.4
	15–18	66	145	176	69	56	1000	10	10	60	1.4
	19–22	70	154	177	70	56	1000	7.5	10	60	1.5
	23–50	70	154	178	70	56	1000	5	10	60	1.4
	51+	70	154	178	70	56	1000	5	10	60	1.2
Females	11–14	46	101	157	62	46	800	10	8	50	1.1
	15–18	55	120	163	64	46	800	10	8	60	1.1
	19–22	55	120	163	64	44	800	7.5	8	60	1.1
	23–50	55	120	163	64	44	800	5	8	60	1.0
	51+	55	120	163	64	44	800	5	8	60	1.0
Pregnant						+30	+200	+5	+2	+20	+0.4
Lactating						+20	+400	+5	+3	+40	+0.5

* The allowances are intended to provide for individual variations among most normal persons as they live in the United States under usual environmental stresses. Diets should be based on a variety of common foods in order to provide other nutrients for which human requirements have been less well defined.
† Retinol equivalents. 1 Retinol equivalent = 1 μg retinol or 6 μg β carotene.
‡ As cholecalciferol. 10 μg cholecalciferol = 400 IU vitamin D.
§ α-tocopherol equivalents. 1 mg d-α-tocopherol = 1 α TE.
‖ 1 NE (niacin equivalent) is equal to 1 mg of niacin or 60 mg of dietary tryptophan.
¶ The folacin allowances refer to dietary sources as determined by *Lactobacillus casei* assay after treatment with enzymes ("conjugases") to make polyglutamyl forms of the vitamin available to the test organism.
** The RDA for vitamin B$_{12}$ in infants is based on average concentration of the vitamin in human milk. The allowances after weaning are based on energy intake (as recommended by the American Academy of Pediatrics) and consideration of other factors such as intestinal absorption.
†† The increased requirement during pregnancy cannot be met by the iron content of habitual American diets nor by the existing iron stores of many women; therefore the use of 30–60 mg of supplemental iron is recommended. Iron needs during lactation are not substantially different from those of nonpregnant women, but continued supplementation of the mother for 2–3 months after parturition is advisable in order to replenish stores depleted by pregnancy.

Table IV-3
Estimate Safe and Adequate Daily Dietary Intakes of Additional Selected Vitamins and Minerals*

	Age (Years)	Vitamins			Trace Elements	
		Vitamin K (μg)	Biotin (μg)	Pantothenic acid (mg)	Copper (mg)	Manganese (mg)
Infants	0–0.5	12	35	2	0.5–0.7	0.5–0.7
Children and	0.5–1	10–20	50	3	0.7–1.0	0.7–1.0
adolescents	1–3	15–30	65	3	1.0–1.5	1.0–1.5
	4–6	20–40	85	3–4	1.5–2.0	1.5–2.0
	7–10	30–60	120	4–5	2.0–2.5	2.0–3.0
	11+	50–100	100–200	4–7	2.0–3.0	2.5–5.0
Adults		70–140	100–200	4–7	2.0–3.0	2.5–5.0

* Because there is less information on which to base allowances, these figures are not given in the main table of the RDA and are provided here in the form of ranges of recommended intake.
† Since the toxic levels for many trace elements may be only several times usual intake, the upper levels for the trace elements given in this table should not be habitually exceeded.

Table IV-3 553

Water-Soluble Vitamins					Minerals					
Riboflavin (mg)	Niacin (mg NE)||	Vitamin B$_6$ (mg)	Folacin^c (μg)	Vitamin B$_{12}$ (μg)	Calcium (mg)	Phosphorus (mg)	Magnesium (mg)	Iron (mg)	Zinc (mg)	Iodine (μg)
0.4	6	0.3	30	0.5**	360	240	50	10	3	40
0.6	8	0.6	45	1.5	540	360	70	15	5	50
0.8	9	0.9	100	2.0	800	800	150	15	10	70
1.0	11	1.3	200	2.5	800	800	200	10	10	90
1.4	16	1.6	300	3.0	800	800	250	10	10	120
1.6	18	1.8	400	3.0	1200	1200	350	18	15	150
1.7	18	2.0	400	3.0	1200	1200	400	18	15	150
1.7	19	2.2	400	3.0	800	800	350	10	15	150
1.6	18	2.2	400	3.0	800	800	350	10	15	150
1.4	16	2.2	400	3.0	800	800	350	10	15	150
1.3	15	1.8	400	3.0	1200	1200	300	18	15	150
1.3	14	2.0	400	3.0	1200	1200	300	18	15	150
1.3	14	2.0	400	3.0	800	800	300	18	15	150
1.2	13	2.0	400	3.0	800	800	300	18	15	150
1.2	13	2.0	400	3.0	800	800	300	10	15	150
+0.3	+2	+0.6	+400	+1.0	+400	+400	+150	††	+5	+25
+0.5	+5	+0.5	+100	+1.0	+400	+400	+150	††	+10	+50

Trace Elements†				Electrolytes		
Fluoride (mg)	Chromium (mg)	Selenium (mg)	Molybdenum (mg)	Sodium (mg)	Potassium (mg)	Chloride (mg)
0.1–0.5	0.01–0.04	0.01–0.04	0.03–0.06	115–350	350–925	275–700
0.2–1.0	0.02–0.06	0.02–0.06	0.04–0.08	250–750	425–1275	400–1200
0.5–1.5	0.02–0.08	0.02–0.08	0.05–0.1	325–975	550–1650	500–1500
1.0–2.5	0.03–0.12	0.03–0.12	0.06–0.15	450–1350	775–2325	700–2100
1.5–2.5	0.05–0.2	0.05–0.2	0.1–0.3	600–1800	1000–3000	925–2775
1.5–2.5	0.05–0.2	0.05–0.2	0.15–0.5	900–2700	1525–4575	1400–4200
1.5–4.0	0.05–0.2	0.05–0.2	0.15–0.5	1100–3300	1875–5625	1700–5100

Appendix V

Exchange Lists for Meal Planning

Foods That Need Not Be Measured (Insignificant carbohydrate or energy)

Diet carbonated beverages	Parsley
Coffee	Nutmeg
Tea	Lemon
Clear broth	Mustard
Bouillon without fat	Chili powder
Unsweetened gelatin	Onion salt or powder
Salt and pepper	Horseradish
Red pepper	Vinegar
Paprika	Mint
Garlic	Cinnamon
Celery salt	Lime
Unsweetened pickles	Other herbs and spices

List 1. Milk Exchange—Nonfat, Low-Fat, and Whole Milk

One nonfat milk exchange contains 8 g protein, trace of fat, 12 g carbohydrate, and 80 kilocalories.

Nonfat fortified* milk

Skim or nonfat milk	1 c
Powdered (nonfat dry before adding liquid)	⅓ c

Canned, evaporated skim milk (undiluted)	½ c
Buttermilk made from skim milk	1 c
Yogurt made from skim milk (plain, unflavored)	1 c

Low-fat fortified* milk

1% fat, fortified milk (103 kilocalories; omit ½ fat exchange)	1 c
2% fat, fortified milk (125 kilocalories; omit 1 fat exchange)	1 c
Yogurt made from 2% fat, fortified skim milk (plain, unflavored; 125 kilocalories; omit 1 fat exchange)	1 c

Whole milk (170 kilocalories; omit 2 fat exchanges)

Whole milk	1 c
Canned, evaporated whole milk (undiluted)	½ c
Buttermilk made from whole milk	1 c
Yogurt made from whole milk (plain, unflavored)	1 c

* Fortified with vitamins A and D

List 2. Vegetable Exchanges

One vegetable exchange contains about 2 g protein, 5 g carbohydrate, and 25 kilocalories. One exchange is ½ c.

Asparagus	Green pepper	Okra
Bean sprouts	Greens*	Onions
Beets	Beet	Rhubarb
Broccoli	Chard	Rutabaga
Brussels sprouts	Collard	Sauerkraut
Cabbage†	Dandelion	String beans, yellow or green
Carrots*	Kale	Summer squash
Cauliflower†	Mustard	Tomatoes†
Celery	Spinach	Tomato juice†
Cucumbers	Turnip	Vegetable juice cocktail
Eggplant	Mushrooms	Zucchini

The following raw vegetables may be used as desired (not to exceed a total of 1½ c per day).

Chicory	Lettuce
Chinese cabbage	Parsley
Endive	Radishes
Escarole	Watercress

* Good source of vitamin A
† Good source of vitamin C

List 3. Fruit Exchanges

One fruit exchange contains 10 g carbohydrate and 40 kilocalories. (This list shows the different amounts of fruits, fresh or processed without the addition of sugar, to use for one fruit exchange.)

Fruit	*Amount to Use*
Apple	1 small
Apple juice	1/3 c
Applesauce (unsweetened)	1/2 c
Apricots, fresh*	2 medium
Apricots, dried*	4 halves
Banana	1/2 small
Berries	
Blackberries	1/2 c
Blueberries	1/2 c
Raspberries	1/2 c
Strawberries†	3/4 c
Cherries	10 large
Cider	1/3 c
Dates, dried	2
Figs, fresh	1
Figs, dried	1
Grapefruit†	1/2
Grapefruit juice†	1/2 c
Grapes	12
Grape juice	1/4 c
Mango	1/2 small
Melon	
Cantaloupe†	1/4 small
Honeydew†	1/8 medium
Watermelon	1 c
Nectarine	1 small
Orange†	1 small
Orange juice†	1/2 c
Papaya†	3/4 c
Peach	1 medium
Pear	1 small
Persimmon, native	1 medium
Pineapple	1/2 c
Pineapple juice	1/3 c
Plums	2 medium
Prunes	2 medium
Prune juice	1/4 c

Fruit	*Amount to Use*
Raisins	2 tbsp
Tangerine[†]	1 medium

* Good source of vitamin A
[†] Good source of vitamin C

List 4. Bread Exchanges

One bread exchange contains about 2 g protein, 15 g carbohydrate, and 70 kilocalories. (This list shows the different amounts of foods to use for one bread exchange.)

Bread, Cereal and Others	*Amount to Use*
Bread	
White (including French and Italian)	1 slice
Whole wheat	1 slice
Rye or pumpernickel	1 slice
Raisin (unfrosted)	1 slice
Bagel	½ small
English muffin	½ small
Plain roll, bread	1
Frankfurter roll	½
Hamburger roll	½
Dried bread crumbs	3 tbsp
Tortilla	1 (6″)
Cereals	
Bran flakes	½ c
Other ready-to-eat unsweetened cereal	¾ c
Puffed cereal (unfrosted)	1 c
Cereal (cooked)	½ c
Grits (cooked)	½ c
Rice or barley (cooked)	½ c
Pasta (cooked)	
Spaghetti, noodles, macaroni	½ c
Popcorn (popped, no fat added)	3 c
Cornmeal (dry)	2 tbsp
Flour	2½ tbsp
Wheat germ	¼ c
Crackers	
Arrowroot	3
Graham (2½″ sq)	2
Matzo (4″–6″)	½

Bread, Cereal and Others	*Amount to Use*
Oyster	20
Pretzels (3⅛″ long, ⅛″ diam)	25
Rye wafers (2″–3½″)	3
Saltines	6
Soda (2½″ sq)	4
Dried beans, peas, and lentils (omit one meat exchange)	
Beans, peas, lentils (dried and cooked)	½ c
Baked beans, no pork, canned	¼ c
High-carbohydrate vegetables	
Corn	⅓ c
Corn on the cob	1 small
Lima beans	½ c
Parsnips	⅔ c
Peas, green (canned or frozen)	½ c
Potato, white	1 small
Potato, mashed	½ c
Pumpkin	¾ c
Winter acorn or butternut squash	½ c
Yam or sweet potato*	¼ c
Prepared foods (omit one fat exchange)	
Biscuits (2″ diam)	1
Cornbread, (2″ × 2″ × 1″)	1
Corn muffin (2″ diam)	1
Crackers, round butter type	5
Muffin, plain small	1
Potatoes, French fried (2″–3½″ long)	8
Pancake (5″ × ½″)	1
Waffle (5″ × ½″)	1
Potato or corn chips (omit two fat exchanges)	15

* Good source of vitamin A

List 5. Meat Exchanges

Lean Meat

One lean meat exchange contains 7 g protein, 3 g fat, and 55 kilocalories. (This list shows the different amounts of foods to use for one lean meat exchange.)

Meat	*Amount to Use*
Beef	1 oz
Baby beef (very lean)	
Steak, chuck, flank, tenderloin, plate	
ribs, round (bottom or top), rump,	
spare ribs, tripe)	
Lamb	1 oz
Leg, rib, sirloin, loin, shank, shoulder	
Pork	1 oz
Leg, whole, rump, center shank, ham,	
center slices	
Veal	1 oz
Leg, loin, rib, shank, shoulder, cutlets	
Poultry (without skin)	1 oz
Chicken, turkey, cornish hen, guinea	
hen, pheasant	
Fish	
Any fresh or frozen	1 oz
Canned salmon, tuna (water packed)	¼ c
Canned mackerel, crab, lobster	¼ c
Clams, oysters, scallops, shrimp	5 or 1 oz
Sardines, drained	3
Cheese	¼ c
Cottage cheese, dry and 2% butter fat	
Dried beans and peas (omit one bread	
exchange)	½ c

Medium-Fat Meat

One medium-fat meat exchange contains 7 g protein, 5 g fat, and 75 kilocalories. (This list shows the different amounts of food to use for one medium-fat meat exchange.)

Meat	*Amount to Use*
Beef	1 oz
Ground (15% fat)	
Corned beef, canned	
Ribeye	
Round, ground (commercial)	
Pork	1 oz
Loin, all cuts	
Shoulder arm, picnic	
Shoulder blade	
Boston butt	

Meat	Amount to Use
Canadian bacon	
Boiled ham	
Organ meats	1 oz
Liver	
Heart	
Kidney	
Sweetbreads	
Cheese	
Cottage cheese, creamed	¼ c
Mozzarella	1 oz
Ricotta	1 oz
Farmer's	1 oz
Neufchatel	1 oz
Parmesan	3 tbsp
Egg	1
Peanut butter (omit two fat exchanges)	2 tbsp

High-Fat Meat

One high-fat meat exchange contains 7 g protein, 8 g fat, and 100 kilocalories. (This list shows the different amounts of foods to use for one high-fat meat exchange.)

Meat	Amount to Use
Beef	1 oz
Brisket	
Corned beef, brisket	
Ground beef, more than 20% fat	
Hamburger, commercial	
Ground chuck, commercial	
Rib roast	
Club and rib steaks	
Lamb	1 oz
Breast	
Pork	1 oz
Spare ribs	
Pork, ground	
Ham, country style	
Deviled ham	
Veal	1 oz
Breast	
Poultry	1 oz
Capon	

Meat	*Amount to Use*
Duck, domestic	
Goose	
Cheese	1 oz
Cheddar types	
Cold cuts	4½″ × ⅛″ slice
Frankfurter	1 small

List 6. Fat Exchanges

One fat exchange contains 5 g fat and 45 kilocalories. (This list shows the different amounts of foods to use for one fat exchange.)

Fat	*Amount to Use*
Polyunsaturated fat	
Margarine, tub or stick (soft)	1 tsp
Oil	1 tsp
Corn	
Cottonseed	
Safflower	
Soy	
Sunflower	
French dressing	1 tbsp*
Italian dressing	1 tbsp*
Mayonnaise	1 tbsp*
Salad dressing, mayonnaise type	2 tsp*
Walnuts	6 small
Monounsaturated fats	
Avocado, 4″ diam	⅛
Oil	1 tsp
Olive	
Peanut	
Olives	5 small
Almonds	10 whole
Pecans	2 large whole
Peanuts	
Spanish	20 whole
Virginia	10 whole
Nuts, others	6 small
Saturated fats	
Margarine, regular stick (hard)	1 tsp
Butter	1 tsp

Fat	Amount to Use
Bacon fat	1 tsp
Bacon, crisp	1 strip
Cream, light	2 tbsp
Cream, heavy	1 tbsp
Cream, sour	2 tbsp
French dressing[†]	1 tbsp
Italian dressing[†]	1 tbsp
Lard	1 tsp
Mayonnaise[†]	1 tsp
Salad dressing, mayonnaise type[†]	2 tsp
Salt pork	¾" cube

[*] If made with polyunsaturated oils such as corn oil
[†] If made with saturated oils such as coconut oil
(Adapted from Exchange Lists for Meal Planning (rev. 1976), American Dietetic Association, 430 North Michigan Avenue, Chicago, IL 60611)

Appendix VI

Protein, Phosphorus, Sodium, and Potassium Exchange Lists

Dairy Exchanges
One serving contains 4 g protein, 100 mg phosphorus, 60 mg sodium, and 175 mg potassium.

Item	g	Amount	Calories	Protein (g)	P (mg)	Na (mg)	K (mg)
Cream, half and half	120	½ c	161	3.8	102	55	154
Cream, heavy	120	½ c	419	2.6	70	38	106
Cream, light	120	½ c	253	3.6	96	52	147
Ice cream (10% fat)	67	½ c	129	3.0	77	42	120
Milk							
Condensed	77	¼ c	245	6.2	105	86	240
Evaporated	63	¼ c	86	4.4	130	75	191
Whole, fresh	120	½ c	80	4.2	114	61	176
Low fat (2%)	120	½ c	68	4.3	117	63	178
Skim	120	½ c	44	4.4	117	64	178
Yogurt, made from partially skimmed milk	120	½ c	62	4.2	115	63	175

Meat Exchanges
One serving contains 7 g protein, 75 mg phosphorus, 25 mg sodium, and 90 mg potassium.

Item	g	Amount	Calories	Protein (g)	P (mg)	Na* (mg)	K (mg)
Beef, rump roast, 75% lean	28	1 oz	98	6.7	55	16	75

(continued)

Meat Exchanges (continued)
One serving contains 7 g protein, 75 mg phosphorus, 25 mg sodium, and 90 mg potassium.

Item	g	Amount	Calories	Protein (g)	P (mg)	Na* (mg)	K (mg)
Beef pattie, 90% lean	28	1 oz	62	7.7	65	19	81
Chicken							
Light meat, without skin	28	1 oz	52	9.1	77	19	120
Dark meat, without skin	28	1 oz	52	8.3	67	25	94
Lamb, 83% lean	28	1 oz	79	7.0	59	18	80
Organ meats							
Beef heart	28	1 oz	53	8.9	51	29	66
Gizzard, chicken	28	1 oz	42	7.6	20	16	60
Tongue, beef	28	1 oz	69	6.1	33	17	47
Liver							
Beef	28	1 oz	65	7.4	135	52	108
Calf	28	1 oz	74	8.3	152	33	128
Chicken	28	1 oz	47	7.5	45	17	43
Peanut butter	32	2 tbsp	188	8.0	122	194	200
Pork, 80% lean	28	1 oz	103	6.9	73	17	78
Seafood							
Flounder, baked	28	1 oz	57	8.5	98	67	166
Haddock, fried	28	1 oz	47	5.6	70	50	99
Halibut, broiled	28	1 oz	48	7.1	70	38	149
Lobster, northern	28	1 oz	27	5.3	54	60	51
Salmon, broiled or baked	28	1 oz	52	7.7	117	33	126
Shrimp, French fried	28	1 oz	64	5.8	54	53	65

(continued)

Meat Exchanges (continued)
One serving contains 7 g protein, 75 mg phosphorus, 25 mg sodium, and 90 mg potassium.

Item	g	Amount	Calories	Protein (g)	P (mg)	Na* (mg)	K (mg)
Tuna, canned, in water							
Without salt	28	1 oz	36	7.9	54	12	79
With salt	28	1 oz	36	7.9	54	212	79
Tuna, canned, in oil							
With salt	28	1 oz	82	7.8	84	227	85
Turkey, without skin	28	1 oz	54	8.9	71	37	104
Veal, rump roast	28	1 oz	66	7.6	65	18	86
Additional Values for Substitutions							
Egg	57	1 large	82	6.5	103	61	65
Cottage cheese	56	¼ c	58	7.6	85	128	48

* These figures represent the average for meats cooked without salt.

Bread Exchanges
One serving contains 2 g protein, 40 mg phosphorus, variable sodium, and 40 mg potassium.

Item	g	Amount	Calories	Protein (g)	P (mg)	Na (mg)	K (mg)
Breads							
Biscuit, baking powder	35	1 (2" diam)	129	2.6	61	219	41

(continued)

Bread Exchanges (continued)
One serving contains 2 g protein, 40 mg phosphorus, variable sodium, and 40 mg potassium.

Item	g	Amount	Calories	Protein (g)	P (mg)	Na (mg)	K (mg)
Bread							
White, regular	25	1 slice	68	2.2	24	127	26
White, without salt	25	1 slice	68	2.2	24	5	26
Whole wheat	28	1 slice	67	2.6	71	148	72
Rye, American	25	1 slice	61	2.3	37	139	36
Doughnut, cake type, plain	25	1 small	98	1.2	48	125	23
Doughnut, yeast	42	1	176	2.7	32	99	34
Graham crackers	14	2 (2½″ squares)	55	1.1	21	95	55
Hamburger or frankfurter bun	40	1	119	3.3	34	202	38
Muffin, plain	40	1 (3″ diam)	118	3.1	60	176	50
Muffin, blueberry	40	1 (3″ diam)	112	2.9	53	253	46
Pancake	27	1 (4″ diam)	61	1.9	70	152	42
Saltines, unsalted tops	14	5	62	1.3	13	5	17
Cooked cereals							
Cream of rice, slow cooking							
With salt	120	½ c	62	1.0	16	216	32
Without salt	120	½ c	62	1.0	16	1	32
Cream of wheat, slow cooking							
With salt	120	½ c	52	1.6	15	177	11
Without salt	120	½ c	52	1.6	15	1	11

(continued)

Bread Exchanges (continued)
One serving contains 2 g protein, 40 mg phosphorus, variable sodium, and 40 mg potassium.

Item	g	Amount	Calories	Protein (g)	P (mg)	Na (mg)	K (mg)
Oatmeal, slow cooking							
With salt	120	½ c	66	2.4	69	262	73
Without salt	120	½ c	66	2.4	69	2	73
Whole wheat, slow cooking							
With salt	120	½ c	55	2.2	64	260	59
Without salt	120	½ c	55	2.2	64	2	59
Dry cereals							
Cornflakes	18	¾ c	72	1.5	7	188	23
Frosted Flakes	30	¾ c	115	1.4	8	200	21
Frosted Mini-wheats	30	4 biscuits	105	2.6	97	5	55
Puffed Rice	11	¾ c	45	0.7	11	1	11
Puffed Wheat	11	¾ c	40	1.7	36	1	38
Raisin Bran	38	¾ c	108	3.2	110	160	116
Rice Krispies	23	¾ c	88	1.4	21	212	22
Shredded Wheat	25	1 biscuit	89	2.5	97	1	87
Starches							
Enriched macaroni, cooked without salt	70	½ c	78	2.4	35	1	43
Enriched noodles, cooked without salt	80	½ c	100	3.3	47	2	35
Enriched rice, cooked							
With salt	102	½ c	112	2.0	29	384	29
Without salt	102	½ c	112	2.0	29	1	29

(continued)

Bread Exchanges (continued)
One serving contains 2 g protein, 40 mg phosphorus, variable sodium, and 40 mg potassium.

Item	g	Amount	Calories	Protein (g)	P (mg)	Na (mg)	K (mg)
Enriched spaghetti, cooked without salt	70	½ c	78	2.4	35	1	43
Popcorn, popped plain, large kernel	6	1 c	23	0.8	17	trace	30

Vegetable Exchanges, Group I
One serving contains variable protein, 25 mg phosphorus, 5 mg sodium, and 100 mg potassium.

Item	g	Amount	Calories	Protein (g)	P (mg)	Na* (mg)	K (mg)
Asparagus, fresh, cooked, cut	73	½ c	15	1.6	73	1	133
Bean, green or wax, fresh, cooked, cut	63	½ c	15	1.0	23	3	95
Beans, green or wax, canned, drained, cut							
Regular	68	½ c	16	1.0	17	160	64
Special diet pack	68	½ c	16	1.0	17	2	64
Beans, green or wax, frozen, cooked, cut	68	½ c	18	1.2	22	1	106

(continued)

Vegetable Exchanges, Group I (continued)
One serving contains variable protein, 25 mg phosphorus, 5 mg sodium, and 100 mg potassium.

Item	g	Amount	Calories	Protein (g)	P (mg)	Na* (mg)	K (mg)
Bean sprouts, mung, fresh	53	½ c	19	2.0	34	3	117
Cabbage, raw, coarsely shredded	35	½ c	9	0.5	10	7	82
Cabbage, cooked, shredded	73	½ c	15	0.8	15	10	118
Cabbage, Chinese, 1" pieces	38	½ c	6	0.5	15	9	95
Carrots, raw, 1 oz	28	6–8 strips	12	0.3	5	13	97
Carrots, canned, sliced, drained							
Regular	78	½ c	24	0.6	17	183	93
Special diet pack	78	½ c	24	0.6	17	30	93
Cauliflower, fresh, cooked	63	½ c	14	1.5	27	6	129
Celery, pascal, fresh, 1 oz	28	6–8 strips	5	0.3	4	36	97
Corn, fresh, cooked	83	½ c	69	2.7	74		136
Corn, canned, drained							
Regular	83	½ c	70	2.2	41	195	80
Special diet pack	83	½ c	70	2.2	41	2	80
Cucumber, fresh, pared, sliced	70	½ c	10	0.4	13	4	112
Endive, fresh, cut in small pieces	50	½ c	5	0.5	14	4	74
Lettuce, fresh, cut in chunks	38	½ c	5	0.4	9	4	66
Onions, green, raw	30	2 medium or 6 small	14	0.3	12	2	69
Onions, mature, dry, chopped	85	½ c	33	1.3	31	9	134
Onions, cooked, drained	105	½ c	31	1.3	31	8	115

(continued)

Vegetable Exchanges, Group I (continued)
One serving contains variable protein, 25 mg phosphorus, 5 mg sodium, and 100 mg potassium.

Item	g	Amount	Calories	Protein (g)	P (mg)	Na* (mg)	K (mg)
Parsley, raw	10	10 sprigs (2½" long)	4	0.2	6	3	37
Peas, canned, drained							
Regular	85	½ c	68	3.9	65	200	82
Special diet pack	85	½ c	68	3.9	65	3	82
Peas, frozen, cooked	80	½ c	55	4.1	69	92	108
Potato, leached, boiled	100	½ c	70	2.0	33	2	120
Peppers, green, raw, cut into strips	50	½ c	11	0.6	11	7	107
Radishes, raw	25	5 medium	4	0.3	7	4	73
Squash, summer, yellow and zucchini, cooked, sliced, drained	90	½ c	21	2.7	23	1	127

* Values for vegetables canned with salt were excluded from calculation of this average.

Vegetable Exchanges, Group II
One serving contains variable protein, 35 mg phosphorus, 20 mg sodium, and 170 mg potassium.

Item	g	Amount	Calories	Protein (g)	P (mg)	Na* (mg)	K (mg)
Asparagus, canned, cut							
Regular	117	½ c	26	2.0	63	277	165
Dietary pack	117	½ c	26	2.0	63	5	165

(continued)

Vegetable Exchanges, Group II (continued)
One serving contains variable protein, 35 mg phosphorus, 20 mg sodium, and 170 mg potassium.

Item	g	Amount	Calories	Protein (g)	P (mg)	Na* (mg)	K (mg)
Asparagus, frozen, cooked, cut	90	½ c	20	2.9	58	1	198
Beets, fresh, cooked, diced	85	½ c	27	1.0	20	37	177
Beets, canned, diced							
Regular	85	½ c	32	0.9	16	200	142
Special diet pack	85	½ c	32	0.9	16	39	142
Broccoli, fresh, cooked	78	½ c	20	2.4	48	8	207
Broccoli, frozen, cooked	93	½ c	24	2.7	52	14	196
Carrots, fresh, cooked, sliced, drained	78	½ c	24	0.7	24	25	172
Cauliflower, raw, flowerbuds	50	½ c	14	1.4	28	7	148
Cauliflower, frozen, cooked	90	½ c	16	1.7	34	9	186
Celery, fresh, diced	60	½ c	10	0.6	17	76	205
Celery, cooked, diced	75	½ c	11	0.6	17	66	179
Corn, frozen, cooked	83	½ c	65	2.5	60	1	152
Eggplant, fresh, cooked, diced	100	½ c	19	1.0	21	1	150
Mushrooms, raw, sliced	35	½ c	10	1.0	41	6	145
Mushrooms, canned, solids and liquid	100	½ c	17	1.9	68	400	197
Mustard greens, fresh, cooked	70	½ c	16	1.6	23	13	154
Okra, fresh, cooked, sliced	80	½ c	23	1.6	33	2	139
Peas, fresh, cooked	80	½ c	57	4.3	79	1	157
Rutabaga, cooked, cubed	85	½ c	30	0.8	27	4	142

(continued)

Vegetable Exchanges, Group II (continued)
One serving contains variable protein, 35 mg phosphorus, 20 mg sodium, and 170 mg potassium.

Item	g	Amount	Calories	Protein (g)	P (mg)	Na* (mg)	K (mg)
Sweet potato, baked (2" diam, 5" long)	73	½ potato	81	1.2	33	7	171
Turnips, raw, cubed	65	½ c	20	0.7	20	32	174
Turnips, cooked, cubed	78	½ c	18	0.6	20	27	146

* Values for vegetables canned with salt were excluded from calculation of this average.

Vegetable Exchanges, Group III
One serving contains variable protein, 40 mg phosphorus, 20 mg sodium, and 280 mg potassium.

Item	g	Amount	Calories	Protein (g)	P (mg)	Na* (mg)	K (mg)
Beet greens, fresh, cooked	73	½ c	13	1.3	18	55	240
Brussels sprouts, fresh, cooked	78	½ c (4 sprouts)	28	3.3	56	8	212
Brussels sprouts, frozen, cooked	78	½ c (4 sprouts)	26	2.5	48	11	229
Chard, Swiss, cooked	87	½ c	16	1.6	21	76	281
Collards, fresh, cooked	95	½ c	32	3.4	50	34	249
Parsnips, cooked, diced	78	½ c	51	1.2	48	6	294
Potato, mashed	105	½ c	99	2.2	51	5	263

(continued)

Vegetable Exchanges, Group III (continued)
One serving contains variable protein, 40 mg phosphorus, 20 mg sodium, and 280 mg potassium.

Item	g	Amount	Calories	Protein (g)	P (mg)	Na* (mg)	K (mg)
Potato, baked (2½" diam, 4½" long)	100	½ potato	73	2.0	51	3	391
Pumpkin, canned, salt added	120	½ c	41	1.3	32	289	294
Spinach, cooked, drained	90	½ c	21	2.7	34	45	292
Squash, winter, acorn, baked	103	½ c	57	2.0	30	1	492
Sweet potato, mashed	128	½ c	138	2.6	53	61	255
Tomato paste, no salt added	33	2 tbsp	27	1.1	23	13	280
Tomato, fresh, not peeled (2⅖" diam)	100	1	20	1.0	25	3	222
Tomatoes, canned							
Regular	120	½ c	25	1.4	23	157	261
Special diet pack	120	½ c	25	1.4	23	3	261
Tomato juice, regular	120	½ c	23	1.1	22	243	276

* Values for vegetables canned with salt were excluded from calculation of this average.

Fruit Exchanges, Group I
One serving contains 0.5 g protein, 15 mg phosphorus, 2 mg sodium, and 85 mg potassium.

Item	g	Amount	Calories*	Protein (g)	P (mg)	Na (mg)	K (mg)
Apple, raw, small	115	1–2½″ diam	61	0.2	11	1	116
Apple juice, canned	120	½ c	59	0.1	11	1	125
Applesauce	120	½ c	116	0.3	7	2.5	83
Blackberries, fresh	72	½ c	42	0.9	14	0.5	123
Blackberries, frozen	72	½ c	42	0.9	14	1	122
Blueberries, fresh	73	½ c	45	0.5	10	0.5	59
Boysenberries, frozen, sweetened	72	½ c	69	0.5	12	0.5	75
Cranberries, raw	48	½ c	22	0.2	5	1	39
Cranberry sauce	138	½ c	202	0.2	6	1.5	42
Cranberry juice	127	½ c	82	0.1	4	1.5	13
Figs, raw	65	1 large	52	0.8	14	1	126
Grapes, white seedless	50	10 whole	34	0.3	10	2	87
Grape juice, frozen, sweetened	125	½ c	67	0.2	5	1.5	43
Grapefruit sections	88	½ c	36	0.5	18	1	118
Lemonade, frozen, diluted	124	½ c	54	tr	1.5	0.5	20
Lime juice, fresh	123	½ c	32	0.4	14	1	128
Limeade	124	½ c	51	tr	1.5	tr	16
Peach, canned, with 1⅔ tbsp syrup	76	1 half	59	0.3	9	2	99
Peach nectar	125	½ c	60	0.3	14	1	97
Pear, raw, Bartlett (2½″ diam, 3½″ high)	90	1 half	50	0.6	9	1.5	107
Pear, canned, with 1 tbsp syrup	48	1 half	36	0.1	3	tr	40
Pear nectar	125	½ c	65	0.4	7	1.5	49

(continued)

Fruit Exchanges, Group I (continued)
One serving contains 0.5 g protein, 15 mg phosphorus, 2 mg sodium, and 85 mg potassium.

Item	g	Amount	Calories*	Protein (g)	P (mg)	Na (mg)	K (mg)
Pineapple, fresh (¾″ thick, 3½″ diam)	84	1 slice	44	0.3	7	1	123
Pineapple, canned, with 1½ tbsp syrup	58	1 medium slice	43	0.2	3	1	56
Plums, raw, damson (1″ diam)	33	3	21	tr	6	0.6	90
Plums, raw, prune (1½″ diam)	60	2	42	0.4	10	tr	96
Strawberries, fresh, whole	75	½ c	28	0.5	16	0.5	122
Tangerine	136	1 large	46	0.8	18	2	127

* Caloric values for canned fruit are based on fruits canned in heavy syrup.

Fruit Exchanges, Group II
One serving contains 0.5 g protein, 15 mg phosphorus, 2 mg sodium, and 170 mg potassium.

Item	g	Amount	Calories*	Protein (g)	P (mg)	Na (mg)	K (mg)
Apricot nectar	120	½ c	72	0.4	15	tr	190
Cherries, raw, sour	78	½ c	45	1.0	15	1.5	148
Cherries, raw, sweet	73	½ c	51	0.9	14	1.5	139
Cherries, sweet, canned	129	½ c	104	1.1	17	1.5	162
Figs, canned	130	½ c	109	0.7	17	2.5	193

(continued)

Fruit Exchanges, Group II (continued)
One serving contains 0.5 g protein, 15 mg phosphorus, 2 mg sodium, and 170 mg potassium.

Item	g	Amount	Calories*	Protein (g)	P (mg)	Na (mg)	K (mg)
Fruit cocktail	128	½ c	97	0.5	16	7	206
Grapes, halves, all varieties	88	½ c	59	0.5	18	2.5	152
Grapefruit, fresh	184	1 half	40	0.5	16	1	132
Grapefruit juice	123	½ c	48	0.6	19	1	200
Lemon juice, fresh	122	½ c	31	0.6	12	1	172
Nectarine (2½″ diam)	75	1 half	44	0.4	17	4	203
Peach, raw, pared (2½″ diam)	115	1	33	0.5	17		177
Pineapple juice	125	½ c	69	0.5	12	1.5	187
Plums, canned	136	½ c	107	0.5	13	1.5	184
Strawberries, frozen, sweetened	128	½ c	136	0.7	22	1.5	143
Watermelon	160	1 c	42	0.8	16	2	160

* Caloric values for canned fruits are based on fruits canned in heavy syrup.

Fruit Exchanges, Group III
One serving contains 1 g protein, 25 mg phosphorus, 5 mg sodium, and 300 mg potassium.

Item	g	Amount	Calories*	Protein (g)	P (mg)	Na (mg)	K (mg)
Apricots, canned	129	½ c	111	0.7	20	1	302

(continued)

Fruits Exchanges, Group III (continued)
One serving contains 1 g protein, 25 mg phosphorus, 5 mg sodium, and 300 mg potassium.

Item	g	Amount	Calories*	Protein (g)	P (mg)	Na (mg)	K (mg)
Apricots, fresh	114	3 whole	55	1.1	25	0.5	301
Banana	88	½ medium	50	0.7	16	0.5	220
Cantaloupe	160	1 c melon balls	48	1.1	26	19	402
Honeydew	170	1 c melon balls	56	1.4	27	20	427
Orange (2⅝″ diam)	180	1	64	1.3	26	1	263
Orange juice	124	½ c	56	0.9	21	1	248
Prunes, cooked and sweetened	140	½ c	205	1.0	36	4	312
Prune juice	128	½ c	99	0.5	26	2.5	301
Rhubarb, cooked and sweetened	135	½ c	190	0.7	21	2.5	274

* Caloric values for canned fruits are based on fruits canned in heavy syrup.

Fat Exchanges
One serving contains 0 g protein, 1 mg phosphorus, 50 mg sodium, and 1 mg potassium.

Item	g	Amount	Calories	Protein (g)	P (mg)	Na (mg)	K (mg)
Butter, salted*	5	1 tsp	45	0	1	48	1
Margarine, salted*	5	1 tsp	45	0	1	48	1

(continued)

Fat Exchanges (continued)
One serving contains 0 g protein, 1 mg phosphorus, 50 mg sodium, and 1 mg potassium.

Item	g	Amount	Calories	Protein (g)	P (mg)	Na (mg)	K (mg)
Mayonnaise, salted	5	1 tsp	34	0	1	30	1
Half and half	30	2 tbsp	40	1	26	14	38
Whipping cream	30	2 tbsp	106	0.6	18	10	26

* Unsalted butter and margarine, and vegetable oil may be used as desired.

Miscellaneous List

Item	g	Amount	Calories	Protein (g)	P (mg)	Na (mg)	K (mg)
Beverages							
Alcoholic (physician's permission)							
Beer	240	8 oz	100	0.7	72	17	60
Gin, vodka, rum, whiskey	90	3 oz	210	0	tr	1	2
Wine							
Dessert	120	4 oz	165	0.1	tr	5	90
Table	120	4 oz	102	0.1	12	6	110
Carbonated							
Coca-Cola	240	8 oz	96	0	40	0	0

(continued)

Miscellaneous List (continued)

Item	g	Amount	Calories	Protein (g)	P (mg)	Na (mg)	K (mg)
Ginger ale	240	8 oz	88	0	0	0	0
Pepsi Cola	240	8 oz	110	0		28	9
Fanta Orange	240	8 oz	128	0	0	8	0
Sprite	240	8 oz	96	0	0	40	0
Bitter lemon	240	8 oz	104	0	0	16	0
Coffee, tea, bouillon							
Coffee	240	8 oz	5	0.3	5	5	135
Tea	240	8 oz	5			5	95
Bouillon							
Salted	4	1 cube	5	0.2		960	4
Unsalted	4	1 cube	11	0.3		2	500
Fruit drinks							
Awake	120	4 oz	51	tr		5	41
Cranberry juice	120	4 oz	78	0.2	3.6	1	12
Grape Tang	120	4 oz	61	tr	40	55	1
Lemonade	120	4 oz	54	tr	2	1	22
Orange Tang	120	4 oz	61	tr	60	13	45
Kool-aid	120	4 oz	45	tr		1	1
Hawaiian Punch	120	4 oz	49	0.4		2	11
Fats							
Bacon, fried	7	1 slice	48	1.5	16	76	17
Butter, margarine							
Salted	14	1 tbsp	102	0.1	2	140	3
Unsalted	14	1 tbsp	102	0.1	2	1	3

(continued)

Miscellaneous List (continued)

Item	g	Amount	Calories	Protein (g)	P (mg)	Na (mg)	K (mg)
Cream cheese	14	1 tbsp	53	1.1	13	35	11
French dressing	14	1 tbsp	66	0.1	2	219	13
Italian dressing	14	1 tbsp	83	tr	1	314	2
Mayonnaise							
Regular	14	1 tbsp	101	0.2	4	84	5
Low sodium	14	1 tbsp	105	0.4	4	3	5
Roquefort dressing	15	1 tbsp	76	0.7	11	164	6
Peanut butter							
Regular	16	1 tbsp	94	4.0	61	97	100
Low sodium	16	1 tbsp	94	4.0	61	2	100
Vegetable oil	14	1 tbsp	120	0	0	0	0
Whipping cream	15	1 tbsp	53	0.3	9	5	13
Low-protein products							
Cornstarch	8	1 tbsp	29	tr	0	tr	tr
Low-protein bread—dp (Henkle Dietary Specialties)	32	1 slice	78	0.3	0	10	8
Low-protein pasta, cooked (Aproten)	100	½ c	91	0.2	0	8	2
Low-protein rusk (Aproten)	12	1 slice	48	0.1		4	5
Wheatstarch (Henkle)	100	1 c	360	0.4	45	60	10
Non-dairy products							
Coffee-Rich, liquid	60	¼ c	94	0.2		24	27
Cool-Whip	18	¼ c	60	0.2		4	tr

(continued)

Miscellaneous List (continued)

Item	g	Amount	Calories	Protein (g)	P (mg)	Na (mg)	K (mg)
Cremora powder (Borden)	12	2 tbsp	66	0.6		1	10
Mocha Mix	60	¼ c	86	0.2		60	35
Rich's Whip Topping, whipped	23	½ c	63	0		13	tr
Poly Perx	60	¼ c	84	0.44	tr	tr	tr
Spices, seasonings, condiments*							
Garlic, fresh	2	1 clove	3	0.1	5	1	11
Green pepper, fresh, chopped	10	1 tbsp	2	0.1	2.2	1	21
Horseradish, prepared	5	1 tsp	2	0.1	1.6	5	16
Lemon juice, fresh	15	1 tbsp	4	0.1	1.5	1	21
Lime juice, fresh	15	1 tbsp	4	0.1	1.7	1	16
Mustard							
Low sodium (Cellu)	5	1 tsp	4	0.2	3.7	1	21
Prepared yellow, regular	5	1 tsp	4	0.2	3.6	63	6.5
Onion, fresh, chopped	10	1 tbsp	4	0.2		1	16
Tabasco sauce	2	½ tsp	tr	tr		11	2
Tomato catsup	15	1 tbsp	16	0.3	7.5	156	54
Tomato, chili sauce	15	1 tbsp	16	0.4	8	201	56
Vinegar, distilled	15	1 tbsp	2		5	2	36
Worcestershire sauce	5	1 tsp	4	0.1	3	105	24

* All dry spices, herbs, and extracts may be used for flavoring.
(From Anderson L, Dipple MV, Turkki PR et al: Nutrition in Health and Disease, 17th ed. Philadelphia, JB Lippincott, 1982)

Appendix VII

Nutrient Composition of Selected Parenteral Solutions

Travasol (Amino Acid) Injections With Electrolytes and Travasol (Amino Acid) Injections Without Electrolytes

Description

Travasol (Amino Acid) Injections are sterile, nonpyrogenic hypertonic solutions of essential and nonessential L-amino acids provided with or without electrolytes for intravenous administration.

Each 100 ml of Travasol (Amino Acid) Injections with Electrolytes and without Electrolytes contains

	5.5%	8.5%
L-amino acids	5.5 g	8.5 g
Total nitrogen	924 mg	1.42 g
Approximate pH	6.0	6.0

Essential Amino Acids

	5.5%	8.5%
L-Leucine	340 mg	526 mg
L-Phenylalanine	340 mg	526 mg
L-Methionine	318 mg	492 mg
L-Lysine (added as the hydrochloride salt)	318 mg	492 mg
L-Isoleucine	263 mg	406 mg
L-Valine	252 mg	390 mg
L-Histidine	241 mg	372 mg
L-Threonine	230 mg	356 mg
L-Tryptophan	99 mg	152 mg

Nonessential Amino Acids

	5.5%	8.5%
L-Alanine	1.14 g	1.76 g
Aminoacetic acid	1.14 g	1.76 g
L-Arginine	570 mg	880 mg
L-Proline	230 mg	356 mg
L-Tyrosine	22 mg	34 mg

In addition to the above, Travasol (Amino Acid) Injections With Electrolytes contain in each 100 ml:

(continued)

Travasol (Amino Acid) Injections With Electrolytes and Travasol (Amino Acid) Injections Without Electrolytes

(continued)

Electrolytes	5.5%	8.5%
Sodium acetate, hydrous, USP	431 mg	594 mg
Dibasic potassium phosphate	522 mg	522 mg
Sodium chloride, USP	224 mg	154 mg
Magnesium chloride, USP	102 mg	102 mg

Travasol (Amino Acid) Injections With Electrolytes contain the following milliequivalents:

Electrolyte	5.5%	8.5%
Sodium	70 mEq/liter	70 mEq/liter
Potassium	60 mEq/liter	60 mEq/liter
Magnesium	10 mEq/liter	10 mEq/liter
Acetate*	100 mEq/liter	135 mEq/liter
Chloride‡	70 mEq/liter	70 mEq/liter
Phosphate (as $HPO_4 =$)	60 mEq/liter	60 mEq/liter
	(30 mM)	(30 mM)

Travasol (Amino Acid) Injections without Electrolytes contain the following anion profiles in mEq/liter:

Anion	5.5%	8.5%
Acetate†	35 mEq/liter	52 mEq/liter
Chloride‡	22 mEq/liter	34 mEq/liter

* Acetate is added as sodium and as acetic acid used for pH adjustment.
† Derives from pH adjustment with acetic acid
‡ Contributed by the L-Lysine Hydrochloride
Approximately 3 mEq/liter sodium bisulfite, USP is added as stabilizer to all Travasol (Amino Acid) Injections.
(Parenteral Products Division, Travenol Laboratories, Inc., Deerfield, IL, 1981)

Appendix VIII

Ideal Urinary Creatinine Values for Adults

Men*		Women†	
Height (cm)	Ideal Creatinine (mg)	Height (cm)	Ideal Creatinine (mg)
157.5	1288	147.3	830
160.0	1325	149.9	851
162.6	1359	152.4	875
165.1	1386	154.9	900
167.6	1426	157.5	925
170.2	1467	160.0	949
172.7	1513	162.6	977
175.3	1555	165.1	1006
177.8	1596	167.6	1044
180.3	1642	170.2	1076
182.9	1691	172.7	1109
185.4	1739	175.3	1141
188.0	1785	177.8	1174
190.5	1831	180.3	1206
193.0	1891	182.9	1240

* Creatinine coefficient (men) = 23 mg/kg of ideal body weight
† Creatinine coefficient (women) = 18 mg/kg of ideal body weight

Formula: Lean Body Mass, Creatinine/Height Index

To compute the creatinine/height index, compare the actual daily creatinine excretion with the ideal values.

$$\text{Creatinine/height index (CHI)} = \frac{\text{Actual urinary creatinine}}{\text{Ideal urinary creatinine}} \times 100$$

Example. The ideal urinary creatinine for a man 177.8 cm high is 1596 mg/day. If his actual daily urinary creatinine loss is 1200, the creatinine/height index is

$$\frac{1200}{1596} \times 100 = 75\%$$

(Blackburn GL: Nutritional assessment: An overview. Clinical Consultations in Nutritional Support 1:10, 1981)

index

An *f* following a page number indicates a figure; a *t* represents tabular material.

stroke, 105–109
subjective information, in nutritional assessment, 6–8, 11
substitution, in diabetes, during illness, 196–197
sugar
  in atherosclerosis, 103
  calorie, sodium, and potassium content, 130*t*
  in prudent diet, 143*t*
  in triglyceride restriction, 331*t*
  substitutes, 223–224
  U.S. dietary goals, 7
sulfonylureas, hypoglycemics, 179*t*
supplements
  composition, 542*t*
  nurse's responsibilities, 74–81*t*
  oral feeding, 52
surface area, burn, 355
surgery
  in cancer, 157–161*t*
  colostomy and ileostomy, 270–271
  in diabetes, 195
  intestinal resection, 264
surgical patient, caloric requirements for, 66*t*
sweeteners, 223–224
Sweet 'n Low, 224
sympathetic depressants, in cardiovascular disease, 116–118*t*, 119*t*

teeth
  in adults, older, 523*t*
  in child, 515*t*
Tenormin (atenolol), 118*t*
therapeutic diets, 42–43
thiazide diuretics
  in hypertension and cardiac dysfunction, 111–113*t*
  in kidney stones, 327
thiazidelike diuretics, in hypertension and cardiac dysfunction, 113*t*
thoracic tubes, 51*t*
thyroid hormones, in breast milk, 447*t*

tissue reserves, nutritional deficiencies and, 5
toxemia, 405
trace elements, recommended intake, 553*t*
tranquilizers
  in human milk, 413, 445*t*
  and nutritional status, 380–381*t*
transferrin, in nutritional status assessment, 13, 37–38*t*
Trauma Cal, composition, advantages, and disadvantages of, 73*t*
triamterene (Dyrenium), 114–115*t*
triceps skinfold measurement, 11, 13, 35*t*
  in pregnancy, 394
  values, 543–546*t*, 547*t*
triglycerides
  age variations of normal limits of, 137*t*
  in atherosclerosis, 103
  for epileptic patients, 363
  in hyperlipoproteinemias, 139*t*
  in liver, 314
  in obesity, 218
  in pancreatitis, 307–308
  in pregnancy, 395
  restriction of, 330, 331, 330–332*t*
tube feedings. *See* enteral feeding
twenty-four hour recall, 11, 32*t*

ulcerative colitis, 268–269, 295–297*t*
ulcers
  in burns, 56
  peptic, 256–258, 285*t*, 286–288*t*
uricosurics, 383–384*t*
urinary creatinine, ideal values, 586
urine analysis, 10, 13
  in diabetes, 182–183, 184, 187
  in GI disorders, 249–250
  infants, 458
  in nutritional status assessment, 38–39*t*
  in pregnancy, 396